Clinical Skills for
Adult Primary Care

Clinical Skills for Adult Primary Care

Editors

Mark E. Silverman, M.D.
Professor of Medicine
Emory University School of Medicine
and
Chief of Cardiology
Piedmont Hospital
Atlanta, Georgia

J. Willis Hurst, M.D.
Consultant to the Division of Cardiology
Emory University School of Medicine and Hospital
(Professor and Chairman
Department of Medicine
1957–1986)

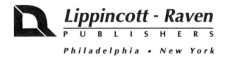 **Lippincott - Raven**
P U B L I S H E R S
Philadelphia • New York

Lippincott-Raven Publishers, Philadelphia, 227 East Washington Square, Philadelphia, PA 19106

Made in the United States of America

Library of Congress Cataloging-in-Publication Data

Clinical skills for adult primary care / edited by Mark E. Silverman and J. Willis Hurst : with 21 contributors.
    p.   cm.
  Includes bibliographical references and index.
  ISBN 0-7817-0327-1
  1. Physical diagnosis—Handbooks, manuals, etc. 2. Medical history taking—Handbooks, manuals, etc. I. Silverman, Mark E. II. Hurst, J. Willis (John Willis), 1920–
  [DNLM: 1. Physical Examination. 2. Physicians, Family. WB 200
C6412 1995
616'.07'5—dc20
DNLM/DLC
for Library of Congress   95-31276
                                     CIP

William Osler (1849–1919) is reverently regarded as the unparalleled master of physical diagnosis and clinical medicine. Born in Bond Head, Canada, and trained at McGill University, he rapidly rose to the highest echelons of American medicine, becoming Chief of Medicine at the University of Pennsylvania in 1884 and then at the newly formed Johns Hopkins Hospital in 1889. At Johns Hopkins Hospital, Osler introduced bedside teaching and an observation clinic; a teaching method that he had observed in Europe but was new to the United States. Many of his disciples became leaders in medicine and carried on this tradition. His textbook, *The Principles and Practice of Medicine,* first published in 1892 and subsequently in 16 editions over 55 years, became the standard reference and enormously influenced the practice of medicine. In addition, he published about 1,500 articles, including many classic essays that are still read and quoted. In 1905, overburdened by the pressures of consultation, teaching, and writing, he accepted the chair of Regius Professor of Medicine at Oxford, where he continued his extraordinarily productive life until his death from pneumonia in 1919.

His personality and style—a blend of high intelligence, charm, wit, effervescence, and warmth—his staunch loyalty to his profession, colleagues, and patients, and his talent at capsulizing medicine into timeless aphorisms of philosophy based on the precepts of humanistic medicine and an appreciation of medical heritage, created an enduring image of the finest attributes of a physician.

Harvey Cushing made the following remark in the dedication to his Pulitzer Prize-winning book, *The Life of Sir William Osler* (1):

> To Medical Students: In the hope that something of Osler's spirit may be conveyed to those of a generation that has not known him; and particularly to those in America, lest it be forgotten who it was that made it possible for them to work at the bedside in the wards.

The editors dedicate this book to the enduring role model of William Osler and to all aspiring bedside diagnosticians who carry on the tradition.

REFERENCE

1. Cushing H. *The life of Sir William Osler.* London: Oxford University Press, 1925.

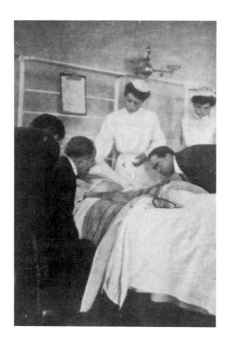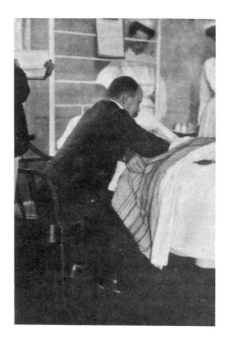

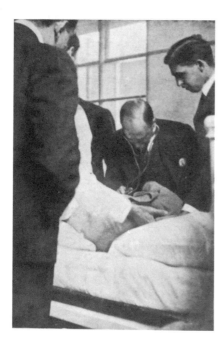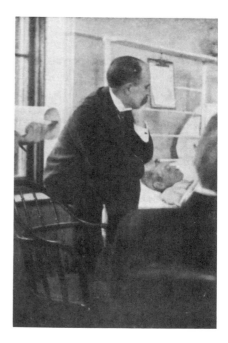

Snapshots ascribed by Harvey Cushing to T.W. Clarke and preserved with the Cushing papers in the Osler Library. Used with permission of the Osler Library of History of Medicine, McGill University and Yale University, Cushing/Whitney Historical Library. From Cushing H. *The life of Sir William Osler.* London: Oxford at the Clarendon Press, 1925.

Contents

Section IV. Indications for Initial Routine Laboratory Testing

CONTENTS

Contributing Authors

Robert S. Allen, M.D. Hematologist, Piedmont Hospital, 1968 Peachtree Road, N.W., Atlanta, Georgia 30309

Stephen M. Barnett, M.D. General Surgeon, Piedmont Hospital, 105 Collier Road, N.W., Suite 1020, Atlanta, Georgia 30309

Jerry D. Cooper, M.D. Internist and Nephrologist, Piedmont Hospital, 1968 Peachtree Road, N.W., Atlanta, Georgia 30309

Dave McAlister Davis, M.D. Psychiatrist, Piedmont Hospital, 1968 Peachtree Road, N.W., Atlanta, Georgia 30309

Sandra Adamson Fryhofer, M.D. Internist, Piedmont Hospital, 1968 Peachtree Road, N.W., Atlanta, Georgia 30309

T. Kirkland Garner, M.D. Internist, Piedmont Hospital, 1968 Peachtree Road, N.W., Atlanta, Georgia 30309

J. Willis Hurst, M.D. Consultant to the Division of Cardiology, Emory University School of Medicine and Hospital, and Professor and Chairman, Department of Medicine (1957–1986), 1462 Clifton Road, N.E., Suite 301, Atlanta, Georgia 30322

Valerie J. Jagiella, M.D. Gastroenterologist, Piedmont Hospital, 1968 Peachtree Road, N.W., Atlanta, Georgia 30309

William H. Jarrett II, M.D. Ophthalmologist and Retina Specialist, Piedmont Hospital, 1968 Peachtree Road, N.W., Atlanta, Georgia 30309

William R. Kenny, M.D. Pulmonologist, Piedmont Hospital, 1968 Peachtree Road, N.W., Atlanta, Georgia 30309

William E. Mitchell, Jr., M.D. Surgeon, Piedmont Hospital, 95 Collier Road, Suite 6015, Atlanta, Georgia 30309

Mark W. Mohney, M.D. Ophthalmologist, Piedmont Hospital, 2004 Peachtree Road, N.W., Atlanta, Georgia 30309

Donald J. Pirozzi, M.D. Dermatologist, Piedmont Hospital, 105 Collier Road, Atlanta, Georgia 30309

William M. Scaljon, M.D. Urologist, Piedmont Hospital, 1968 Peachtree Road, N.W., Atlanta, Georgia 30309

Wyman P. Sloan III, M.D.   Internist, Piedmont Hospital, 1968 Peachtree Road, N.W., Atlanta, Georgia 30309

Mark E. Silverman, M.D.   Professor of Medicine, Emory University School of Medicine, and Chief of Cardiology, Piedmont Hospital, 1968 Peachtree Road, N.W., Atlanta, Georgia 30309

Douglas S. Stuart, M.D.   Neurologist, Piedmont Hospital, 105 Collier Road, Suite 5000, Atlanta, Georgia 30309

Bruce F. Walker, M.D.   Pathologist, Piedmont Hospital, 1968 Peachtree Road, N.W., Atlanta, Georgia 30309

Jonne B. Walter, M.D.   Pulmonologist, Piedmont Hospital, 1938 Peachtree Road, Suite 408, Atlanta, Georgia 30309

N. Spencer Welch, M.D.   Internist and Endocrinologist, Piedmont Hospital, 35 Collier Road, Suite 625, Atlanta, Georgia 30309

Kimberley E. Wilson, M.D.   Rheumatologist, Piedmont Hospital, 2001 Peachtree Road, N.W., Suite 205, Atlanta, Georgia 30309

W. Hayes Wilson, M.D.   Rheumatologist, Piedmont Hospital, 2001 Peachtree Road, N.E., Suite 205, Atlanta, Georgia 30309

Randy J. Yanda, M.D.   Gastroenterologist, Piedmont Hospital, 35 Collier Road, Suite 350, Atlanta, Georgia 30309

Preface

"Observe, record, tabulate, communicate. Use your five senses. . . . Learn to see, learn to hear, learn to feel, learn to smell, and know that by practice alone you can become expert. Medicine is learned by the bedside and not in the classroom. Let not your conceptions of disease come from words heard in the lecture room or read from the book. See, and then reason and compare and control. But see first."

William Osler, quoted by Thayer WS. Osler, the teacher. *Bull Johns Hopkins Hosp* 1919;30:198–200.

"As the role of the primary care physician as 'gatekeeper' expands in the future, so will the importance of a careful history and physical examination. . . . Continuing medical education in the 21st century should include offerings directed toward improving the already excellent clinical skills of experienced practitioners. After all, even top professional golfers use video feedback and coaching to stay on top of their game."

James T.C. Li. *Arch Intern Med* 1994;154:22–24. Copyright 1994, American Medical Association. Used with permission.

The diagnostic ability of William Osler, represented in the four familiar snapshots, "Osler at the Bedside," inspired generations of physicians. Until recently, this tradition of the bedside diagnostician was held in high esteem, and physicians took great pride in their ability to establish a diagnosis from a comprehensive clinical history, bedside examination, and simple testing. With the advent of highly sophisticated testing, physicians now devote less time to low technology data collection, and their interest and skills at bedside data collection have atrophied. In addition, there has been a corresponding decline of interest in the teaching of bedside skills to students and house staff at many academic centers, as well as in the use and interpretation of routine tests, such as the chest X-ray film and resting electrocardiogram. It is the premise of Clinical Skills For Adult Primary Care that future practice guidelines and restrictions on costly tests will renew an interest and satisfaction in the intrinsic value of starting with a careful history and examination before embarking on expensive high technology procedures.

This book was developed from a 3 month, twice a week course given for primary care physicians at Piedmont Hospital, a community hospital in Atlanta, Georgia. The course was designed in collaboration with practicing primary care physicians and consultants who were believed to be expert and experienced in problems that confront primary care physicians. Each clinician–teacher was asked to provide a one-hour discussion and demonstration of useful bedside skills pertinent to primary care based on their extensive experience and training. Common problems were emphasized, but infrequent findings and diseases that may appear were also included. The course was well received and it was felt that other primary care physicians might appreciate and benefit from a book reviewing these basic skills. A subsequent course on "Clinical Guidelines" led to a third section on routine testing. This section emphasizes that the basic clinical skills of primary care require thoughtful deliberation before ordering even a simple laboratory test because this may lead to an unwarranted cascade effect and an escalation in testing.

This book is directed to primary care physicians to be used as a handbook to review techniques, expand into areas that may not have been emphasized in their training, and for rethinking the utilization of routine laboratory testing. Medical students, nurse-clinicians, professional associates, and others on the front line should also find the material of interest and help in their training and in the care of patients.

Mark E. Silverman, M.D.
J. Willis Hurst, M.D.

Acknowledgments

We thank the contributors who have transferred their practical experience to paper while maintaining heavy practice responsibilities and cheerfully responded to nudging, editing, and deadlines. We thank Linda Mason for her invaluable skills and unfailing good cheer at putting this book together and Michelle Glazer, Mike Moseley, Jan Mulder, and Patsy Bryan for their talented photography and illustrations. We are most grateful to Lisa Berger at Lippincott-Raven Publishers and Helen Shaw at Colophon for their commitment to a quality book.

Clinical Skills for Adult Primary Care
edited by M. E. Silverman and J. W. Hurst.
Lippincott-Raven Publishers, Philadelphia © 1996.

1

The Role of the Primary Care Physician

J. Willis Hurst, M.D.

Emory University School of Medicine and Emory Hospital, Atlanta, Georgia 30322

*"There are, in truth, no specialties in medicine, since to know fully many of the most im-
portant diseases a man must be familiar with their manifestations in many organs."*
William Osler. *Army Surgeon Med News* 1894;64:318.

The "winds of change" are blowing strongly, and the delivery of primary care is
the centerpiece of the new era. The primary care physician will be called on to
give more definitive care than is currently practiced and will be expected to be an
expert in preventive medicine and cost containment.

This being true, the educational programs for medical students and house of-
ficers will change considerably in order to meet the needs of the future practicing primary care physician.

This book, *Clinical Skills for Adult Primary Care*, has been created with the
primary care physician in mind. In fact, many of the chapters were written by primary care physicians. The specialists who wrote the remainder of the book are in
daily contact with primary care physicians and recognize their needs. The book
does not cover everything that a primary care physician does. Rather, it emphasizes those areas that we, the editors, believe have been neglected.

WHAT DO PRIMARY CARE PHYSICIANS DO?

Primary care physicians should care for all of the medical needs of their patients. They are the patient's medical advisor, advocate, and friend. This does not
imply that they know everything or do everything. It does mean that they are trusted
to diagnose and manage those medical problems that they are trained to diagnose
and manage and that they arrange for consultation of those conditions requiring
the attention of a specialist. This approach gives the patient an anchor and elimi-
nates the need for "doctor shopping."

A list of the duties that primary care physicians are expected to perform are de-
picted in Table 1. These duties are discussed below.

TABLE 1. *Types of medical care provided by primary care physicians*

Comprehensive care
Follow-up care
Episodic care
Preventive care for sick patients
Preventive care for well patients
Paramedical care

See text description of each type of "care."

Comprehensive Care

Primary care physicians are interested in all of the patient's medical problems. Properly trained primary care physicians are capable of deciding if a headache is caused by a brain tumor or is a migraine headache. If the former is suspected, they know whom to call for help. Properly trained primary care physicians are capable of differentiating noncardiac chest pain from angina pectoris or myocardial infarction. Should help be needed to manage the latter, they arrange it. They are skilled in the recognition of the emotional and psychiatric state of the patient. They know when to seek the help of a psychiatrist.

Excellent primary care physicians become skilled at what they are doing. They become expert at history taking and the analysis of symptoms. They extract a great deal of diagnostic clues from the physical examination. They become proficient at interpreting electrocardiograms and other necessary laboratory data.

Comprehensive care requires that the primary care physician extract information about all of the body systems using the history, physical examination, and carefully selected routine laboratory tests. When the clues from each technique are reviewed, the primary care physician formulates a set of medical problems that characterize the entire patient (1). These medical conditions, or problems, should be listed on a special sheet and placed on the front of the medical record (1). Some of the medical problems will be a complete diagnosis, whereas others will need additional investigation before a complete diagnosis can be made.

The type of information that primary care physicians should gather from the history, physical examination, and routine laboratory tests are discussed in the subsequent chapters of the book. The type of workup used for initial comprehensive care is, of course, very different from the workup used in follow-up care or episodic care.

Above all, the patient knows to call the primary care physician whenever he or she is ill.

Follow-up Care

Well Persons

Should the primary care physician find no medical problems on the initial examination of the patient, the "well" person should be instructed in preventive care.

The follow-up care of the patient is individualized according to need. When a change in diet, the discontinuation of smoking, or the need for more exercise is recommended, the physician must assess the personality of the patient and make a judgment regarding the need for and timing of the follow-up visit. If there is a family history of diabetes and the level of the patient's blood glucose is currently normal, the physician may wish to determine the level of blood glucose every 6 months.

The blood pressure of persons with borderline hypertension should be checked on several visits to the physician's office (by nonphysicians as well as physicians). The physician should then judge how often the patient should be checked.

The point is that the physician must judge when the well patient should be seen again based on the data collected during the initial examination. The idea of checking "everything" annually is no longer the appropriate approach.

Sick Persons

The follow-up of patients in whom one or more medical problems are identified during the initial visit must also be individualized. The time of the follow-up visit and what to look for at the time of the visit is determined by the nature of the problem, the natural history of the problem, the possible modification of the problem with treatment, the side effects of the drugs used to treat the problem, and the anxiety of the patient. The data to be collected at the time of the follow-up should be predetermined to identify those items that permit the physician to ascertain whether the patient is recovering properly.

Episodic Care

The patient may develop an illness that is unrelated to the medical problems that were identified at the time of the initial illness. For example, the patient may develop acute cholecystitis. The primary care physician should be called. The primary care physician knows the patient and is familiar with the patient's list of medical problems, and arranges for surgical consultation for the condition.

Preventive Care for Sick Patients

The concept of preventive care is changing. Not only should primary care physicians make arrangements for the patient to receive the vaccines recommended to prevent influenza and pneumococcal pneumonia, but they should also extend their view of prevention to include the prevention of stroke in patients with atrial fibrillation, hypertension, or a carotid bruit; inoperable colon cancer; advanced cancer of the cervix; advanced prostate cancer; pulmonary emphysema and lung cancer; and pulmonary embolism in certain patients. In fact, the complications of many illnesses can be postponed or prevented, and primary care physicians should be aggressive in their efforts to prevent them.

Preventive Care for Well Persons

The primary care physician should be aggressive in his or her efforts to convince apparently well persons that appropriately prescribed exercise is useful; excessive exposure to the sun is dangerous; smoking will kill them; and that the person should always know their numbers, including weight, blood pressure, level of total cholesterol, and low-density lipoprotein and blood glucose levels. They should have a sigmoidoscopy and rectal examination at prescribed intervals (Chapter 28); mammograms after age 40 (Chapter 30), cervical smears for cancer (Chapter 17), and so forth.

Primary care physicians should make every effort to analyze the current medical literature and implement those preventive measures that they believe are worthwhile.

Paramedical Care

This term is used here to identify the type of medical workup required by the legal profession, the insurance industry, and for certain occupations. The primary care physician may be recruited to answer certain health questions related to these paramedical activities.

THE VALUE OF THE COMPREHENSIVE WORKUP

The comprehensive workup of a patient should enable the physician to either make a diagnosis or to establish a differential diagnosis in almost all patients. This statement is true if the primary care physician defines the data he or she plans to collect that will screen the population of patients he or she sees for conditions known to be prevalent in that population. The idea of a *thorough* or *complete* workup is a euphemism that is noncommunicative. The data to be collected must be defined. The physician must then become skilled at collecting the data. If it is important to examine the retina of the eye or to interpret an electrocardiogram, then it is necessary for the clinician to become proficient in doing so.

Today it is mandatory for the primary care physician to state the medical problem(s) as precisely as possible after the comprehensive (but defined) examination. This is necessary because the need for high-technology procedures is determined by the careful statement of the health problem that has been identified by using low technology (history, physical examination, and "routine" laboratory tests). Stated another way, those who use low technology poorly also use high technology poorly. They also waste a lot of money.

The Diagnostic Value of the History, Physical Examination, and the Routine Laboratory Tests

Several decades ago the medical masters of the day were prone to say that 70% of the diagnoses could be made by the analysis of symptoms (the history); 20% of the diagnoses could be made by interpreting the results of the physical examination; and 10% of the diagnoses could be made by analyzing the results of routine laboratory tests. As discussed in Chapter 2, a 1975 study indicated that the medical history provided the diagnoses in 66 of 80 patients in a British medical clinic, whereas seven patients were diagnosed by the physical examination and the remainder were diagnosed by laboratory tests (2). Although this was true in that setting, one must look at the population being served because the disease process itself predetermines the low-technology procedure that provides the diagnostic information, be it the history, the physical examination, or results of routine laboratory tests. For example, angina pectoris due to atherosclerotic coronary heart disease can be identified only in the history; faint aortic valve regurgitation can be identified only by physical examination; preexcitation of the ventricles can be documented only by the electrocardiogram; and an elevated blood level of low-density lipoprotein or blood glucose level can be discovered only by laboratory testing.

In many instances a clue to the diagnosis is found in the history, another clue is found in the physical examination, and still another clue in the results of routine laboratory tests. The clinician's analytical ability is challenged because the definitive diagnosis can be made only if he or she is highly skilled in adding up the clues.

The History

The details of the history that are related to each body system are not covered in this book. The technique of history taking is discussed at length in Chapter 2, and the often neglected recognition of mental illness is discussed in Chapter 3.

As discussed in Chapters 2 and 3, it is important to permit the patient to "tell his or her story," so the physician must develop listening skills. If patients are given an unlimited amount of time to tell their stories, many of them will give the clues to a diagnosis (if the physician is a skilled listener). Unfortunately, practical considerations do not permit this leisurely pace of data gathering and the physician must guide the interview without misleading or leading the patient. This is true because some patients may spend considerable time on irrelevant information. The legendary Paul Wood, one of the great diagnosticians of the mid-20th century, wrote, "It is scarcely too much to say that the best history-taker is he who can best interpret the answer to a leading question" (3).

I also recommend the occasional approach of the famous Sam Levine, who taught the value of the leading question (4). He pointed out that when he had difficulty obtaining a definite answer as to when a patient had chest discomfort that might be angina, he would ask, "I suppose the discomfort is improved when you walk up a hill." If the patient said, "No, no, it is worse when I walk up a hill," Dr. Levine believed he had reached a definite diagnosis of angina because the patient corrected him rather than passively agreeing with his leading question.

There is another gentle admonition that I wish to impart regarding the history. The words "chief complaint" bother me because they are sometimes viewed by the physician as the most important complaint. We must remember that it is the patient's complaint; however, the patient is hardly qualified to determine which is the most important medical problem he or she has when experiencing several symptoms. If the physician accepts the patient's chief complaint as meaning the chief problem, the physician may be led astray from the identification of a far more serious illness that is not bothering the patient to any serious degree at that time. For example, the patient's chief complaint may be caused by esophageal reflux, whereas in addition to the symptoms of esophageal reflux the patient has mild angina pectoris of recent onset (unstable angina) that may be the forerunner of a myocardial infarction.

Finally, the examining physician must always be aware of the clinical setting in which he or she sees the patient. For example, a pulmonary embolus should be considered in a patient with acute dyspnea who 3 days before experiencing symptoms had surgery for fracture of the hip.

History taking has two objectives: to collect scientific information and to establish a relationship of trust between the physician and patient. It takes a lifetime of intense effort to learn to take an excellent medical history.

Physical Examination

The physician must define in advance the types of data he or she wishes to collect on the physical examination. The words *thorough* and *complete* have no communicative value. The physician must then develop the skill to identify (and understand) the abnormalities that are discovered.

There must be no pretense. If the stethoscope is used to examine the heart, the examiner must listen specifically for certain defined abnormalities. When this is not done, the murmur of mitral stenosis is missed or gallop sounds are not heard.

The examiner must not write in the record that the "EENT examination is essentially normal" when the word *essentially* is not defined and the examiner has not checked the patient's vision or hearing or has not examined the retina, etc. The examiner must record exactly what was examined and discovered. The medical record is no place for a hazy entry.

The physical examination as discussed in this book is not intended to cover everything. However, the information offered will be useful to the primary care physician.

Routine Laboratory Tests

Routine laboratory tests must be carefully defined. Routine laboratory tests should screen the patient for certain illnesses that cannot be identified by the history or physical examination. Furthermore, the results should be positive often enough to make the testing worthwhile. It is this latter requirement that creates the controversy. No one doubts the value of knowing the level of blood glucose or lipoproteins in asymptomatic subjects, but one can question the value of knowing the level of serum calcium in an asymptomatic subject.

These issues are discussed in Chapter 32.

THE COST OF MEDICAL CARE

There is little hope that medical care in the future will cost less than it costs now. Gene therapy, for example, will not be cheap. However, the primary care physician can help enormously because an excellent, defined examination may decrease the cost of unnecessary and costly high-technology procedures. When Will Strunk wrote *The Elements of Style*, his little book on grammar, he emphasized "Omit needless words." He was not urging his readers to write briefly, but he was asking them to be sure every word counted (5). The same is true with the use of high technology. No thinking person should say that high technology is not valuable because, after all, it is why medical care has improved. Thinking persons would say that there should be specific indications for the proper use of high-technology procedures. For example, a physician should not order an echocardiogram to determine if there is a heart murmur because he or she is not skilled in auscultation. The information gained by high technology must assist in the improvement of the care of the patient. The high-cost test must not be performed because the result will be interesting or make the patient care seem more "complete" or just to document findings that will not be acted upon. In fact, this approach may document an extraneous benign finding that is harmful to the patient's insurance rating or future employment. Excellent clinical judgment is often manifested in the discipline of knowing when not to order a test.

The thesis here is that the primary care physician is in a position to identify all of the patient's medical problems and, when the problems are formulated properly, he or she should know when to obtain consultation (if needed) or when to use properly selected high-technology procedures.

THE MEDICAL RECORD

An organized medical record with a well thought out problem list is basic to good medical care, proper thinking, proper communication, and the proper teaching of all concerned with the care of the patient. I favor the Weed system, which is better known as the problem-oriented system (1). The problem-oriented record can be manually generated or created using a computer.

FINAL COMMENT

It is hoped that this book will stimulate a good bit of thinking and serve as a refresher course for those who engage in primary care for adults.

REFERENCES

1. Weed LL. *Medical records, medical education, and patient care.* Chicago: Year Book Medical; 1969.
2. Hampton JR, Harrison MJ, Mitchell JR, et al. Relative contributions of history taking, physical examination, and laboratory investigations to a diagnosis and management of medical outpatients. *Br Med J* 1975;2:486–9.
3. Wood P. *Diseases of the heart and circulation.* Philadelphia: Lippincott; 1956:1.
4. Sam Levine, communicated in teaching sessions.
5. Strunk W Jr, White EB. *The elements of style.* New York: Macmillan; 1959:IX.

SUGGESTED READING

Hurst JW. Ten reasons why Lawrence Weed is right. *N Engl J Med* 1971;284:51–2.
Hurst JW. *The bench and me.* New York: Igaku-Shoin; 1992.
Hurst JW. The value of a patient problem list. *Emory Univ J Med* 1989;4:293–5.

Clinical Skills for Adult Primary Care
edited by M. E. Silverman and J. W. Hurst.
Lippincott-Raven Publishers, Philadelphia © 1996.

2

The General History

T. Kirkland Garner, M.D.

Piedmont Hospital, Atlanta, Georgia 30309

"In taking histories follow each line of thought; ask no leading questions; never suggest. Give the patient's own words in the complaint."

William Osler, quoted in Bean WB. *Sir William Osler: Aphorisms.*
Springfield, IL: Charles C Thomas, 1968:41.

The historical interview provides the data from which many diagnoses are made, initiates a medium by which a therapeutic bond is formed with the patient, and creates a forum for education, thereby improving adherence with therapy (1). The history alone provided the correct diagnosis in 66 of 80 patients in a British medical clinic. An additional seven patients were diagnosed by physical examination (most had heart disease). The remaining patients were diagnosed by laboratory tests (2). The average physician, in a professional lifetime of 40 years, may perform 120,000 to 160,000 histories. Even assuming a brief 5 minutes, this will amount to a minimum of 10,000 hours (1). Considering efficiency as well as patient and physician satisfaction, this interaction often falls short of the ideal. This can lead to widespread dissatisfaction manifesting as patient noncompliance and clinician burnout. This may be partially attributed to a lack of respect by the physician for the information obtained from the history compared with the glittering array of sophisticated laboratory tests that have been developed over the past 30 years.

The courtroom-style series of yes/no questions used by many physicians has been criticized. One study of internists found that the patient was able to complete their response to the opening question in only 23% of the interviews. In 69%, the patient was interrupted to follow up on a stated problem after an average of only 15 seconds. For the 31% of the patients who were allowed to continue, none took more than $2^{11}/_{42}$ minutes to complete their opening statement (3). Patients' perceptions that their emotions were ignored has resulted in dissatisfaction that may often lead to doctor shopping. In addition, physicians were found to be more satisfied when they were able to respond to their patient's emotional distress.

9

TECHNIQUE

Better interviewing techniques can lead to a "win–win" situation for both physician and patient. Steven Cohen-Cole and Julian Bird have developed an approach to the patient interview that serves the following three functions (1):

- Gathering information
- Developing rapport with the patient and responding to the patient's emotions
- Educating the patient and motivating the patient to cooperate with therapy

This technique is neither a license for letting a patient ramble on nor for taking the patient on an emotional roller coaster ride. Physicians who master the three-function interview find that the reward outweighs the drawbacks and requires only minor changes in their previous approach.

Chief Complaint and History of Present Illness (HPI)

After welcoming the patient and introducing yourself, open with a question that gets to the reason for the visit; either of the following or some variation has been found to work well: "What brought you here?" or "How can I help you?" To get to the origin of the present illness, ask "When was the last time you felt perfectly well?" Another way to show that the physician is genuinely interested in the patient is to start by saying "Tell me about yourself." As Osler said, "Care more particularly for the individual patient than for the special features of the disease" (4). The physician should sit at eye level with the patient, preferably at a nonauthoritarian angle with a relaxed habitus, leaning forward, making eye contact, and lis-

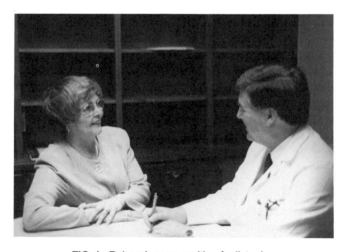

FIG. 1. Relaxed, open position for listening.

tening—just listening (5) (Fig. 1). As we have seen, most patients' opening statements take no more than $2^{11}/_{42}$ minutes. Minimal notes are taken, pausing only to jot down important details with minimal loss of eye contact. If the patient is hesitant, a nod, other nonverbal cues, an "uh-huh" or "yes" should prompt the patient to continue. Silence on the part of the physician will often encourage the patient to drop his or her guard and reveal a hidden reason for the visit. Open-ended questions are useful in eliciting valuable information; for example, instead of asking "Are you short of breath?" it may be better to ask "Tell me about your breathing."

Characterization of Symptoms

It is important to refine the history of the present illness as much as possible and to search for relevant details. This is helped by exploring the following eight elements that may distinguish a symptom of one disease from another:

- Body location: the location of maximal intensity or origin. Diagrams that the patient completes may be helpful, especially in chronic pain.
- Quality: try to record the patient's own words, or, if vague or contradictory, record this as well.
- Quantity: a zero to ten scale, with zero being no pain and ten being completely unbearable, is useful. One experienced physician used a "dollar's worth of pain" to help follow pain levels in a patient. ("If it was a dollar's worth of pain then, how much is it now?")
- Chronology: the precise date of onset and its development over time.
- Setting: the time of day, the activity level, the fasting or eating state, the work or social context, the emotional setting.
- Aggravating or alleviating factors: what was done or taken to get relief, the effect of body position, respiration, and movement.
- Associated symptoms: before, during, and after the symptom being clarified.
- Previous episodes: patients will often remember these if asked.

It is important that the physician convey to the patient that he or she is interested, sympathetic, and nonjudgmental, even with difficult interviews when the patient may become upset or hostile. It is usually helpful to use reflection to help create a therapeutic bond by verbally acknowledging the patient's emotional state; for example, "You seem sad" or "This seems to be difficult for you." Most patients find these kind of remarks reassuring for they indicate concern with the patient's whole being, not just the physical illness. Physicians, being human, are likely to filter the data through their own experience and values. A study of the effect of presentation style of a 40-year-old woman with chest pain showed that internists who were randomized to view a videotape of a "businesslike" presentation by an actress were more likely to order a cardiac workup (93%) than were the internists who viewed a videotape of the same actress with the same symptoms but with a "histrionic" portrayal (53%) (6).

Nonverbal Communication

The impact of the social encounter is often communicated nonverbally. This nonverbal communication influences the physician's assessment of the credibility of the data (as in the above example), the severity of the illness, and the generation of diagnostic hypotheses and their proof or repudiation (5). Examples of nonverbal communication include paralanguage (the pitch, intensity, and tempo of language), physical appearance (clothing, adornments, make-up, hairstyle, gender, ethnic origin), kinesis (gestures, posture, trunk and limb movement), visual behavior (eye contact behavior), and proxemics (interpersonal distance and spacing relationships).

Recapitulation

When the history of the present illness is completed, recapitulation is a useful technique to employ. The physician should summarize the history and repeat it to the patient, saying something like "Let's see if I understand your problem. You were well until 3 days ago when you began to have a dull continuous pain in your lower stomach. . . ." This is a self-checking device that will improve the accuracy of data collection and will also let the patient know that the physician has listened carefully.

Patient's Perception of the Problem

A question that will often yield useful information is "What do you think is wrong?" This allows the patients to present their ideas about the cause and sometimes the cure of their problem as they perceive it. It is sometimes important to understand the patient's cultural and folk medicine beliefs and behaviors and how they might influence the patient's diagnosis and adherence to therapy (7). The present illness can be turned from a chronicle to a more patient-centered story by eliciting, then documenting in a sentence or two, what the illness has been like for the patient (8).

EFFICIENCY AND THE PROBLEM OF TIME

Efficiency and negotiation are the answers to the problem of time. Efficiency in this context means letting patients tell the story in their opening statement which, as we have stated, usually takes less than 3 minutes if there are no interruptions. The physician should follow up on the symptoms with open-ended questions phrased "Tell me about . . ." and then, "What else is bothering you?" To get a psychosocial insight, ask "What is going on in your life?" If the patient has a large number of nonacute problems, negotiate with the patient about which problems can be handled at the next visit. After a brief and efficient physical examination of the pertinent areas, provide patient education, remembering to address the patient's concerns, while enlisting the patient's cooperation in the therapy chosen.

Many physicians use questionnaires to supplement their history taking. These may be derived for the physician's defined population and problems or by using a commercially prepared version. In general, questionnaires are most useful to supplement, not replace, the careful oral interview. Computerized history taking has been studied in The Netherlands, where there is widespread use and availability of personal computers in medical practice (9). Patient acceptance of computerized history taking is excellent, with 92% of the patients finding it useful. However, the patient's complaint was expressed in the oral interview much better than in the computerized version. The history obtained from the computerized questionnaire will produce 40% more clinical data, but the clinician must refine it and determine its usefulness. The authors of the study concluded that computerized history taking is suitable for certain patients but not as a replacement for the careful oral interview.

Review of Systems

When the patient appears to have finished giving the history of the present illness, and you have completed the follow-up questions, ask "What else is bothering you?" Then use the data-gathering techniques described above. By doing this, you create a data base of information and a patient-driven review of systems. Some feel that the traditional review of systems using a series of closed-ended questions may produce as many blind trails and false-positive results as an indiscriminately ordered serum multichannel analysis (10).

FAMILY HISTORY

The family history deserves emphasis for it can provide useful information that leads to advice on preventing genetically determined illnesses. It may also elicit fears from the patient that he or she is concerned about sharing a terrible disease with a family member. The age (or age at death), state of health, and diseases present should be ascertained for at least the parents and siblings. The patient should be asked, "Are there any diseases that run in your family?" It is particularly important to ask about the familial occurrence of diabetes mellitus, hypertension, kidney disease, heart disease or stroke, cancer of the breast or colon, sudden death, and depression. Slang is appropriate such as "Did anyone have hardening of the arteries? . . . sugar diabetes . . . high blood pressure?" The patient should be specifically questioned about birth defects, retardation of growth, and mental development. If there is a history suggesting a genetically determined disorder, an extensive pedigree of the family members should be recorded on a diagram (11).

PSYCHOSOCIAL HISTORY AND OCCUPATIONAL HISTORY

A pertinent psychosocial history can be elicited by asking "What else is going on in your life?" The answer to this question gives a window of opportunity for the patient to express concerns that they might otherwise be too ashamed or preoccupied to express (12). Other useful questions are "Tell me about your day," "What do you do to relax?" and "Are there things that you do that cause you to be embarrassed or you would not want others to know?" Work and hobbies are important. A useful question is "Have you ever had any job or hobby that might cause you to be exposed to toxic gases, dusts, fumes, or chemicals?"

SEX AND SUBSTANCES

Alcohol and tobacco use, illicit drug use, and the sexual practices of the patient are important areas to discuss. These issues must be discussed frankly, openly, and in a nonjudgmental manner. A useful general question for opening these areas is "Tell me about your marriage (or relationship)." Follow up with ". . . and your sexual relations?" "Do you engage in any activities that might place you at risk for AIDS?" "Do you donate blood?" (A patient who has donated blood has been tested for the human immunodeficiency virus and hepatitis A, B, and C.) "Are there things that you do that you feel are harmful?" If the patient answers yes to tobacco use, quantitate the type and amount of tobacco (pipe, cigars, cigarettes, or "smokeless"). If the patient answers yes to alcohol use, try to quantitate the type and amount. The "CAGE" test is a useful screen. An affirmative answer to two or more questions identifies problem drinkers with a 75% accuracy (13):

- Have you ever thought that you should **C**ut down on your drinking?
- Have people **A**nnoyed you by criticizing your drinking?
- Have you ever felt bad or **G**uilty about your drinking?
- Have you ever had a drink first thing in the morning to steady your nerves or to get rid of a hangover (**E**ye opener)?

This may be an appropriate time to counsel the patient regarding life-style issues (14) (Table 1).

PAST MEDICAL HISTORY

Questions such as "Tell me about any times you were in the hospital" and "Tell me about any surgery you have had" are useful ways to obtain a past medical history. Ask the patient specifically about childhood diseases, as well as hepatitis, rheumatic fever, polio, tuberculosis, diabetes, cancer, arthritis, seizures, stroke and vascular disease, heart, lung, or liver disease, and peptic ulcer.

TABLE 1. *Elements of periodic counseling of adults about health matters, according to three expert panels*

Health issue	Focus of counseling	ACP	CTF	USTF
Nutrition counseling	Follow diet and exercise to maintain desirable weight; total fat intake, <30% of calories, and saturated fat, <10%; cholesterol intake, <300 mg/day; high fiber, low sodium	Yes	NC	Yes
Calcium and iron levels	Maintain adequate dietary intake	NC	NR (C)	Yes
Physical activity	Explain role of exercise in disease prevention (USTF); tell women >40 yr about immobility and bone mass (CTF)	NC	Yes (C)	Yes (A)
Breast and testes self-examination	Counsel patients to perform self-examination	NC	NR (C)	NR (C)
Sexual practices	Advise patients about barrier contraception (B); transmission of sexually transmitted diseases (C); avoidance of anal intercourse (C) and needle-sharing behavior (A)	NC	NC	Yes
Tobacco use	Counsel quitting, especially if at high risk for coronary artery disease or lung cancer	Yes	Yes (A)	Yes (A)
Alcohol	Apply case-finding approach for problem drinking (CTF); stop alcohol use during pregnancy (USTF); limit alcohol use	Yes	Yes (B)	Yes (A)
Intravenous drugs	Counsel about dangers; advise to quit	Yes	NC	Yes
Injury prevention	Encourage use of seat belts	Yes	Yes (C)	Yes (A)
	Avoid back injuries; protect against violence and firearm injuries	NC	NC	Yes
	Teach fire safety (install smoke detectors; do not smoke in bed)	NC	Yes (C)	Yes
	Teach the elderly to avoid falls	NC	Yes (C)	Yes
	Store firearms unloaded in locked container	NC	NC	Yes
Dental hygiene	Encourage daily oral hygiene	NC	Yes (A)	Yes (A)
Functional assessment	Elicit marital and sexual problems	Yes	Yes (B)	Yes
	Assess cognitive and physical function in elderly	Yes	Yes (B)	Yes
Prevention of unwanted pregnancy	Advise use of contraceptives	NC	Yes (B)	Yes (A)

ACP, American College of Physicians; CTF, Canadian Task Force; USTF, U.S. Preventive Services Task Force; A, favorable recommendation based on strong evidence; B, favorable recommendation based on weak evidence; C, intermediate recommendation in which the evidence is too weak to support a positive or a negative recommendation; D, unfavorable recommendation based on weak evidence; E, unfavorable recommendation based on strong evidence; NC, not considered, meaning that the expert panel did not review the topic or withheld comment.

The task forces occasionally make a recommendation despite grade C evidence (Yes (C) or No (C)), but the usual recommendation with grade C evidence is NR (no recommendation). The American College of Physicians did not grade its recommendations, and the U.S. Task Force did so only for selected topics. Reprinted from Sox HC. Preventive health services in adults. *N Engl J Med* 1994;330:1592 by permission of the New England Journal of Medicine, Copyright 1994. Massachusetts Medical Society. All rights reserved.

ALLERGIES

Ask the patient "Have you ever had any allergies or reactions to any medications, foods, or substances?" Any positive responses must be followed up in detail. Determine the nature of the reaction, whether the patient was seen by a physician, and ask specifically about penicillin, sulfa drugs, and radiocontrast media.

MEDICATIONS

"Tell me about your medications." Ask the patient specifically about over-the-counter medications, vitamins, supplements, eye drops, ear drops, topical medications, hormone supplements, and home remedies. Inquire about medications at each visit. Many patients are seeing multiple physicians and receiving medications from all of them. Advise the patients to bring all medications on each visit.

ADHERENCE

Praise the patient for what they have done to adhere to therapy. This includes the family members and significant others. An example of this involves an older woman who was having severe life stress due to her husband's progressive Alzheimer's disease. The physician said, "You are to be commended for the way you are looking after your husband. I know that it is very difficult for you." At this, the patient burst into tears and said, "You know, in all this time, you are the first person to recognize this." After this, the patient and her physician had excellent communication about herself and her husband. Expressing empathy such as this will enhance the physician–patient bond and adherence to instructions.

EDUCATION

Find out what the patient thinks is causing the illness. Later, when all the data have been collected and a conclusion reached, it is important for the physician to tell the patient in brief and precise terms what is wrong. Find out what the patient already knows about the diagnosis. Answer the patient's questions and make sure the patient can express a reasonable understanding of the illness, according to his or her level of education. Negotiate goals with the patient and discuss a plan with the patient for reaching those goals.

CONCLUSION

Listening must be active and the interviewing clinician must be willing to let the patients tell their stories, with little interruption, in a helpful, open, nonjudgmental way. The physician "must follow the patient, much as one follows a dance partner" (15). So be like Ginger Rogers, not like Fred Astaire.

REFERENCES

1. Cohen-Cole SA. *The medical interview: the three function approach.* St. Louis: Mosby, 1991.
2. Hampton JR, Harrison MJ, Mitchell JR, et al. Relative contributions of history taking, physical examination, and laboratory investigation to diagnosis and management of medical outpatients. *Br Med J* 1975;2:486–9.
3. Beckman HB, Frankel RM. The effect of physician behavior on the collection of data. *Ann Intern Med* 1984;101:692–6.
4. Osler W. Address to the students of the Albany Medical College. *Albany Med Ann* 1899;20:307.
5. Nardone DA, Johnson GK, Faryna A, et al. A model for the diagnostic interview: nonverbal, verbal, and cognitive assessments. *J Gen Intern Med* 1992;7:432–7.
6. Birdwell BG, Herbers JE, Kroenke K. Evaluating chest pain: the patient's presentation style alters the physician's diagnostic approach. *Arch Intern Med* 1993;153:1991–5.
7. Prachter LM. Culture and clinical care: folk illness beliefs and behaviors and their implications for health care delivery. *JAMA* 1994;271:690–4.
8. Donnelly WJ. Righting the medical record: transforming chronicle into story. *JAMA* 1988;260:823–5.
9. Quaak MJ, Westerman RF, van Bemmel JH. Comparisons between written and computerized patient histories. *Br Med J* 1987;295:184–90.
10. Hoffbrand BI. Away with the system review: a plea for parsimony. *Br Med J* 1990;298:817–9.
11. Walker HK, Hall WD, Hurst JW. *Clinical methods: the history, physical, and laboratory examinations.* 3rd ed. Boston: Butterworths, 1990.
12. Branch WT, Malik TK. Using "windows of opportunities" in brief patient interviews to understand patient concerns. *JAMA* 1993;1667–8.
13. Mayfield D, McLeod G, Hall P. The CAGE test for alcohol use. *Am J Psychiatry* 1974;131:1121–3.
14. Sox HC. Preventive health services in adults. *N Engl J Med* 1994;330:1589–95.
15. Smith RC, Hoppe RB. The patient's story: integrating the patient- and physician-centered approaches to interviewing. *Ann Intern Med* 1991;115:470–7.
16. Hayward RSA, Steinberg EP, Ford DE, et al. Preventive care guidelines: 1991. *Ann Intern Med* 1991; 114:758–83. [Erratum, *Ann Intern Med* 1991;115:332.]

SUGGESTED READING

Meador CK. *A little book of doctor's rules.* Philadelphia: Mosby Year Book, 1992.
Morgan WL, Engel GL. *The clinical approach to the patient.* Philadelphia: W.B. Saunders, 1969.

Clinical Skills for Adult Primary Care
edited by M. E. Silverman and J. W. Hurst.
Lippincott-Raven Publishers, Philadelphia © 1996.

3

The Recognition of Mental Illness

Dave McAlister Davis, M.D.

Piedmont Hospital, Atlanta, Georgia 30309

"Care more particularly for the individual patient than for the special features of the disease."

William Osler. Address to the students of the Albany Medical College.
Albany Med Ann 1899;20:307.

At any given time, between 30 and 45 million Americans, nearly one in five people, are experiencing some form of mental illness that requires professional treatment (1). Twenty percent of these individuals will seek care in the non–mental health-care sector (2). At least one third of all patients who present to the primary care physician will have a psychiatric disorder that is important to address. Strikingly, it was found that the lifetime prevalence for any diagnosable psychiatric disorder was 48% and the 12-month prevalence 29.5%. The lifetime prevalence of affective disorders was 19%; of anxiety disorders, 25%; and of substance abuse, 27% (3).

The main tasks of the primary care physician are as follows:

- To obtain a history that covers relevant psychiatric material.
- To formulate a diagnosis.
- To provide a supportive atmosphere for discussion and therapy.
- To treat those psychiatric conditions that he or she is competent to treat.
- To make a decision if a referral to a psychiatric colleague is indicated and to prepare the patient properly for the psychiatric consultation.

INTERVIEW

In order to assess a patient for an emotional disturbance, the physician should obtain the following information in addition to that obtained in the usual medical interview.

Developmental History

Screening Questions

- Are there experiences from your childhood or adolescence that are bothering you today?
- Were you ever abused as a child?
- Did you grow up in a loving home?
- Was your family life nurturing as a child?
- What were the three worst things that happened to you as a child?

A developmental history is essential. It is important to know who reared the patient and what type of parenting the patient received. Were the parents available, loving, affirming, and did they provide accurate information? Was there ridicule, abandonment, emotional or physical separations, or excessive shaming? Do they know what their parents' philosophy of child rearing was? Was there verbal, physical, or sexual abuse?

Was there any family history of psychiatric illness or psychiatric treatment, addiction, psychiatric hospitalization, suicide, homicide, or jailings? Ask specifically about each immediate family member and their current state of mental health. Did the family move around?

Early behavioral history is important. As a child or adolescent, were they ever in trouble for lying, stealing, shoplifting, fire-setting, cruelty to animals, fighting, truancy, destruction of property, or cruelty to people? Have they ever been in juvenile court or in a foster home? Obtain an educational history. What was the highest grade the patient completed? Why did they stop school? Were there any adolescent pregnancies? What kind of grades did they receive, were they in special education, and were they ever expelled or suspended from school? Did they receive any honors or participate in extracurricular activities?

It is helpful to ask, "What were the three worst things that happened to you as a child?"

Marital History

Screening Questions

- How is your marriage now?
- How are you and your spouse getting along?
- Is your current sexual life satisfactory?

The marital history should include information about the course of the marriage and the quality of the relationship. Have there been previous marriages, divorces, or separations? If so, are there child support payments and parental visits? Obtain information about the course of all marriages. Include a sexual history to learn when the individual became interested in sexuality, when they began intercourse, number of pregnancies, number of partners, and sexual orientation and experience. Additional helpful information is to know if the patient has been in trouble because of their sexual behavior, and information about masturbation and their masturbatory fantasies.

Occupational History

Screening Questions

* How are things at work now?
* How is your spouse's job?

Occupational history can be extremely helpful. When did the individual begin working? What is the philosophy about work? Do they enjoy work? Obtain a history of all jobs and their outcomes. What is the longest period of continual employment with one company? Have they ever been fired from a job? Have they ever been on worker's compensation or unemployment? What is their level of income?

Legal History

Screening Question

* Have you ever been in trouble with the law or other authorities?

Has the patient ever been arrested, convicted of a crime, filed bankruptcy, or lost their driver's license? Have they ever spent time in jail or prison? Have they ever filed bankruptcy or paid child support? Have they ever filed a lawsuit or been sued? Do they participate in risky or impulsive behaviors?

Adult History

Screening Question

* Has your adulthood turned out like you had hoped?

It is very helpful to know about the patient's current living situation. Do they have religious beliefs and are they active? Are they members of any civic, social, political, or occupational organizations? What are their hobbies and how do they spend their leisure time? Does the patient drink, smoke, or use recreational drugs? What has been their experience in the past?

Psychiatric History

Screening Question

- Have you ever had psychiatric, psychological, or other types of psychiatric counseling?

Patients are often reluctant to admit previous treatment, so they must be questioned closely. Have they ever seen a marriage counselor, school counselor, or minister for help? Have they ever been in a psychiatric hospital or been on any type of psychiatric medication? Have they ever had a physician or anyone else give them a psychiatric diagnosis?

MENTAL STATUS EXAMINATION

A complete mental status examination should be performed. When there is a question of any organic brain disorder, the Mini Mental Status Exam should also be completed (see Chapter 19).

Screening Examination

- Orientation
- Cooperation
- Alertness and concentration
- General appearance and grooming
- Rapport
- Speech (rate, tone, volume, inflection)
- Mood
- Anxiety level (panic attacks, phobias)
- Appropriateness
- Anger level
- Vegetative signs (sleep, energy, appetite, libido)
- Cognition (hallucinations, delusions, ideas of reference)
- Obsessions or compulsions
- Memory
- Intelligence and general fund of information
- Spontaneity
- Sense of humor
- Common sense

All patients with mood, anxiety, or substance abuse disorders should be questioned about suicidal thoughts. If any such thoughts are present, question them about a plan, availability of methods, previous attempts. Refer all such patients immediately to a psychiatrist and record this carefully in your records.

DIAGNOSTIC APPROACH

The current criteria for psychiatric diagnoses are delineated in the *Diagnostic and Statistical Manual of Mental Disorders* (4th ed.) (DSM-IV) of the American Psychiatric Association published in 1994 (4). DSM-IV uses a multiaxial system composed of five axes: axis I includes the clinical (psychiatric) disorders; axis II includes the personality disorders and mental retardation; axis III is for general medical conditions; axis IV relates to psychosocial and environmental problems; and axis V rates the global assessment of function on a scale.

The primary care physician should be generally familiar with the DSM-IV, but an in-depth knowledge of making psychiatric diagnoses is a formidable undertaking. The most common errors made in diagnoses are discussed below.

Diagnosing Symptoms Instead of Syndromes

Anxiety may manifest itself in terms of anticipatory anxiety, phobias, panic attacks, or compulsions, all of which have different treatment. Depression may be due to bipolar illness, major depression, or chronic personality characteristics.

Not Diagnosing Axis II (Personality Disorders and Mental Retardation) Disorders

Personality disorders exist in at least 35% of the population and often significantly impact the presentation of both physical and mental disorders. The personality disorder itself may be the major cause of the patient's difficulty. Although the patient may present with symptoms of depression—anxiety, fatigue, insomnia, etc.—the personality disorder, not a clinical syndrome, may be the major cause.

Not Diagnosing Comorbid Disorders

Comorbid conditions are common in psychiatric patients. For example, there is an extremely high rate of alcoholism and other substance abuse in patients with anxiety disorders. Comorbidity rates of addictive disorders in psychiatric patients vary, but have been reported to be 80% in antisocial personality disorders, 50% in bipolar and schizophrenic disorders, 30% in depressive and anxiety disorders, and 25% in phobic disorders (5–8). The reverse also is often true: that patients seen in addiction settings frequently have psychiatric diagnoses (9). The setting in which a patient goes for treatment is important in determining what prevalence rates are found for comorbidity; this would be true whether the patient is seen in a primary care, psychiatric care, or addiction setting (10). Additionally, there is a high rate of comorbidity between a depressive disorder, obsessive compulsive disorder, generalized anxiety disorder, and phobias. A patient who has one of these has a high likelihood of having one or more of the others.

Not Diagnosing Substance Abuse

Alcohol abuse and drug usage are so common in the population that all patients should be carefully screened.

Using Outdated Diagnoses

DSM-IV replaced previous psychiatric nomenclature; such terms as reactive depression, endogenous depression, and manic-depressive illness are no longer used.

Not Obtaining Outside Histories from Family and Others

Family members are especially helpful in terms of gathering information on substance abuse, personality changes, violent behavior, and suicidal tendencies.

Not Obtaining Old Psychiatric Records

If the primary care physician contemplates prescribing any psychiatric medication, he or she should try to obtain records of all previous psychiatric treatment.

MALPRACTICE RISKS

When a primary care physician undertakes the care of a psychiatric patient, they may be held to the same standard of care as a psychiatrist. Psychiatric experts, testifying for plaintiffs, tend to hold that a physician who undertakes psychiatric treatment should do so with the same level of knowledge and competence as a psychiatrist. The most likely reasons for a law suit against a primary care physician are as follows:

- Suicide
- Improper diagnosis
- Drug reactions
- Failure to refer to a psychiatrist
- Failure to hospitalize
- Tardive dyskinesia

REFERRAL AND PREPARATION

Often the primary care physician is in the best position to learn about an individual's emotional problems. The patient may present the symptoms directly or indirectly. In most cases, a presumptive diagnosis can be made and a referral arranged, if indicated. The primary care physician should be familiar with several psychiatrists in the community, including psychiatrists who do family work, treat children, and handle substance abuse problems.

A good psychiatrist should be board certified, kind and empathic, and trained at an institution with a good psychiatric residency program. It is a good sign if the psychiatrist is a member of the county medical association and/or active with hospital medical staff or other community organizations. It is also often a plus if the psychiatrist has been involved in some type of personal therapy. This frequently makes the psychiatrist a more empathic therapist.

All serious psychiatric disorders should be immediately referred to a psychiatrist. This includes any complicated condition such as psychosis, organic brain syndrome, bipolar illness, schizophrenia, obsessive-compulsive disorder, or patients with suicidal or homicidal tendencies. Moderate cases of depressive anxiety or panic disorder also should be referred, especially if the illness has begun to impact the patient's daily functioning at home or work. Mild or moderate cases of anxiety or depression may be treated, but if the patient has not significantly improved by 4 to 6 weeks, then they should be referred. Most primary care physicians only know one or two treatment approaches, and patients are likely to become discouraged and/or noncompliant by their third treatment trial. Because new therapeutic techniques are rapidly being developed for psychiatric disorders, the primary care physician may wish to obtain a "curbside" consultation by phone before beginning any medication or treatment.

It is important to prepare the patient appropriately for the referral. Those patients who come well prepared from their primary care physician do much better. They are better motivated for therapy, form a bond and rapport much more quickly, and tend to get down to work from the beginning. The patient should be informed that psychiatric evaluations are confidential, and that all information presented to the psychiatrist is privileged. However, primary physicians should inform the patient of their desire to remain apprised of the diagnosis, treatment plan, and progress so as to be able to deliver the highest level of overall medical care to the patient.

It frequently helps for physicians to tell the patient that they know the psychiatrist personally and to give the patient a few facts about the psychiatrist's involvement in the medical community. This helps to decrease the patient's stereotypes about psychiatrists and allows the patient to see the psychiatrist as an overall part of the medical support system. It is also helpful to let the patient know that the psychiatrist may need one or more interviews to gather enough information to set up a treatment plan. The patient should be reassured that the psychiatrist will want to get to know them well before beginning any medication, unless the need for medication is urgent. The patient generally appreciates this. The primary care physician should ask if it would be okay to call the psychiatrist in the patient's presence to make the referral. This often helps to establish a three-way bond.

REFERENCES

1. American Psychiatric Association. *Facts about: mental illness.* Washington, DC: American Psychiatric Press, 1987.
2. American Psychiatric Association. *Principles/national health care reform press.* Washington, DC: American Psychiatric Association, 1993.
3. Kessler RC, McGonagle KA, Zhao S, et al. Lifetime and 12 month prevalence of DSM-III-R psychiatric disorders in the United States. *Arch Gen Psychiatry* 1994;51:8–19.
4. *American Psychiatric Association: diagnostic and statistical manual of mental disorders.* 4th ed. Washington, DC: American Psychiatric Press, 1994.
5. Regier DA, Farmer ME, Rae DS, et al. Comorbidity of mental disorders with alcohol and other drug abuse. *JAMA* 1990;264:2511–9.
6. Drake RE, Wallach MA. Substance abuse among the chronically mentally ill. *Hosp Commun Psychiatry* 1989;40:1041–6.
7. Brady K, Casto S, Lydiard RB. Substance abuse in an inpatient psychiatric sample. *Am J Drug Alcohol Abuse* 1991;17:389–98.
8. Pepper B, Kirshner MC, Ryglewicz H. The young adult chronic patient: overview of a population. *Hosp Commun Psychiatry* 1981;32:463–74.
9. Helzer JE, Pryzbeck TR. The co-occurrence of alcoholism with other psychiatric disorders in the general population and its impact on treatment. *J Stud Alcohol* 1991;49:219–24.
10. Miller NS. Prevalence and treatment models for addiction in psychiatric populations. *Psych Ann* 1994; 24:399–406.

SUGGESTED READING

Gabbard GO. *Psychodynamic psychiatry in clinical practice.* Washington, DC: American Psychiatric Press, 1994.
Scheiber SC. The psychiatric interview, psychiatric history and mental status examination. In: Hales RE, Yudofsky SC, Talbott JA. *Textbook of psychiatry.* 2nd ed. Washington, DC: American Psychiatric Press, 1994.
Spitzer RL, Gibbon MG, Skodol AE, et al. *DSM-IV casebook.* 1st ed. Washington, DC: American Psychiatric Press, 1994.

Clinical Skills for Adult Primary Care
edited by M. E. Silverman and J. W. Hurst.
Lippincott-Raven Publishers, Philadelphia © 1996.

4

A Five-Step Approach to an Efficient Physical Examination

Mark E. Silverman, M.D.

*Emory University School of Medicine, Atlanta, Georgia 30322
and Piedmont Hospital, Atlanta, Georgia 30309*

"Make a thorough inspection. Never forget to look at the back of a patient. Always look at the feet. Looking at a woman's legs has often saved her life."
William Osler, quoted in Bean WB. *Sir William Osler: Aphorisms.*
Springfield, IL: Charles C Thomas, 1968:104.

The examination should be designed with the following goals in mind.

- Establishing normal baselines
- Finding abnormalities that may or may not require further investigation
- Correlating the findings on the examination with the clinical history
- Interacting with the patient in such a way that the patient is assured that the physician is thorough, competent, and has a sensitive, gentle bedside manner

In order to achieve these goals, the examiner needs to follow a rote method that will not overlook anything of importance yet be economical in the time required. The following is a five-step approach using a regional approach with minimal patient movement. Individual patients will require different approaches, and parts of the examination may be eliminated, modified, or expanded depending on the clinical history or the findings discovered at examination. It is extremely important to explain to the patient what you are planning to do next.

STEP 1. THE PATIENT IS SITTING ON THE SIDE OF THE BED OR EXAMINING TABLE FACING THE EXAMINER

- Take the blood pressure in both arms if measured the first time.
- Examine the nails, fingers, and both sides of each hand. Move up both arms from the hands to the axillae, feeling for lumps and checking skin turgor.

- Examine the head from the front. Begin with the eyes. Include funduscopic, vision, visual fields, and cranial nerves II, III, IV, and VI. Check the ears next, looking into the ear canals and testing for hearing acuity, then the nose and mouth, looking at the teeth, tongue, and pharynx. Complete checking cranial nerves V, VII, IX, X, XI, and XII.
- Examine the breasts from in front.
- Check arm and leg reflexes, strength, position sense, sensory exam, cerebellum.
- Listen with the stethoscope to the lungs in front.
- Listen to the heart with the diaphragm of the stethoscope.

STEP 2. MOVE BEHIND THE SITTING PATIENT

- Complete the head and neck examination. Look at the scalp. Feel for cervical and submandibular nodes. Palpate the thyroid. Feel both carotids simultaneously.
- Look at the posterior chest, including the skin. Observe respiratory movements. Look at, feel, and percuss the spine. Check for flank pain, if indicated.
- Check for fremitus. Percuss the chest. Listen to the lungs with the stethoscope.

STEP 3. THE PATIENT IS ASKED TO LIE DOWN IN A RELAXED FASHION. THE CHEST IS ELEVATED TO 30 DEGREES

- Inspect and palpate the chest wall, breasts, and cardiac impulses.
- Examine the jugular veins for venous pressure and palpation.
- Listen for carotid, abdominal, and femoral bruits sequentially with the stethoscope.
- Listen to the heart while looking at the jugular venous waves and feeling the carotid arterial pulse. Count the pulse and respirations if not already done. Turn the patient 30 degrees leftward and feel the apex with the left hand while listening to the apex with the bell of the stethoscope held in the right hand.
- Lower the trunk so that the patient is lying flat. Auscultate, then inspect and palpate the abdomen and groin.
- Examine the legs, inspecting and feeling the skin, joints, veins, and feet. Feel for the pedal arterial pulses (and popliteal arterial pulses if no pedal pulses are present). Check for edema. Test leg strength, sensation, position sense, and plantar reflexes in the legs.

STEP 4. THE PATIENT IS ASKED TO STAND WITHOUT SUPPORT

- Check standing blood pressure.
- Listen to the heart standing, squatting, and after squatting, if indicated.

- Look for varicosities and skin coloration of the feet.
- Evaluate Romberg sign and gait, including heel to toe.
- Examine the male genitalia, rectum, and prostate. Check for hernia.
- Repeat standing blood pressure if indicated.

STEP 5. PELVIC EXAMINATION

A complete description of a pelvic examination can be found in Chapter 17.

Clinical Skills for Adult Primary Care
edited by M. E. Silverman and J. W. Hurst.
Lippincott-Raven Publishers, Philadelphia © 1996.

5

General Inspection of the Patient

Mark E. Silverman, M.D.

*Emory University School of Medicine, Atlanta, Georgia 30322
and Piedmont Hospital, Atlanta, Georgia 30309*

"There is no more difficult art to acquire than the art of observation."
William Osler. On the educational value of the medical society.
Boston Med Surg J 1903;148:278.

TECHNIQUE

General inspection of the patient begins immediately. Experienced clinicians are remarkably adept in observing gait, color, posture, breathing and talking patterns, grimaces and gestures, resting motions, and the external signs of disease that lead to an early and often correct diagnosis. After the history has been obtained, the general inspection continues throughout the physical examination, searching for supportive evidence elicited during the interview. This is done best by examining the patient in the sitting position, squarely in front of the searching eyes of the physician, to permit easy observation and comparison of both sides of the body. This section will focus on the external manifestations of more frequent diseases that will present to the primary care physician as well as some less common problems that should not be overlooked.

ENDOCRINE DISEASES

The skin of a *diabetic* is often tight and has less elasticity when pinched together on the forearm. Necrobiosis diabeticorum, an atrophic expanding skin lesion with an erythematous border and central telangiectasis, can develop on the legs and precede or follow the onset of diabetes. *Hyperlipidemia* may be discovered by the presence of xanthelasma on the upper eyelids, arcus senilis in a person under age 40, or tendinous xanthoma, a nodular thickening of the dorsal tendons of the hands, knuckles, or Achilles tendons (Fig. 1). The stare and prominent eyes produced by *hyperthyroidism* secondary to Graves disease is well known (Fig. 2). Pretibial myxedema and clubbing are rare findings. With *hypothyroidism*, the

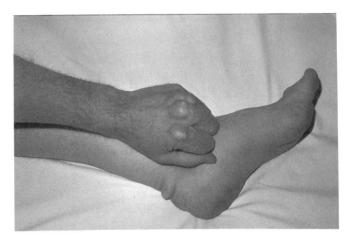

FIG. 1. Xanthoma. Nodular growths on the metacarpal and Achilles tendons associated with hyperlipidemia and coronary artery disease.

facial features are coarse and the skin dry and puffy. An unsightly *thyroid goiter* jutting from the neck is obvious. Hirsutism may be a cosmetic problem but when new or inappropriate, leads to a search for *tumor* and *ovarian* or *adrenal disease.* The familiar manifestations of *Cushing's syndrome* include central obesity with thin extremities, acne, purple striae, and a ruddy, inflated-appearing face (Fig. 3). *Addison's disease* causes darkening of the skin over the neck, palmar creases, arms, and gums. In *acromegaly,* the forehead and lower jaw enlarge and the fa-

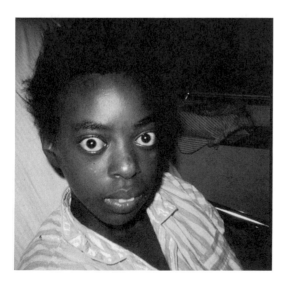

FIG. 2. Hyperthyroidism. Exophthalmos and stare typical of Grave's disease.

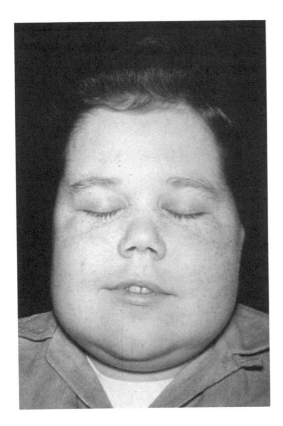

FIG. 3. Cushing's syndrome. Moon face due to steroids. Reprinted from Silverman ME and Hurst JW. In: Hurst JW ed. The heart, 2nd ed. New York: McGraw-Hill, 1970. Used by permission of McGraw-Hill.

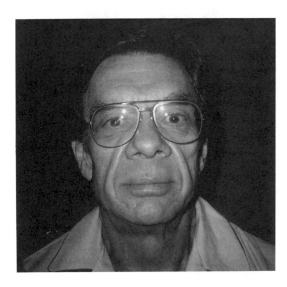

FIG. 4. Acromegaly. Prominent forehead, nose, and chin as well as thickened redundant skin due to excessive growth hormone. Reprinted from Silverman ME. Series on visual clues to the diagnosis. In: *Primary cardiology.* Reprinted with permission from Physicians World Communications Group.

cial features become coarse with a thickened, grooved skin and an enlarged tongue, nose, and lips (Fig. 4). The fingers become sausagelike. *Hypopituitarism* produces a smooth, soft skin, although fine wrinkling of the forehead may occur. Axillary and pubic hair is sparse or absent.

HEART DISEASE

The patient with advanced *right heart failure* may have distended neck veins, ascites, and marked edema. *Constrictive pericarditis* can produce similar findings. A number of congenital heart–related diseases or syndromes may be detected by examining the hands. These include cyanosis and clubbing with right-to-left shunts, a transverse crease in *Down syndrome*, arachnodactyly and lax joints in *Marfan syndrome* (Fig. 5), a fingerized thumb in *Holt-Oram syndrome* (Fig. 6), and polydactyly. Endocarditis, on rare occasions, may be detected by the finding of splinter hemorrhages, tender, purplish Osler nodes on the finger pads, and petechiae (Fig. 7). Women with *mitral valve prolapse* may share in common hypomastia and a Marfanoid skeletal appearance. A *straight back* and marked *pectus excavatum* may be the explanation for a systolic murmur. Body fat distribution producing an apple shape has been linked with *coronary disease* and *hypertension*. A diagonal ear lobe crease is a curious finding linked with *coronary disease* and *stroke* (Fig. 8). *Multiple lentigines* are small, darkbrown frecklelike skin lesions seen in large numbers on the trunk and arm and associated with hypertrophic cardiomyopathy (Fig. 9).

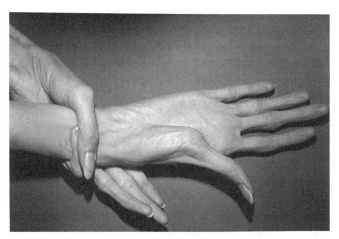

FIG. 5. The Marfan syndrome. Arachnodactyly and "wrist sign" with thumb and fifth fingers overlapping the wrist. Reprinted from Silverman ME, Hurst JW. In: Hurst JW (ed). *The heart.* 4th ed. New York: McGraw-Hill, 1978. Used by permission of McGraw-Hill.

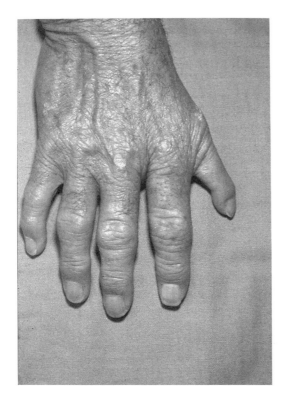

FIG. 6. Holt-Oram syndrome. Finger-ized thumb associated with atrial septal defect. Reprinted from Silverman ME, Hurst JW. The hand and the heart. *Am J Cardiol* 1968;22:718–28. Used by permission.

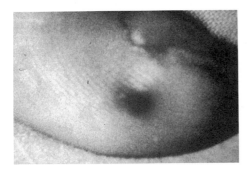

FIG. 7. Endocarditis. A purple, painful "Osler's node" on the finger pad.

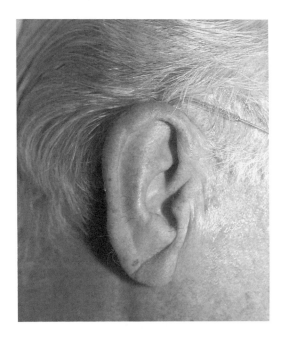

FIG. 8. Coronary disease. A diagonal ear lobe crease in a patient with coronary disease.

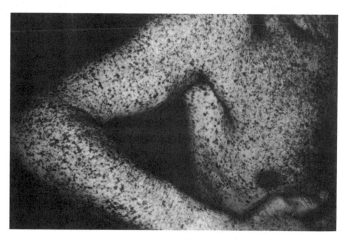

FIG. 9. Multiple lentigines syndrome. Multiple, dark macular lesions associated with hypertrophic cardiomyopathy. Reprinted from Silverman ME. Series on visual clues to the diagnosis. In: *Primary cardiology*. Reprinted with permission from Physicians World Communications Group.

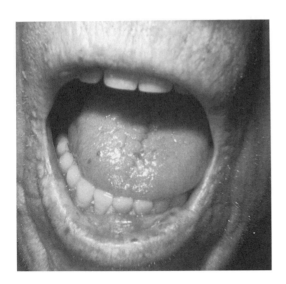

FIG. 10. Hereditary telangiectasia. Telangiectasia on tongue and lower lip associated with gastrointestinal bleeding and arteriovenous fistulae.

GASTROINTESTINAL DISEASE

Spider angioma, jaundice, ascites, and a gaunt facial appearance are stigmata of *cirrhosis*. Telangiectasia on the lips and under the nails as seen in *hereditary hemorrhagic telangiectasia* may explain gastrointestinal bleeding (Fig. 10). In the *Peutz-Jehger syndrome*, pigmented spots are present on the lip and hamartomatous polyps in the intestine, predominately the small bowel. Arthritis can be a manifestation of *inflammatory bowel disease*. Purpura, generalized hyperpigmentation most prominent around scars, and arthritis are signs of *Whipple's disease*.

NUTRITION

An assessment of nutritional status is an important part of general inspection. Obesity and cachexia will be obvious. The skin, mouth, teeth, eyes, and hair are the best places to look for *protein and vitamin deficiency. Protein deficiency* can cause pitting edema of the legs and arms, fine, brittle hair, a moon face, and muscle wasting. Signs of various *vitamin deficiencies* include petechiae, purpura, pigmented areas, gingivitis, cheilosis, glossitis or a scarlet tongue, and follicular hyperkeratosis.

CANCER

Cutaneous metastases may be the presenting sign of an internal malignancy. The scalp is a favorite area. The metastases are often nodular, usually hard, and

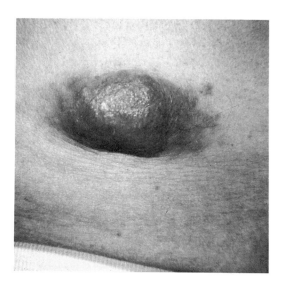

FIG. 11. Cutaneous cancer. A firm, purple nodule due to lymphoma.

may be colored or pigmented (Fig. 11). Diffuse hyperpigmentation can occur with *metastatic melanoma* and tumors that produce an *ectopic adrenocorticophic hormone (ACTH) syndrome* (Fig. 12). Recent onset of clubbing of the fingers should always prompt a search for a *neoplasm of the lung* or *lymphoma* (Fig. 13). Repeated attacks of flushing of the head and upper chest and the subsequent development of cyanosis and telangiectasia point to the *carcinoid syndrome*. Various skin eruptions, including erythema multiforme, dermatomyositis, herpes zoster,

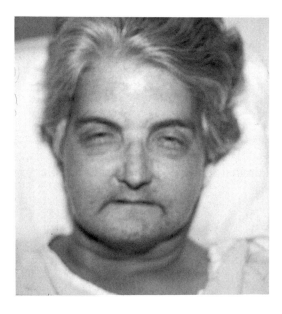

FIG. 12. ACTH-producing tumor. Patient with Cushinoid face and hyperpigmentation caused by ACTH-producing lung neoplasm.

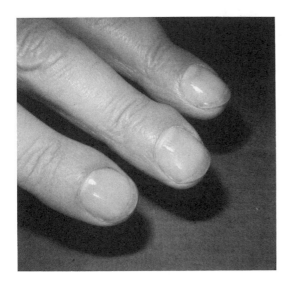

FIG. 13. Clubbing. New onset clubbing in a patient with asymptomatic cancer of the lung.

erythema gyratum repens, hyperkeratosis of the palms and soles, and exfoliative dermatitis have been associated with *malignancy*. Acanthosis nigricans, a velvety, dirty-appearing exaggeration of the skin folds of the neck, axillae, groin, and antecubital areas, is found with various tumors as well as more benign conditions. Migratory phlebitis may herald a silent malignancy, often pancreatic.

COLLAGEN AND RHEUMATOLOGIC DISORDERS

A butterfly-shaped eruption in a malar distribution, characterized by hyper- and hypopigmentation, scaling, and telangiectasia, immediately brings *systemic lupus erythematosus* to mind (Fig. 14). Other evidence for lupus includes reddish-purple, elevated plaques (discoid lupus), areas of atrophy, telangiectasia, alopecia, diffuse erythema, Raynaud's phenomenon, photosensitivity, and a variety of other cutaneous findings. A heliotropic hue and edema of the upper eyelids is almost pathognomonic for *dermatomyositis* (Fig. 15). An erythematous, scaly eruption over the interphalangeal joints (Gottron's sign) is also typical. In *scleroderma*, the skin is taut and cannot be pinched; the normal skin creases are absent; the fingers may be curled into a claw; and hyper- and hypopigmentation may occur (Fig. 16). Telangiectasia may be seen in the nail fold and on the cheeks and linear creases known as rhagades may surround the lips. Raynaud's phenomenon is common. Calcium deposits may be found in the *CREST (Calcinosis, Raynaud's, Esophageal, Sclerodactyly, Telangiectasia)* variant of scleroderma. A collapsed nasal cartilage and/or cauliflower type ears raises the possibility of *polychondritis. Rheumatoid arthritis*, in its advanced stages, is recognized by ulnar deviation of the fingers, interosseal wasting, boxing of the wrists, and thickened metacarpophalangeal and

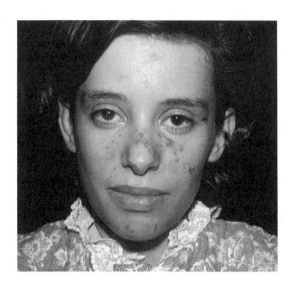

FIG. 14.   Lupus erythematosus. Telangiectatic rash in malar distribution.

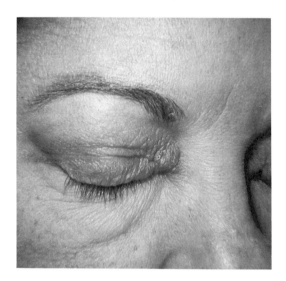

FIG. 15.   Dermatomyositis. Heliotropic discoloration and edematous eyelid in a patient with dermatomyositis.

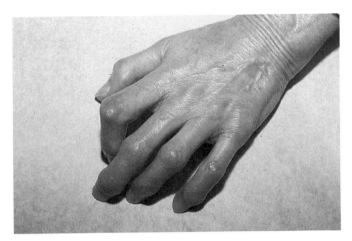

FIG. 16. Scleroderma. Tight shiny skin and clawlike deformity.

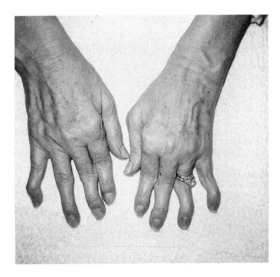

FIG. 17. Rheumatoid arthritis. Thickened joints, subluxated fingers, and interosseal wasting are present. Reprinted from Silverman ME. Series on visual clues to the diagnosis. In: *Primary cardiology.* Reprinted with permission from Physicians World Communications Group.

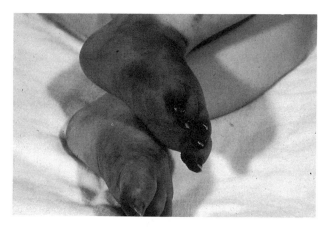

FIG. 18. Polyarteritis. Gangrenous feet due to necrotizing polyarteritis in a child with myocardial infarction.

proximal interphalangeal joints (Fig. 17). Early signs include spindle-shaped swelling of the proximal interphalangeal joints, palmar erythema, and arthritis of the knees and toes. *Polyarteritis* may present with gangrene of the fingers and toes, livedo reticularis, urticaria, erythema nodosum, and superficial skin ulcerations on the legs (Fig. 18). Patients with ankylosing spondylitis walk with a stiff and halting gait. In advanced stages, the fused spine forces the patient into a permanently hunched-over stature (Fig. 19). *Gout* often presents as acute inflamma-

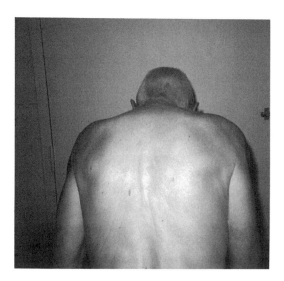

FIG. 19. Rheumatoid spondylitis. Hunched over appearance due to fused spine. Reprinted from Silverman ME. Series on visual clues to the diagnosis. In: *Primary cardiology.* Reprinted with permission from Physicians World Communications Group.

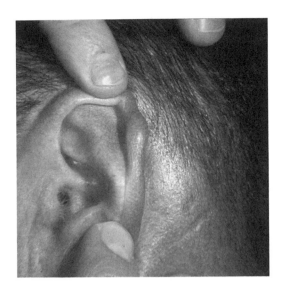

FIG. 20. Gout. Tophus on the earlobe.

tion of the great toe (podagra), instep, heel, or ankle (Fig. 20). Subsequent attacks involve the fingers, shoulders, and other joints and can result in gross deformity.

INFILTRATIVE DISEASES

Amyloidosis may be diagnosed by noting an enlarged tongue, purpura of the eyelids or skin when pinched, waxy papules, or enlarged submandibular nodes (Fig. 21). *Hemochromatosis* causes bronzed, slate gray, or speckled pigmentation of the skin, and arthritis. *Sarcoidosis* should be considered when the lachrymal glands are enlarged, nasolabial plaques (lupus pernio) are present, or erythema nodosa

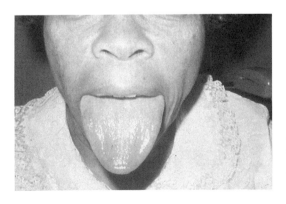

FIG. 21. Amyloidosis. Enlarged, rubbery feeling tongue in a patient with myeloma and amyloidosis. Reprinted from Silverman ME. Series on visual clues to the diagnosis. In: *Primary cardiology.* Reprinted with permission from Physicians World Communications Group.

erupts. A Kayser-Fleischer ring—a golden or greenish-brown circle of pigmentation along the corneal edge—points to *Wilson's disease* as the cause for cirrhosis.

LUNG DISEASE

The patient with severe obstructive *lung disease* is easily recognized by the increased anteroposterior diameter of the chest, the use of extrarespiratory muscles to aid breathing, pursed lips, and cyanotic hue. Clubbing is well known to be associated with lung disease, especially *pulmonary fibrosis* and *lung abscess*. Yellow staining of the fingernails is a common finding in heavy smokers. *Kyphoscoliosis* is an obvious cause of restrictive lung disease.

INHERITED CONNECTIVE TISSUE DISEASES

In the *Marfan syndrome,* the patient exhibits tall stature, elongated fingers and toes, an arched palate, pectus excavatum, dislocated lenses, sparse subcutaneous skin, and poor muscular development. The skin in *pseudoxanthoma elasticum* has a yellowish, scored appearance over the neck and antecubital area described as a "plucked chicken" appearance (Fig. 22). The skin may be redundant. The skin is hyperelastic and soft in the *Ehlers-Danlos syndrome* (Fig. 23). Scar formation is poor. Blue sclerae and multiple bone fractures are evidence for *osteogenesis imperfecta.* Clinical features seen in *mucopolysaccharidosis* include coarse facial appearance, corneal clouding, stiff joints, and short stature.

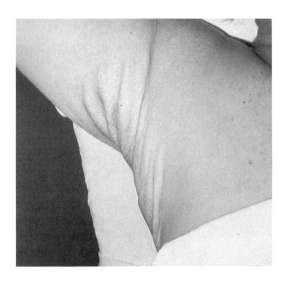

FIG. 22. Pseudoxanthoma elasticum. Scored, yellowish axillary folds of the skin.

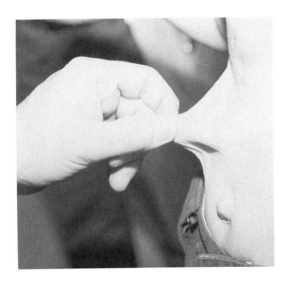

FIG. 23. Ehlers-Danlos syndrome. Crepelike, elastic skin associated with mitral valve prolapse.

RENAL DISEASE

Patients with *chronic renal disease* often appear cachectic, sallow, and pigmented. Ecchymoses are common. Cutaneous calcifications and uremic frost are rarely present. The nails may display a white band proximally and red band distally. *Fabry's disease* is an X-linked recessive disorder that can cause renal failure or angina. The diagnosis can be made by finding small red to dark blue papules (angiokeratomas) on the scrotum, penis, umbilicus, or trunk.

IMMUNODEFICIENCY

Patients with immunodeficiency, especially those with *AIDS*, develop serious opportunistic infections when the T-helper cell population falls to 150 cells/mm^3 or less. Herpes simplex infections, often confined to fever blisters in normal people, can erupt as widespread pustules, deep ulcerations with secondary infection, angular cheilosis, and perirectal infection. Warts with severe condyloma may be seen on the genitalia. Shingles, due to herpes zoster, can be widespread, cause scarring, nerve damage, and blindness, and can be recurrent. Molluscum contagiosum is frequent, and numerous lesions may appear on the face and genitalia. Oral lesions include hairy leukoplakia on the side of the tongue from an Epstein-Barr virus, thrush from candida, and Kaposi's sarcoma. Candida may also involve the nails and hands. Other telltale skin lesions are ichthyosis, seborrheic dermatitis, erythroderma, and Kaposi's sarcoma.

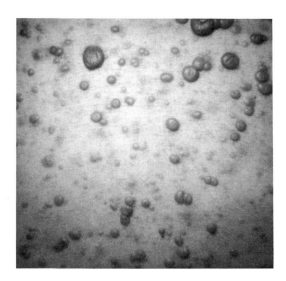

FIG. 24. Neurofibromatosis. Multiple neurofibromas on the chest.

NEUROLOGIC DISEASES

Neurofibromatosis, a genetically determined disorder, is characterized by six or more café au lait spots seen on the trunk and axilla, as well as multiple fibroma, which are sometimes confluent and pendulous. Gross hypertrophy of affected parts may occur (Fig. 24). In *Friederich's ataxia*, kyphoscoliosis, pes caves, and an arched palate are seen. Tremors may indicate *Parkinson's disease*, a form of *chorea*, or may be familial.

SUGGESTED READING

Belkin BM, Neelon FA. The art of observation: William Osler and the method of Zadig. *Ann Intern Med* 1992;116:863–5.
Braverman IM. Skin signs of systemic disease. 2nd ed. Philadelphia: W.B. Saunders, 1981.
Holzburg M, Walker HK. A systematic approach to nail examination. *Hosp Pract* 1985;20:21–8.
Hurst JW. Physical examination. In: Hurst JW. Cardiovascular diagnosis: the initial examination. St. Louis: Mosby, 1993:71–125.
Silverman ME. Inspection of the patient. In: *The heart.* 7th ed. New York: McGraw-Hill, 1990:135–49.

Clinical Skills for Adult Primary Care
edited by M. E. Silverman and J. W. Hurst.
Lippincott-Raven Publishers, Philadelphia © 1996.

6

Examination of the Skin

Donald J. Pirozzi, M.D.

Piedmont Hospital, Atlanta, Georgia 30309

"Don't touch the patient—state first what you see; cultivate your powers of observation."
William Osler, quoted in Bean WB. *Sir William Osler: Aphorisms.*
Springfield, IL: Charles C Thomas, 1968:37.

Patients presenting for answers to dermatologic questions usually have a specific complaint: a rash; a rash that itches or hurts; a sore spot that is new, changing color, or increasing in size, or that will not heal; or any combination of the above. Because these changes are readily apparent, being easily seen when looking in a mirror, immediate attention is often requested. The physician examining the patient, whether as part of a general physical examination or more specifically to answer an individual question, must try to distinguish between various lesions in order to make an accurate diagnosis. A skin examination should always be part of a general physical examination.

TECHNIQUE

Examination of the skin, unlike examination of other organs, is relatively easy. No tests of blood or other fluids are needed initially because the conditions are clearly visible to the careful observer. Inspection of the skin should involve the entire body so that one may see individual surface changes and how they relate to different body areas. This is important because skin diseases can be classified according to the type of lesion and its location. A knowledge of pathological changes also helps distinguish lesions that can be dismissed as having no serious health consequence. An adequate skin examination should take no more than 10 minutes unless some unusual changes are noted. Dermatology is a visually oriented specialty, and past masters have used configuration and morphology of skin lesions to make a diagnosis. Palpation of individual lesions, generally not available when examining other organs, provides a secondary method of examination (1). As Robert Wilan, the first modern dermatologist, said, "We should endeavor . . . to constitute general division of orders of diseases, from leading and peculiar circumstances in their appearance, to arrange them into distinct genera, and to describe at large their specific forms or varieties" (2).

To make a dermatologic diagnosis, one needs to consider the following:

- The characteristics of the individual lesion. This includes color, scaling, ulcerations, erosion, vesiculation, smoothness, palpability, and itchiness. Table 1 and Fig. 1 provide a helpful algorithm.
- The grouping and location of the lesions. Where are they located? Are they on sun-exposed areas such as the face, neck, and backs of the hands? How many are present?
- The medical history, the physical examination, and the results of laboratory studies.
- A skin biopsy should be performed in difficult cases.

TABLE 1. *The problem-oriented algorithm: match the patient's finding on the left and the correct category of lesion will be found on the right.*

I. No apparent lesions
  A. Symptoms only
    Pruritus   1. Pruritus
    Pain   2. Pain, paresthesia, and anesthesia
II. Skin-colored lesions
  A. Epidermis intact and attached
    Scale absent   3. Smooth skin-colored lesions
    Scale present   4. Scaling skin-colored lesions
  B. Epidermis lifted (blisters)
    Blister fluid clear   5. Vesiculobullous lesions
    Blister fluid white/yellow-white   6. Pustular lesions
  C. Epidermis missing
    Defect shallow   7. Erosions
    Defect deep   8. Ulcers
III. Nonblanchable, abnormally colored lesions
  A. Melanin pigment
    Hypopigmentation   9. White lesions
    Hyperpigmentation   10. Brown-black lesions
  B. Heme pigment
    Nonpalpable   11. Nonpalpable purpuras
    Palpable   12. Palpable purpuras
  C. Other pigments
    Blue-gray hues   13. Blue-gray lesions
    Yellow hues   14. Yellow lesions
IV. Blanchable, red (inflammatory) lesions
  A. Nonscaling red lesions
    Flat and flat-topped lesions   15. Vascular reactions
    Rounded and slope-shouldered lesions   16. Red papules and nodules
  B. Scaling, red lesions
    Epithelium intact   17. Papulosquamous lesions
    Epithelium disrupted   18. Eczematous lesions

From Sams WM, Lynch PJ. *Principles and practice of dermatology.* New York: Churchill-Livingstone, 1990. Used by permission of Churchill Livingstone.

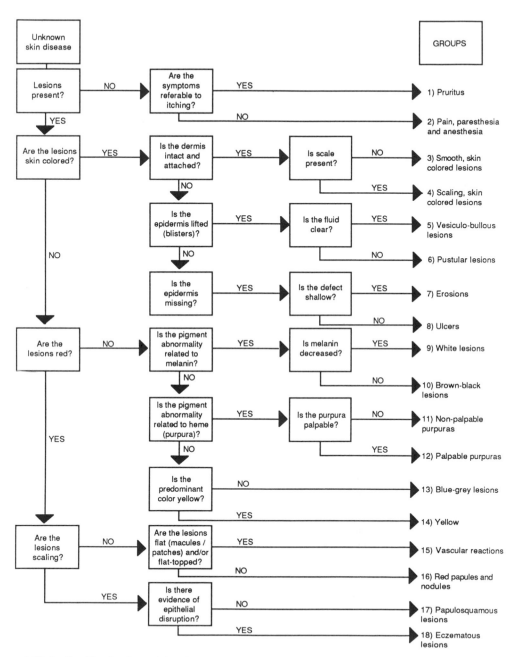

FIG. 1. Algorithm for determining the diagnosis of dermatologic diseases. From Sams WM, Lynch PJ. *Principles and practice of dermatology.* New York: Churchill-Livingstone, 1990. Used by permission of Churchill-Livingstone.

NORMAL FINDINGS

The normal skin is a homogeneous, smooth surface that differs in thickness in different areas of the body. The appendages, including the hair, hair follicles, sweat glands, and oil glands, are noted directly or by the products they produce. When the skin is functioning normally, this is usually taken for granted. However, when skin disease compromises the function of these structures, the skin usually responds with noticeable surface changes.

The skin is divided into three layers: the epidermis, the dermis, and the subcutaneous tissue. The outermost layer of the epidermis is the horny layer of stratum corneum consisting of cells that form the first protective layer of skin and aid in its semipermeable nature. The epidermis is a complex layer that produces the keratinocytes, which form the horny cells of the stratum corneum. The skin appendages, including the sweat glands, oil glands, and hair, are a component of the dermal layer. The dermal–epidermal junction contains cells that help anchor the epidermis to the dermis and melanocytes in various quantities that impart the different colors of the skin. The dermis consists of many nerve fibers, elastic fibers, and collagen that support the skin. The subcutaneous fat provides insulation, shock absorption, and mobility for the epidermis. The skin differs in thickness in different areas of the body. For example, the skin of the back is much thicker than the skin on the face. This difference in thickness may cause the appearance of similar skin lesions to vary in different areas of the body.

Benign/Aging Changes

Some findings, although not normal, are benign and can be a manifestation of aging or previous injury. *Scars* are nodules of connective tissue that form after an injury to the dermal–epidermal junction. Seborrheic, so-called *senile keratoses*, are hyperpigmented collections of keratin found on most individuals over the age of 50 (Fig. 2). *Cherry hemangiomas* are red, raised papules derived from blood vessels and found on the trunk of the majority of middle-aged people. *Skin tags* or *papillomas* occur in areas of friction, such as the axillae or the neck, and occur in mature adults. These changes and acute problems such as bruising can be easily recognized, and the patient can be reassured.

DISEASES OF THE SKIN

Individual lesions or changes of the skin in disease are divided into primary or secondary lesions. *Primary lesions* are the changes in the skin caused by an immunologic event, disease, or infection. *Secondary lesions* are changes resulting from a reaction to the primary lesions and are created by the patient through scratching or secondary infection.

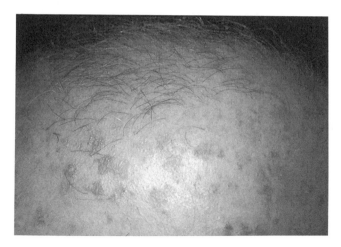

FIG. 2. Seborrheic keratosis. Example of multiple seborrheic keratoses showing the "stuck on" appearance.

Primary Lesions

Macules

Macules are discrete changes in the color of the skin. These lesions can be seen but not felt. They may be brown, blue, red, or hypopigmented.

- *Nevi* are the most obvious example of a macule. They are usually light brown to black in color and represent a collection of pigmented nevus cells within the epidermis or dermis.

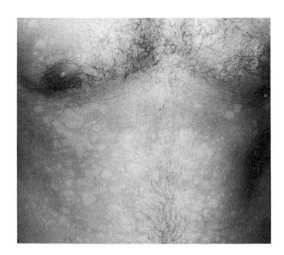

FIG. 3. Tinea versicolor. A papulosquamous hypopigmented eruption on the trunk.

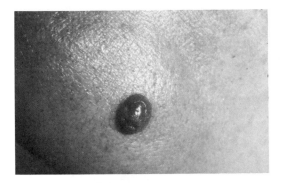

FIG. 4. Nevus. A hyperpigmented nodular lesion.

- *Purpura* are red to purple collections of blood in the skin due to hemorrhage.
- *Tinea versicolor* is a fungus infection consisting of hypopigmented or brown macules that occur on the back or chest and are usually more obvious in the summer months when the skin is unable to tan because of the fungal infection (Fig. 3).

Palpable Lesions

Papules, nodules, and tumors are solid, elevated lesions that are palpable. The terms differ only in size and involvement of subcutaneous tissue. Papules may become confluent and form plaques. Papules are solid lesions up to 0.5 cm in diameter.

- *Dermal nevi*, a collection of pigmented cells a bit deeper in the skin, are examples of papules. Their color may range from light to dark brown (Fig. 4).
- Closed *comedones*, which are the hallmark of acne vulgaris, are small papules, usually red in color, found on the face, chest, and back.
- *Flat warts* are seen on the face. They measure 1 to 3 mm in diameter and are usually skin colored. These lesions are caused by a virus and tend to spread rapidly, especially in men who shave.

Nodules

Nodules are solid lesions over 0.5 cm in diameter; tumors are large nodules.

- *Basal cell carcinoma* (Fig. 5) and *squamous cell carcinoma* are examples of nodules. In their initial stages, they may be red and solid. Later they may ulcerate.
- *Lipomas* are collections of fat cells, usually palpable, and occasionally painful.
- *Epidermal cysts* occur on the scalp or other hairy areas of the body and represent invaginations of the skin into which stratum corneum cells are secreted.

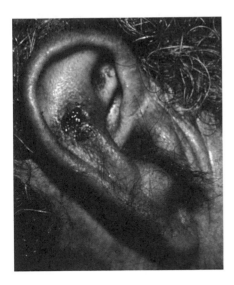

FIG. 5. Basal cell carcinoma. A nodular, ulcerated lesion typically found on a sun-exposed area.

This creates the characteristic white, cheesy substance with a peculiar odor that is usually easily expressed.

• *Melanomas* can occur anywhere on the body, although they are often found on sun-exposed areas. They may arise from previously diagnosed junctional nevi. They are usually irregular in shape, palpable, and display a spectrum of color from light brown to black, all within the same lesion (Fig. 6). A change of color in a previously monochromatic nevus to multi-shade or dark black is an ominous diagnostic change. A change in the symmetry of the edge of the lesion is another.

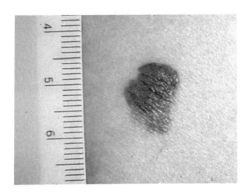

FIG. 6. Malignant melanoma. A hyperpigmented, papular lesion with uneven pigmentation.

- *Warts* or *verruca vulgaris* can occur on any part of the body. Sometimes they appear like flowers growing rapidly on the skin. They are caused by a virus and are easily traumatized, occasionally causing a frightening amount of bleeding.
- *Lymphomas* and other tumors, some types of *eczema, hemangiomas,* and *dermatofibromas*, are other conditions characterized by nodules or tumors.

Wheals

Wheals are unusual papules or plaques resulting from extravasation of fluid into the dermis. They are edematous and often ephemeral, lasting only several hours. They are often red and can occur on any part of the body.

- *Urticaria*, or hives, is the best example of a wheal. These can be allergic or psychogenic in etiology. They are usually very itchy.
- *Insect bites* are another extremely pruritic example of a wheal.

Pustules

A pustule is a circumscribed collection of white blood cells and fluid that may vary in size. It is a superficial abscess of the skin that may be sterile or infectious.

- The pustule found on the face in *acne vulgaris* is a classic example.
- The skin manifestation of *gonococcemia* is an infected pustule that can be found anywhere on the body.
- *Impetigo* is a superficial infection of the skin caused by staphylococcus or streptococcus organisms and often manifested by a pustule (Fig. 7).
- *Dyshidrotic eczema*, found on the hands and the feet, manifests pruritic pustules.

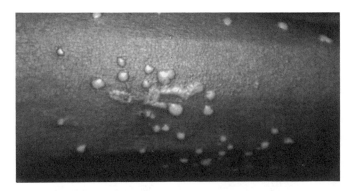

FIG. 7. Impetigo. Multiple pustules are the hallmark.

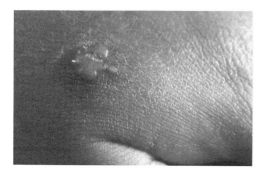

FIG. 8. Herpes simplex. Grouped vesicles on an erythematous base.

Vesicles and Bullae

A vesicle is a circumscribed collection of fluid under 0.5 cm in diameter, whereas a bulla is over 0.5 cm in diameter. Vesicular disorders can occur anywhere within the epidermis and at the dermal–epidermal junction.

- *Herpes simplex* and *varicella/zoster* are viral conditions that often manifest as vesicles. Herpes simplex can occur anywhere on the body (Fig. 8). More commonly, lesions occur around the mouth or genital area. The lesions are usually groups of small vesicles sitting on an erythematous base. Varicella is seen as a generalized eruption of small vesicles. Zoster causes a group of vesicles on an erythematous base along a dermatome (Fig. 9). Zoster and herpes simplex are usually painful, whereas varicella is pruritic.

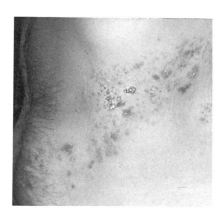
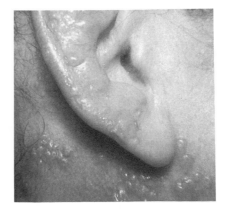

FIG. 9. Herpes zoster. Grouped vesicles on an erythematous base occurring along a dermatome distribution.

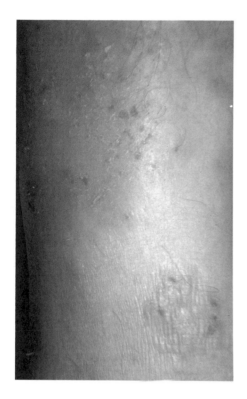

FIG. 10. Atopic dermatitis. Erythema, scaling, and lichenification typically occur on antecubital and popliteal surfaces.

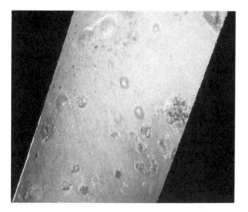

FIG. 11. Pemphigus. Large vesicles and bullae are seen.

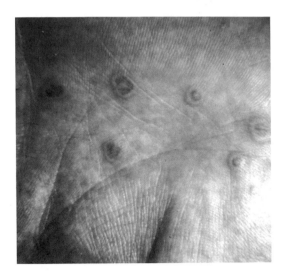

FIG. 12. Erythema multiforme. Target-like vesicles on the hand due to a drug eruption.

- Any of the eczemas, including acute contact dermatitis and atopic dermatitis, may display vesicles or bullae. Generally, these are pruritic and may be asymmetrical, seen on only one hand or leg (Fig. 10).
- *Dermatitis herpetiformis, pemphigoid,* and *pemphigus* are more unusual bullous disorders. They are immunologic diseases that occur within the epidermis or at the dermal–epidermal junction (Fig. 11). They all have the bulla as their primary lesion. Immunologic studies are usually needed to differentiate one from the other.
- *Erythema multiform* is a reaction to a drug, infection, or topical substance. The lesion is a vesicle with a central umbilication resembling a target (Fig. 12). The individual lesions can occur anywhere on the body, but most often start on the extremities.

Secondary Lesions

Scales

Scales are accumulated, excess, dead epidermal cells produced by abnormal keratinization and lack of shedding.

Papulosquamous Disorders

Many of the more common dermatological conditions have been grouped under this heading, which implies that they have characteristics of both papules and scales.

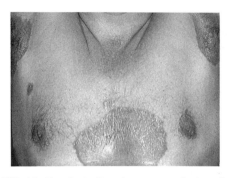 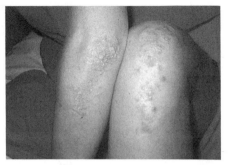

FIG. 13. Psoriasis. Papulosquamous lesions that coalesce into plaques. Classically occurs on the knees and elbows.

- *Psoriasis* characteristically occurs on the knees, elbows, and scalp. Papules that may coalesce into plaques with noticeable scales are the hallmark of the disease (Fig. 13).
- *Pityriasis rosacea* is a common condition, usually occurring in the spring or fall. The lesions are papulosquamous and generally occur in a Christmas tree pattern on the back or the chest. The initial lesion is usually larger than the rest and is known as a "herald" plaque.
- *Lichen planus* is an unusual papulosquamous disorder usually manifest as violaceous papules on the anterior tibial areas and flexor aspect of the arms. It is pruritic and tends to be both chronic and scarring.
- *Seborrheic dermatitis* is a common scaling eczema found on the scalp, central part of the face, and sternal area. Erythema, scaling, and a certain greasiness of the skin are characteristic (Fig. 14).
- *Tinea corporis*, caused by a dermatophyte infection, can occur anywhere on the body. In its chronic form, it is usually very scaly. Acutely, however, vesicles may be obvious (Fig. 15).

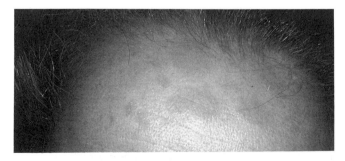

FIG. 14. Seborrheic dermatitis. A common papulosquamous disorder occurring on the face.

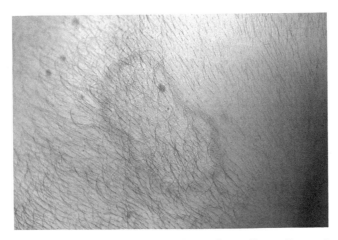

FIG. 15. Tinea corporis. So-called ringworm, which usually manifests with papules and scales, but in the acute stage peripheral vesicles are evident.

- *Secondary syphilis*, known as the great imitator, can look like any other papulosquamous disorder. Generally, it has a violaceous hue and, unlike the other diseases, it involves the palms and soles. The individual lesions are very infectious, teeming with treponema pallidum.
- *Drug eruptions.* Many medications can cause allergic reactions that are both papular and scaly. These tend to develop quickly and are generalized and very pruritic. Penicillin, sulfa drugs, aspirin, and diuretics are common offenders (Fig. 16).

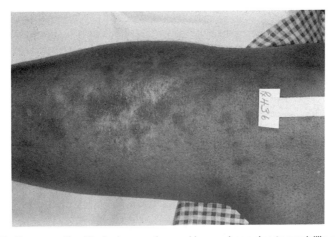

FIG. 16. Drug eruption. Vesicular reaction and hemorrhage due to penicillin allergy.

Crusts

A crust is synonymous with a scab, which is a collection of serum and dead cells. Crusts are often superimposed on chronic eczemas, impetigo, and fungal infections.

Erosions and Ulcers

Erosions are due to a superficial loss of epidermis that does not penetrate to the dermal–epidermal junction and does not cause a scar. Various eczemas, candida and fungal infections, and the vesiculobullous disorders can all produce erosions. Ulcers are caused by a localized loss of epidermis as well as dermis and heal with scar formation. Decubiti, syphilitic chancres, some neoplasms, and various self-induced injuries can show secondary changes of ulceration.

Atrophy

Atrophy is a thinning of the epidermis or dermis caused by a loss of supporting structure. The aging process, including actinic keratoses, which is facilitated by excess sun exposure, lupus erythematosus, morphea, or excessive use of topical corticosteroids, which can all cause atrophy. Actinic keratoses are one of the more common skin changes manifesting atrophy, especially in people who have engaged in excessive sun exposure. They occur on the face, chest, and the dorsum of the hands and arms. Atrophic lesions are usually hyperpigmented, scaling, and premalignant.

Excoriation

Excoriations are a particular type of erosion induced by scratching the skin. They are seen with any primary lesion. As the scratching continues, ulceration may result.

Lichenification

Lichenification is also secondary to rubbing or scratching primary lesions. This is a chronic, not a short-term manifestation, and represents a thickening of the epidermis, which then resembles a lichen or a washboard.

The terms discussed above are used in any consideration of skin disorders; even a cursory knowledge of their definition will allow one to understand and make a basic dermatologic diagnosis.

Configuration of the Lesions

Once the characteristics of the lesion are identified, then a consideration of their configuration helps in differentiating them from similar conditions. If a group of papulosquamous lesions that coalesce into plaques are found on the elbows, knees, and scalp, psoriasis is the most likely diagnosis. If individual lesions are found on sun-exposed areas, such as the face, dorsum of the arms, or chest, then actinic keratoses or possibly basal cell carcinomas are the differential diagnoses. The arrangement of grouped vesicles on an erythematous base found with herpes simplex or zoster is a perfect example of configuration helping to make a diagnosis.

Lesions also have a uniformity within their configuration: vesicles and bullae are obviously fluid-filled, whereas epidermal cysts are solid, but movable. They must be closely examined in sections to determine which particular lesion is present and in what groupings they occur.

GENERAL MEDICAL HISTORY

In dermatology, the examination is usually more important than history. For instance, an ulcerated papule with a pearly border on the face is easily diagnosed by visualization. However, one would never be able to make a diagnosis of contact dermatitis without some type of exposure history. Also, a diagnosis of dermatitis herpetiformis is more easily made when one is aware of the patient's intermittent diarrhea (sprue). Pemphigoid is often accompanied by or is the first sign of an internal malignancy. A patient manifesting the classic bullous target lesions of erythema multiforme may have a history of recent antibiotic use. The patient with classical childhood atopic dermatitis, with scaling and erythema in the antecubital and popliteal fossae, may have a history of asthma or a family history of hay fever or eczema. Therefore, a general medical history can be helpful in establishing the cause of the dermatologic problem.

General Physical Examination

The skin may provide the first and best location to diagnose a systemic disease, such as a collagen–vascular disease or endocarditis. Skin manifestations of systemic disease are covered in Chapter 5.

DIAGNOSTIC AIDS

Most diagnostic procedures in dermatology are usually confirmatory of an initial visual assessment. A fungus infection can be confirmed by scraping the scaly border, placing it on a microscopic slide, applying KOH solution, and examining it under the microscope. A scraping and Tzanck preparation from the base of a vesicle can help make the diagnosis of herpes simplex. A scraping of pruritic vesicles on the hand can, by visualizing a mite under the microscope, make or break a diagnosis of scabies. Finally, if all principles of diagnosis fail to justify an unequivocal judgment, a biopsy is recommended. The results of a shave biopsy with a scalpel or a simple punch biopsy should confirm the presumptive diagnosis or at least eliminate less likely possibilities.

REFERENCES

1. Witkowski J, Parish LC. The touching question. *Int J Dermatol* 1981;20:426.
2. Willan R. *On cutaneous diseases.* London: J. Johnson, 1808.

SUGGESTED READING

Braverman IM. *Skin signs of systemic disease.* 2nd ed. Philadelphia: W.B. Saunders, 1981.
Callen JP, Jorizzo J, Greer KE, et al., eds. *Dermatological signs of internal disease.* Philadelphia: W.B. Saunders, 1988.
Fitzpatrick TB, Eisen AZ, Wolf K, et al., eds. *Dermatology in general medicine: textbook and atlas.* 3rd ed. New York: McGraw-Hill, 1987.
Sams WM, Lynch PJ. *Principles and practice of dermatology.* New York: Churchill-Livingstone, 1990.

Clinical Skills for Adult Primary Care
edited by M. E. Silverman and J. W. Hurst.
Lippincott-Raven Publishers, Philadelphia © 1996.

7

Examination of the Eye

William H. Jarrett II, M.D., and Mark W. Mohney, M.D.

Piedmont Hospital, Atlanta, Georgia 30309

"Half of us are blind, few of us feel, and we are all deaf."
William Osler, quoted in Bean WB. *William Osler: Aphorisms.*
Springfield, IL: Charles C Thomas, 1968:37.

A basic ophthalmic evaluation can easily be performed by the primary care physician with minimal instrumentation. A simple history and examination of the eyes and surrounding tissues with a penlight and an ophthalmoscope provides valuable clues to the diagnosis of ocular disease.

VISION

Examination of Visual Acuity

It has been estimated that nearly 20% of the cerebral anatomy correlates with visual pathways and processing. Our understanding of the anatomy far exceeds our understanding of "how we see."

Technique

Typically, distance acuity is checked both with and without glass correction. A Snellen chart will gauge visual acuity. This is listed as a numerator and a denominator. The numerator represents the testing distance, which is standardized at 20 feet. The denominator corresponds to the level of acuity on the chart that the patient can perceive. A recording of 20/40 means that the patient is reading at 20 feet what a normal person could read at a distance of 40 feet. Independent recordings of both the right and the left eye are noted. By convention, for ophthalmic evaluations, the right eye is usually recorded first. If the visual acuity is less than 20/20, a pinhole can be used to try to improve the recorded vision. A pinhole placed in front of the eye will eliminate all of the rays emanating from

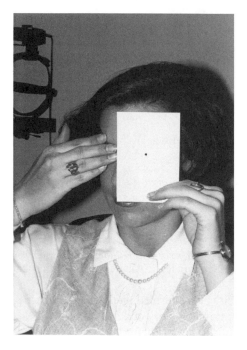

FIG. 1. Technique for using pinhole.

the target that originate off the visual axis (Fig. 1). The effect of the pinhole is to compensate for any imperfections in the visual pathway and the need for further glasses without having to perform a refraction. An uncorrected refractive error will generally improve by pinhole testing. A pinhole is available through local medical supply stores. It also may be fashioned simply by passing the tip of a pencil through a 3 × 5–inch card and asking the patient to fixate through the hole placed in front of the glasses or the uncorrected eye. The pinhole vision is also noted in the patient's chart. When distance acuity is not possible, such as in a hospital setting, a "near" card can be used to check vision.

People over age 40 often are developing presbyopia and may need glass correction to allow them to see a near card.

If the patient is unable to identify any letters on a Snellen acuity chart or near card, visual acuity is noted as "counts fingers" at whatever distance the patient is able to perceive fingers held in front of their eyes. If the patient is unable to perceive even the gross fingers, visual acuity is recorded as "hand motion" or "light perception." If severe trauma precludes patients from easily opening their eyes, a drop of sterile anesthetic agent such as proparacaine may be placed in the eyes before asking the patient to fixate. If they are still unable to do so, a flashlight shown through the closed lid will indicate some presence of light perception, and, therefore, some degree of visual function.

Normal Findings

Normal visual acuity is judged as 20/20 for both the right and left eyes. If a glass correction is needed to perceive the 20/20 line, the vision is still considered normal.

Abnormal Findings

Any acuity of less than 20/20 indicates that the visual acuity, whether corrected or uncorrected, is less than normal. A thorough ophthalmic evaluation should provide justification for the recorded decrease in acuity.

Testing for Color Vision

Technique

The integrity of color vision in each eye should be addressed. This is especially important when decreased central visual acuity is noted. It aids in the diagnosis of optic neuropathies, either inflammatory or compressive, drug toxicities, or early macular disease. Color vision is routinely checked through the polychromatic

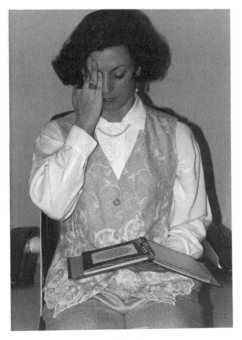

FIG. 2. Testing color vision.

plates of Ishihara or Hardy-Rand-Ritter (Fig. 2) In a well-illuminated room, each eye is checked independently while the other eye is occluded. The number of incorrect responses are noted and compared with the fellow eye. If formal color plates are not available, color perception or intensity can be judged from one eye to the fellow eye using any brightly colored objects, especially red. Cola cans, eyedrop containers, or other similar common utensils can be used to help assess the quality of vision in one versus the fellow eye. The test needs to be performed in a well-illuminated setting.

Normal Findings

A person with normal color vision can usually discern fine degrees of difference of hue. Patients should have no difficulty discerning the color plates on recorded tests.

Abnormal Findings

Approximately 8% of males and 0.5% of females are color weak or color blind. The most common difficulties for these patients will be decreased vision in the red/green axis of color. People who are color blind still do perceive differences in color hue or variation.

EXAMINATION OF THE EXTERNAL EYE AND ADNEXA

Extraocular Muscle Function

Technique

Eye movement in all fields of gaze is easily assessed. Straight ahead vision refers to the primary position of gaze. A penlight held in front of the eye should cause a symmetric reflex off the cornea to be seen slightly nasal to the visual axis. The patient is then asked to look to the right, up and right, up and left, left, down and left, and down and right.

Normal Findings

The eye should move symmetrically and with equal excursions in all fields of gaze.

Abnormal Findings

Sudden onset of misalignment of one eye in any field of gaze will result in double vision. This may be eliminated by the patient's head position or gaze direction. The report of diplopia during testing of the extraocular movements likely represents an abnormal finding. Misalignment of the eyes without awareness of diplopia often indicates a long-standing history of strabismus. The patient has compensated for the misalignment by suppressing one of the images centrally, and thereby eliminating the diplopia.

Trauma to the orbits may induce fractures of the orbital walls. If this results in entrapment of the extraocular tissues or muscles, the patient may experience a sudden pain on extraocular movement and a limitation of gaze. This is especially true with blowout fractures of the orbital floor causing limitation of up-gaze. Medial wall fractures may entrap the medial rectus, limiting abduction.

Abducens Nerve (Sixth Cranial Nerve)

Normal Findings

The sixth cranial nerve supplies the ipsilateral lateral rectus muscle. The function of this nerve is to produce abduction, an outward movement of the globe.

Abnormal Findings

A sixth nerve palsy will result in esotropia, or crossing of the eyes. This can be compensated for by an abnormal head position. The patient will report a horizontal diplopia, or side-by-side double vision. A sixth nerve palsy will produce a head turn toward the side of the weak sixth nerve so that gaze position shifts out of the field of action; for example, a right sixth nerve palsy will often produce a right head turn so that the patient fixates in left gaze. The sixth nerve may be affected on an isolated basis due to vascular disease. Elevated intracranial pressure may also isolate the abducens nerve.

Trochlear Nerve (Fourth Cranial Nerve)

Normal Findings

The fourth cranial nerve supplies the ipsilateral superior oblique muscle. The primary function of the superior oblique is to lower the eye as well as rotate it.

Abnormal Findings

Paresis of the superior oblique muscle will cause a concurrent elevation of the affected eye. The patient will report vertical diplopia. The fourth nerve is especially prone to trauma along its course so that vertical diplopia after head injury often indicates a fourth nerve palsy. This is especially true if there is no entrapment present. The patient often tilts the head to the opposite side so that a right fourth nerve palsy will often present with the patient tilting the left ear toward the left shoulder. This removes the eye from the field of action of the weakened fourth nerve, eliminating the double vision.

Trauma producing bilateral fourth nerve palsies may produce vertical misalignment in all fields of gaze. However, rather than just one eye being elevated, the elevated eye may change with different fields of gaze so that with right shoulder tilt, the right eye is elevated and with left shoulder tilt, the left eye is elevated.

The fourth nerve is also susceptible to ischemic mononeuropathies due to diabetes or other vascular events. Herpes zoster also may affect this nerve, causing isolated neuropathy and concurrent strabismus.

The Oculomotor Nerve (Third Cranial Nerve)

Normal Findings

This nerve supplies the remaining ocular muscles as well as the levator aponeurosis of the eyelids. This nerve does branch, producing a superior division to the superior rectus and levator aponeurosis, and an inferior division to the inferior rectus, inferior oblique, and medial rectus. Passing along with the path of the third nerve are the pupillomotor fibers to the ipsilateral pupil. These fibers lie in the outer layer of the nerve close to the blood supply, producing constriction of the pupil.

Abnormal Findings

Patients with a third nerve palsy will usually present with ptosis and an exotropia or outward rotation of the eye, yielding horizontal diplopia. Eighty percent of pupillomotor fibers are spared in ischemic third nerve palsies but are affected in 95% of compressive third nerve palsies. A posterior communicating artery aneurysm is the most common cause of an isolated third nerve palsy with pupillary involvement.

TESTING FOR VISUAL FIELD ABNORMALITIES

Technique

The integrity of the peripheral visual field is easy to assess in the clinical setting. Confrontation visual field is the method most commonly used. The unoccluded eye of the patient is compared with that of the examiner by moving fingers or targets in the peripheral field and comparing the visual field with that of the examiner (Fig. 3). Each eye is tested independently. The patient is simply asked to identify when fingers are first seen moving or asked to count the number of

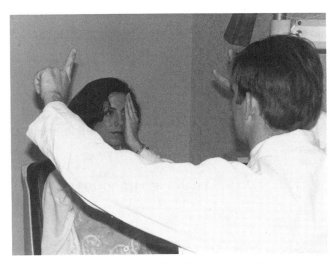

FIG. 3. Testing visual fields by confrontation.

fingers in the visual field. If a defect is suspected, a more definitive confrontational field can be performed using a small, red test object. The top of a typical bottle of dilating drops works well for this.

With the patient looking centrally at the examiner's nose or eye, the test object is brought in from the periphery and the patient is simply asked to report when it is first seen. The object is moved from the periphery toward the central visual field until it is identified. This is performed in multiple different meridians along the full 360 degrees of visual field. If a deficit is suspected by the examiner, the size and intensity can be estimated against the field of both the examiner and the fellow eye of the patient.

Normal Findings

The normal visual field extends nearly 180 degrees on the horizontal meridian and approximately 100 degrees on the vertical meridian. The field extends farthest in the temporal direction. There is greater sensitivity in the central visual field than in the peripheral field for both fine acuity and light perception.

Abnormal Findings

The visual pathway is long and complex. However, there are a few salient and simple points to remember. Lesions or interruptions of the visual pathway posterior to the optic chiasm produce bilateral visual field deficits. The closer the lesion approaches the occipital lobe of the cerebral cortex, the more congruous or symmetric the visual field deficit becomes between the two eyes. Lesions anterior to the optic chiasm typically produce a visual field deficit in the field of only one eye. Therefore, if the field defect seems to be isolated to one confrontational field, a lesion in the globe or optic nerve anterior to the chiasm is suspected. Ischemic optic neuropathy and glaucoma produce a visual field deficit that respects the horizontal meridian. Lesions producing visual field deficits at the chiasm typically produce bitemporal visual field loss. These lesions usually respect the vertical meridian. They may be congruous or varied and still represent lesions in the region of the chiasm.

EXAMINATION OF THE PUPILS

Technique

The pupil is easily evaluated with a simple penlight shining into one eye and then the other. This reflex produces both a direct response to light in the ipsilateral eye as well as a consensual response in the contralateral eye.

The pupil is best examined in slightly subdued lighting, especially if pathology or an abnormal reflex is suspected. Glass correction is not needed, and it often aids the examiner to have the subject's eyeglasses removed. With the patient gazing across the room, a penlight is brought from the side to shine on the patient's right eye. This should produce a brisk reaction of both the left and right pupils. After confirming this by testing the right eye a few times, the left eye is tested in a similar fashion.

The pupils not only respond to light but also constrict when the eye is focused on a near object. The light response typically exceeds the near response. If the pupils react minimally to direct light stimulation, they should be checked for a light-near dissociation. In a well-illuminated room, the patient is asked to look closely at the edge of the examiner's fingernails while they are held approximately 9 inches in front of the eye. If the pupil's response to this reaction produces a greater degree of constriction than that elicited from a direct or consensual light reaction, this represents a light-near dissociation of the pupil.

Normal Findings

A bright light illuminating one eye will typically produce a brisk reaction of the ipsilateral and contralateral pupil. When the light is removed, the pupil will dilate. The overall size of the pupil and the amount of reaction typically decrease with increasing age. The light response should normally be greater than the near response.

Abnormal Findings

If swinging a penlight from the right eye to the left eye and back to the right causes one pupil to dilate slightly with the light shining in this eye and then constrict when the light is shining in the other eye, an abnormal response is documented. Pathology in the visual system in one eye anterior to the optic chiasm will often produce a relative afferent pupillary defect or "positive Marcus-Gunn" (see Chapter 19). The visual system has judged the light to be brighter to a consensual response than to a direct response, indicating pathology on the side of the poor response. When there is a relative afferent pupillary defect, both pupils enlarge when the light is directed into the abnormal eye and become smaller when the light is directed into the unaffected or normal eye. The size of this asymmetry can be quite small or rather dramatic. The larger the deficit present, the greater the degree of pathology in the affected visual pathway. Opacities of the optical media do not produce a Marcus-Gunn defect. Pupillary abnormalities are discussed below.

Adie's Tonic Pupil

Adie's tonic pupil represents a benign lesion of the ciliary ganglion or post-ganglionic nerves. Most commonly, it is unilateral and results in a brisk light-near dissociation. Over time, these pupils become small.

Argyll-Robertson Pupil

An Argyll Robertson pupil also produces light-near dissociation. The pupils are noted to be small and usually irregular. They often dilate poorly. Twenty percent of people with neurosyphilis may demonstrate this abnormality.

Horner's Syndrome

Horner's syndrome is a deficit of the efferent branch of pupillary fibers. This results in a smaller than normal pupil. Because sympathetic fibers also supply Mueller's muscle of the eyelids, a mild ptosis of the upper lids and reverse ptosis of the lower lids is seen. Most noticeable is a dilation lag of the pupil. It dilates slowly when the lights are turned on.

EXAMINATION OF THE LIDS AND CONJUNCTIVA

Technique

The anterior segment of the eye is examined under good illumination with the aid of a penlight or a direct ophthalmoscope. The inspection begins with the lids and lashes and proceeds posteriorly in an orderly fashion. The lower palpebral conjunctiva can easily be examined using the thumb or forefinger to lightly pull the lower lid inferiorly, thereby producing a marked ectropion of the lid. To view

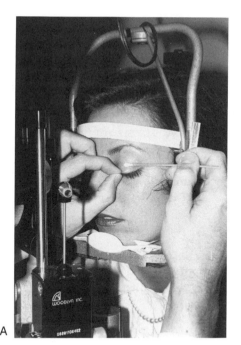
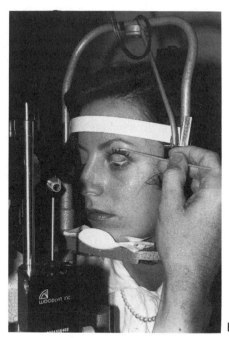

A   B

FIG. 4. Technique for everting upper lid. **A:** Lashes are grasped and the lid is pulled anteriorly and inferiorly. **B:** Cotton-tipped applicator is used to roll the lid posteriorly and superiorly.

the superior palpebral conjunctiva, the eyelid needs to be everted. To accomplish this, the patient is asked to look down while the lashes of the upper lid are grasped. The lid is pulled anteriorly and inferiorly while a cotton-tipped applicator is used to push firmly into the middle of the upper lid (Fig. 4A). The upper lid is then quickly rolled posteriorly and superiorly, exposing the conjunctival surface (Fig. 4B). This procedure can be performed without the use of topical anesthesia.

Normal Findings

The upper lid usually rests at the level of the cornea, covering the cornea for approximately 1 to 2 mm superiorly. The lower lid usually just touches the lower limbus of the cornea. The conjunctiva covers the eyeball over the sclera. It then everts upon itself to cover the inner aspect of the eyelids. The conjunctiva overlying the globe, or bulbar conjunctiva, is normally thin, transparent tissue appearing nearly white. The blood vessels are typically arranged in a radial pattern. A slight prominence of the medial vessels in each eye is common. The conjunctiva should not extend onto the surface of the cornea.

Abnormal Findings

The lash line is examined for the presence of focal or diffuse inflammation. Blockage of the glands along the lash line may produce localized or diffuse redness or flaking of the skin. Trichiasis—lashes misdirected against the globe—may become apparent. Focal loss of lashes also should be noted. The presence of any skin lesions along the lash line or lids should next be recorded. Basal cell carcinomas are the most frequent type of malignant tumor of the eyelids and are most frequently found along the lower lids and medial canthal region. Ptosis, ectropion, or entropion all may affect the visual field or function of the eyes.

A pterygium, a growth of conjunctiva tissue onto the cornea, usually at the medial aspect of the globe, is abnormal. The pattern of the vascular abnormality can aid in the diagnosis of anterior ocular disease. Uveitis or iritis will cause injection of the conjunctiva and scleral vessels at the limbus. Episcleritis often causes a sectorial localization of conjunctival hyperemia. Conjunctivitis most commonly produces a diffuse injection over the four quadrants of the conjunctiva, as well as the palpebral conjunctiva. If a foreign body is present in the conjunctiva, a moistened cotton-tipped applicator can be used to brush against the conjunctival surface A drop of topical anesthetic, such as Pontocaine, may facilitate removal if the patient notes discomfort.

EXAMINATION OF THE CORNEA

Technique

The cornea is examined with either a penlight or the aid of magnification of a direct ophthalmoscope. Illumination of the cornea tangentially also may show abnormalities such as abrasions or foreign bodies. Fluorescein dye applied topically to the cornea will stain any erosion or abrasion of the epithelium. A cobalt blue filter over the tip of a penlight or through the illuminating source of a direct ophthalmoscope will cause the fluorescein dye to appear green. This will illuminate epithelial defects of the cornea or conjunctiva.

Normal Findings

The cornea typically has a smooth contour and a glistening surface. Its diameter is slightly larger horizontally than vertically.

Abnormal Findings

Imperfections of the corneal surface will produce an abnormal light reflex or a break in the image as the light reflects off the cornea. Arcus senilis, a gray ring surrounding the cornea at the limbus, appears with frequency with advancing age; however, it does not affect visual acuity. Rust within the cornea often produces a localized inflammatory response yielding a white ring around a dark object imbedded in the corneal surface. A perforation of the cornea will produce an abnormal light reflex due to a break in the corneal epithelium. Fluorescein dye instilled on this defect will often proceed to stream away from the wound, indicating a break in the corneal integrity.

EXAMINATION OF THE ANTERIOR CHAMBER

Technique

The anterior chamber is examined using a penlight to illuminate the depth of the angle. If the light is illuminated from the temporal aspect of the eye parallel to the plane of the iris, a deep anterior chamber will allow the light to pass across the entire iris and illuminate its surface. A shallow chamber will cause light to strike the iris as it bows forward, casting a shadow over the nasal half of the iris.

Normal Findings

The anterior chamber should be symmetric with its fellow eye. This is especially important after trauma. It is filled with clear fluid, and its depth should be discernably separate from the cornea.

Abnormal Findings

A shallow anterior chamber can lead to narrow angle glaucoma. This is usually a symmetric condition. It is more common with increasing age and in farsighted patients. If the iris falls into a shadow with temporal illumination, a narrow angle is suspected. A shallow anterior chamber after trauma may indicate a rupture of the eye or possible penetrating foreign body. Hyphema, or blood within the anterior chamber, is abnormal and may follow trauma. The amount of hyphema is judged in proportion to the amount of anterior chamber that it fills.

MEASUREMENT OF INTRAOCULAR PRESSURE

Technique

An approximate estimate of the intraocular pressure can be made by simply judging the firmness of the eyeballs through the closed and relaxed lids of the patient. With the patient looking slightly down and the eyes closed, one or two fingers of the examiner can be placed on the upper lid of each eye independently. Firm pressure is applied just to the point of slight indentation of the globe and released quickly.

This should be a painless procedure unless the eye is inflamed. Rigidity of the globe is assessed and compared with the fellow eye. Asymmetry of ocular firmness can be a sign of glaucoma. A more accurate recording of the intraocular pressure requires instrumentation such as an applanation tonometer or a Schiotz tonometer.

Normal Findings

Normal intraocular pressure is considered to be 10 to 21 mm Hg.

Abnormal Findings

An intraocular pressure of less than 4 mm Hg indicates hypotony of the globe and might be a sign of ocular perforation or a retinal detachment. An intraocular pressure of greater than 21 mm Hg increases the risk for glaucoma. The incidence of glaucoma does increase along family lineage as well as beyond the age of 40.

EXAMINATION OF THE OCULAR FUNDUS AND OTHER STRUCTURES

With the invention of the ophthalmoscope by von Helmholz in 1851, it became possible for the first time to visualize the ocular fundus (1). This invention was a vitally important milestone in the development of modern scientific medicine; it allowed physicians to observe blood vessels in the living human eye, to study intrinsic diseases of the retina, and to observe the numerous ocular manifestations of systemic disease.

Technique

Every clinician should be familiar with the direct ophthalmoscope and understand the basic principles of ophthalmoscopy and, more importantly, what can be derived from an examination of the eye grounds. Ophthalmoscopes have a dial containing plus and minus lenses, which allow the examiner to compensate for refractive error. One begins the examination with a +10 lens, holding the ophthalmoscope approximately a foot from the patient's eye. A brilliant red reflex should be seen in the pupil; opacities in the media, such as cataract or vitreous hemorrhage, will diminish this brilliant red reflex. The examiner then dials down the lenses until the ocular fundus is in focus. The direct ophthalmoscope gives a two-dimensional, nonstereoscopic view of the ocular fundus. For the advanced student of ophthalmoscopy, there is a variety of other ways of examining the fundus, including binocular stereoscopic indirect ophthalmoscopy, the use of a fundus contact lens with a slit lamp, fundus photography using a specially developed fundus camera, and fluorescein angiography, which yields valuable information about the status of the retinal and choroidal circulation.

It is difficult to obtain a decent view of the ocular fundus through a small, undilated pupil. In most instances, useful information can be obtained only with pupillary dilatation. As in every clinical situation, the physician must balance the benefits of the information to be obtained by dilating the pupils versus the potential complications. Pupillary dilatation will render the patient photophobic in bright sunlight because the dilated iris is unable to constrict to block out excess light. In addition, if a cycloplegic is used, reading will be impossible until the effect wears off. As a rule, these do not constitute significant contraindications to pupillary dilatation. The major ophthalmic complication of dilating the pupil is the possible provocation of an attack of pupillary block glaucoma, which occurs in the setting of an anatomically narrow anterior chamber angle. This is a rare condition that usually occurs spontaneously in the anatomically predisposed eye but can be induced by dilating the pupil. Should it occur, it is a definite ocular emergency, which causes severe pain, an acutely inflamed eye, and loss of vision.

Ideally, every new patient should have their pupils dilated as part of a routine physical examination. Failing this, patients who are at high risk for vascular disease, such as those with diabetes mellitus or hypertension, should have dilated funduscopic examinations at least yearly in order to detect the earliest changes of diabetic retinopathy or to ascertain the adverse affects of hypertension on the circulation. In addition, patients with human immunodeficiency virus (HIV) may present with acquired immunodeficiency syndrome (AIDS) microvasculopathy (hemorrhages, cotton-wool spots) as well as cytomegalovirus (CMV) retinitis, which can be diagnosed with direct ophthalmoscopy.

There are two classes of drugs that can be used to dilate the pupil: cycloplegics and mydriatics. Cycloplegic drugs paralyze the smooth muscle in the ciliary body, thereby preventing accommodation for the duration of the drug's action. Consequently, a patient whose pupils have been dilated with a cycloplegic is unable to read until the effects of the drug wear off. Commonly used short-acting cycloplegics include Mydriacyl and Cyclogyl (Alcon Laboratories, Fort Worth, Texas). Atropine and homatropine are more long-lasting cycloplegics and are usually not used to dilate the pupils for examination. They are useful in cycloplegic refraction of children.

The second category of drugs, mydriatics, dilate the pupil without paralyzing the ciliary body. A commonly used mydriatic is Neosynephrine (2.5%) (Alcon Laboratories, Fort Worth, Texas). A combination of Neosynephrine (2.5%) and Mydriacyl (1%) should provide adequate pupillary dilatation in a short period of time, allowing a good examination of the fundus.

EXAMINATION OF THE LENS AND VITREOUS

Normal Findings

In evaluating the eye grounds, the examiner should have a specific checklist in mind (Table 1). By starting with a +10 lens and moving toward the patient, the

---

TABLE 1. *Systematic evaluation of the ocular fundus*

A. Lens and vitreous
   1. Clear
   2. Hazy
B. Optic disk
   1. Color
   2. Contour
   3. Cupping
C. Retinal vessels
   1. Caliber
     a. ? dilated
     b. ? narrowed
     c. ? beaded
   2. Light reflex of arterioles
     a. Copper wiring
     b. Silver wiring
   3. Lipid exudates
   4. Retinal hemorrhages (see Table 2)
   5. Cotton-wool spots (see Table 3)
D. Macula
   1. Abnormal pigmentation
   2. Presence or absence of fluid
   3. Presence or absence of hemorrhage
   4. Macular hole

---

examiner should detect a brilliant red reflex in the pupil. In the normal patient, the lens and vitreous should be crystal clear and allow a sharp distinct view of the posterior pole of the eye.

Abnormal Findings

The most common cause of hazy media is a cataractous lens. The usually clear vitreous may become opacified from disease processes causing vitreous hemorrhage (diabetes, retinal tear) or vitreous inflammation (uveitis). In children, a white reflex (leukocoria) may be the earliest sign of retinoblastoma or could indicate an inflammatory process such as toxoplasmosis or ocular toxocariasis.

EXAMINATION OF THE OPTIC NERVE HEAD

Normal Findings

The optic nerve head is located at the posterior pole of the eye and is a vertically elongated oval structure, measuring 1.75 mm in its vertical length. The normal optic nerve is flat, with sharp distinct margins, sometimes surrounded by a crescent of pigment. It has a pinkish hue from capillaries nourishing the tissues comprising the disk (see Color Fig. 5 following page 80).

Abnormal Findings

The examiner should carefully observe the optic nerve head, noting its color, contour, and the presence or absence of cupping. A pale (atrophic) optic nerve is indicative of a pathologic process such as prior inflammation (retrobulbar neuritis, syphilis), or a space-occupying lesion compressing the nerve (craniopharyngioma). If the intracranial pressure is elevated, the nerve may appear swollen, with hazy, indistinct margins (papilledema). Even though the disk is swollen and edematous, such patients initially have normal visual acuity. However, long-standing, unrelieved elevated intracranial pressure will eventually cause optic atrophy and loss of vision. Papillitis refers to inflammatory swelling and edema of the nerve, caused by a condition such as ischemic optic neuritis or temporal arteritis. Patients with papillitis usually experience a profound loss of vision. It is not possible to distinguish between papillitis and papilledema on the basis of the appearance of the disk alone; both are serious findings and need expert evaluation. Optic nerve cupping refers to the depression of tissue in the center of the disk and is measured by the fraction (percentage) of the disk occupied by the cup, the cup/disk (C/D) ratio. A C/D ratio of 0.2 to 0.4 is considered normal; increased intraocular pressure (glaucoma) slowly but steadily erodes healthy nerve tissue and increases the C/D ratio. A C/D ratio of 0.7 to 0.8 means that the nerve has been badly damaged by glaucoma; the affected patient will have visual field loss as a result.

EXAMINATION OF THE RETINAL VASCULATURE

Normal Findings

The ocular fundus offers the only opportunity to observe and study the vascular system in vivo. The central retinal artery enters the eye via the optic nerve, where it bifurcates, sending arteriolar branches into the four quadrants of the retina. The vessels observed in the eye are therefore arterioles, rather than arteries. By definition, an artery possesses an internal elastic lamina and a well-developed muscular coat. In contrast, arterioles lack the internal elastic lamina, and the mus-

TABLE 2. *Causes of retinal hemorrhages*

Hypertension
Diabetes
AIDS
Anemia
Venous occlusion
Sickle-cell disease
Blood dyscrasias
Endocarditis

TABLE 3. *Causes of cotton-wool spots*

Hypertension
Diabetes
AIDS
Collagen vascular disease
Venous occlusive disease
Arterial occlusion
Anemia
Blood dyscrasias; leukemia
Cardiac valvular disease
Radiation retinitis

cle layer is not continuous. One can easily distinguish arterioles from venules by the darker color of the venules. As the blood flows through the vessel, the normal arteriole reflects the light from the ophthalmoscope, creating the light reflex.

Abnormal Findings

In retinal vascular disease, the examiner looks for changes in the caliber of the vessels, the light reflex from the walls of the arterioles, and the presence of retinal hemorrhages, cotton-wool spots, and yellow lipid exudates (Tables 2 and 3). Retinal hemorrhages located in the nerve fiber layer of the retina are arranged in a linear fashion, paralleling the nerve fibers, and are referred to as flame-shaped hemorrhages. Hemorrhages located deeper in the retinal tissue are round and are referred to as dot and blot hemorrhages. Both are indicative of systemic disease and must be further investigated. Cotton-wool spots, sometimes called soft exudates, are white fluffy lesions, usually one-third to one-half the size of the optic disk, scattered around the posterior pole of the fundus. Histologically, they are infarcts in the nerve fiber layer of the retina. As a rule, neither retinal hemorrhages nor cotton-wool spots give rise to visual symptoms, but their presence indicates systemic disease, and they are therefore of diagnostic significance. Lipid exudates, often called hard exudates, are glistening yellowish deposits in the retina, often seen in the macular region. These exudates indicate leakage of protein and lipid from the vascular system and are frequently found in diabetic macular edema.

EXAMINATION OF THE MACULA

Normal Findings

The macula is that specialized part of the retina necessary for clear central vision. It contains the highest concentration of cones in the retina. Its center, the fovea, is marked by a tiny depression in the retina.

Abnormal Findings

Any disease of the macula may result in loss of central visual acuity and render the patient unable to read or to drive a car. Signs of macular disease include edema of the macula, hemorrhage, lipid exudates, or pigmented scar tissue.

SPECIFIC DISEASES OF THE RETINA

Diabetic Retinopathy

The single most important retinal disease encountered in clinical practice and the one most responsible for adult-onset blindness is diabetes mellitus. The physician must be familiar with the ocular manifestations of this disease. Diabetic retinopathy is essentially a microvasculopathy that produces characteristic, readily recognizable ocular changes. The earliest sign of diabetic retinopathy is the appearance of microaneurysms (see Color Fig. 6 the following page). These are saccular out-pouchings of the capillary wall, typically 15 to 60 microns in diameter. They are recognized as round red dots on funduscopic examination. Early on, microaneurysms do not cause visual loss. With time, however, the diseased vessels develop increased permeability, allowing leakage of lipid, plasma, and protein into the surrounding tissue, causing retinal edema and subsequent loss of vision. Eventually, arteriolar and capillary closure occurs, leading to ischemia of the retina. The ophthalmoscopic signs of retinal ischemia include retinal hemorrhage, venous beading, cotton-wool spots, and intraretinal vascular abnormalities. The appearance of numerous hemorrhages in the diabetic fundus is an ominous sign because the severity of retinal hemorrhage parallels the severity of the retinopathy. With progressive retinal ischemia, proliferative diabetic retinopathy supervenes, representing a grave threat to vision. In proliferative diabetic retinopathy, abnormal new blood vessels proliferate on the surface of the retina or on the surface of the optic nerve head. Once these new blood vessels appear, the diabetic eye is at great risk for vitreous hemorrhage and consequent catastrophic loss of vision. It is exceedingly important that any diabetic patient showing evidence of neovascularization receive prompt ophthalmologic referral for possible laser therapy.

The final and most severe stage in the evolution of diabetic retinopathy is characterized by the formation of sheets of fibrovascular connective tissue on the surface of the retina. The connective tissue eventually contracts, shrinks, and bleeds, causing traction retinal detachment and vitreous hemorrhage. This will lead to irrevocable blindness unless corrected surgically by means of pars plana vitrectomy surgery.

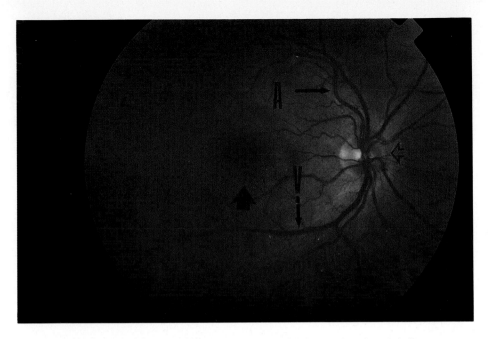

FIG. 5. Normal ocular fundus. Open arrow points to optic disk. Large, closed arrow indicates macula. A, points to arteriole; V, points to vein.

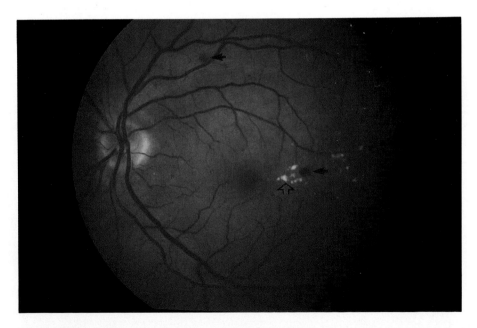

FIG. 6. Diabetic retinopathy. Open arrow points to lipid deposits. Closed arrows point to retinal hemorrhages.

The American Academy of Ophthalmology recommends that insulin-dependent diabetics (juvenile onset diabetes) have ophthalmic evaluation at 5 years after the onset of their disease and at yearly intervals thereafter. Non–insulin-dependent diabetics should have funduscopic evaluation at the time of the diagnosis and yearly thereafter. Because of the adverse affect of pregnancy on diabetic retinopathy, a pregnant diabetic should be examined in the first trimester of pregnancy and thereafter at frequent intervals until the termination of the pregnancy.

Hypertension

High blood pressure causes profound changes in the retinal vasculature that are readily recognized with the ophthalmoscope. Hypertension causes constriction and narrowing of the retinal arterioles, along with some irregularity in the caliber of the arterioles. Eventually, the restricted blood flow damages the capillary walls, resulting in bleeding into the surrounding tissues, recognized as flame-shaped or dot and blot retinal hemorrhages. Cotton-wool spots represent localized infarcts in the nerve fiber layer of the retina. This is caused by hypertensive ischemia in the tissue. In severe and advanced cases of hypertension, papilledema can occur and is an ominous sign.

Arteriolosclerosis

Hypertensive changes in the retinal arterioles may occur when the hypertension is of sudden onset, as occurs with acute glomerulonephritis or toxemia of pregnancy. Long-standing hypertension, on the other hand, leads to the changes of arteriolosclerosis. In arteriolosclerosis, hyaline material is deposited in the endothelium, followed by progressive thickening of the vessel wall. Arteriolosclerosis is a generalized disease involving arterioles throughout the body in a uniform fashion. If the retinal vessels show changes of arteriolosclerosis, it is highly likely that arterioles in the brain, kidney, and other organs will likewise be afflicted. The normal arteriole displays a characteristic light reflex as the blood flows through the vessels. In arteriolosclerosis, the wall of the vessel becomes hardened and more opaque as the disease progresses. The light reflex becomes brighter and wider. This is called copper wiring when the vessel wall has the appearance of burnished copper. In extreme arteriolosclerosis, the vessel wall becomes so thickened that the artery appears as a white cord, and the blood column is obscured. This is referred to as silver wiring of the arterioles. Also, in arteriolosclerosis, progressive changes at arteriovenous crossings are observed. Ordinarily, there is no deflection of the vein at such crossings, but as the adventitial covering of the arteriole becomes harder and denser, the underlying vein becomes bent, distorted, and deflected from its path. Such changes are referred to as arteriovenous (AV) crossing defects, or AV nicking. Branch vein occlusions usually occur at the site of a pathologic AV crossing defect.

AIDS

In patients infected with HIV, a retinal vasculopathy occurs, resulting in the appearance of flame-shaped hemorrhages and cotton-wool spots. Such changes are often transitory and may clear between examinations. In the late stages of AIDS, when the CD4 count is reduced to 50 or below, CMV retinitis may occur. This is an opportunistic infection seen in patients with AIDS or in others who are iatrogenically immunosuppressed. In CMV retinitis, patchy areas of white, granular retinal infiltrate appear, often accompanied by retinal hemorrhage.

Age-related Macular Degeneration (ARMD)

Macular degeneration is the most common cause of visual disability among older Americans and results from senescent changes in the choriocapillaris (Bruch's membrane) retinal pigment epithelial complex at the posterior pole of the eye. There are two forms of ARMD: "dry" and "wet." In the former, the examiner notes increased pigmentation at the posterior pole, along with drusen, which are yellowish-white excrescences on Bruch's membrane. There is often an oval-shaped area of retinal pigment epithelial atrophy in the center of the macula. In the wet form of ARMD, a subretinal new vessel membrane forms that eventually leaks fluid, blood, and lipid into the macular tissues, causing an exudative macular detachment and eventual loss of central visual acuity.

Vitreous Hemorrhage

The most common causes of intraocular (vitreous) hemorrhage are hemorrhagic proliferative diabetic retinopathy, retinal tear with overlying blood vessels, and retinal neovascularization secondary to retinal vein occlusion. In cases of vitreous hemorrhage, the patient experiences rapid loss of vision, sometimes proceeded by flashing lights and vitreous floaters. The media are hazy on ophthalmoscopic examination to the point where the disk and retinal vessels are not visible because of the blood. In most such cases, the hemorrhage will clear spontaneously; if not, vitrectomy may be indicated.

Retinal Detachment

Detached retina is caused by a tear or hole in the retina, which then allows vitreous fluid to gain access to the subretinal space, detaching the retina from the underlying choroid and retinal pigment epithelium. The symptoms of retinal detachment include flashing lights, vitreous floaters, photopsia, and the sensation of a curtain being drawn across the affected visual field. Should the macula become involved with the detachment, central visual acuity is lost. Prompt surgical repair usually results in restoration of the peripheral visual field.

Central Retinal Artery Occlusion

Occlusion of the central retinal artery occurs in the clinical setting of hypertensive arteriosclerotic vascular disease. Sudden, massive loss of central vision and most of the visual field is the presenting symptom. Many patients will retain a small island of vision temporally. The classical ophthalmologic finding is that of a cherry red spot in the macula, caused by cloudy swelling of the retina in the macular area. The swollen edematous retina turns white, accentuating the normal reddish appearance of the fovea. No treatment has been found to be effective for central retinal artery occlusion.

Central Retinal Vein Occlusion

Obstruction of the central retinal vein results in a "blood and thunder" fundus, characterized by extensive intraretinal hemorrhage in all four quadrants of the retina. Cotton-wool spots, swollen, dilated veins, and macular edema complete the clinical picture of central retinal vein occlusion. Such patients describe a central blur in their vision, although the onset of the disease may be insidious. The disease is caused by a thrombus in the central retinal vein.

REFERENCE

1. von Helmholtz H. *Beschreibung eines augenspiegels Z. Untersuch. d. Netzhaut Im Iebenden Auge.* Berlin, 1851.

SUGGESTED READING

Diabetic Retinopathy Education Study Group. *Detection and referral of diabetic eye disease: a guide for practicing physicians.* Washington, DC: The Worthen Center for Eye Care Research, Georgetown University Medical Center, 1992.
Diabetic Retinopathy: Slide/Script Program. The American Academy of Ophthalmology, 1992.
Duke-Elder, S. *System of ophthalmology.* London: Henry Kimpton, 1971.
Scheie HG. Evaluation of ophthalmoscopic changes of hypertension and arteriolar sclerosis. *AMA Arch Ophthalmol* 1953;49:117–38.
Walsh FB. *Clinical neurophthalmology.* 2nd ed. Baltimore: Williams & Wilkins, 1957.
Wise GN, Dollery CT, Henkind P. *The retinal circulation.* New York: Harper & Row, 1971.

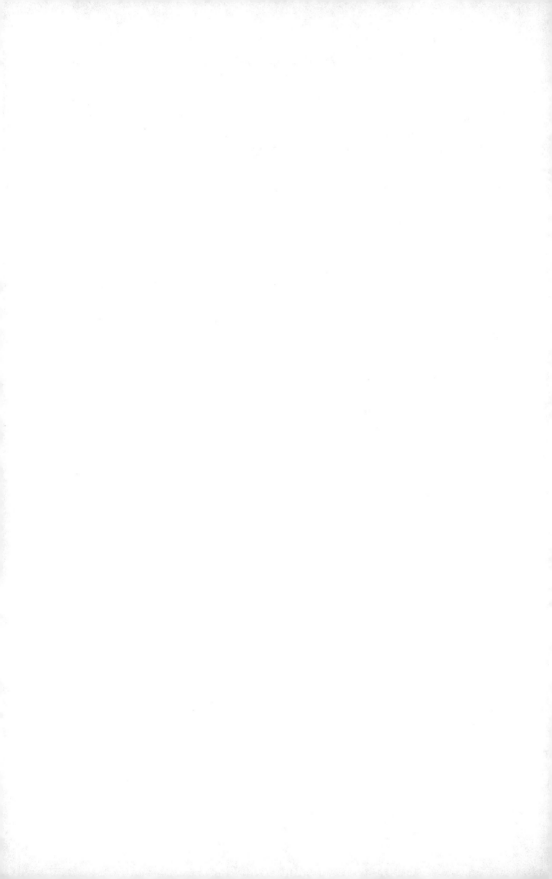

Clinical Skills for Adult Primary Care
edited by M. E. Silverman and J. W. Hurst.
Lippincott-Raven Publishers, Philadelphia © 1996.

8

Examination of the Mouth

Wyman P. Sloan III, M.D.

Piedmont Hospital, Atlanta, Georgia 30309

"Failure to examine the throat is a glaring sin of omission, especially in children. One finger in the throat and one finger in the rectum makes a good diagnostician."
William Osler, quoted in Bean WB. *Sir William Osler: Aphorisms.*
Springfield, IL: Charles C Thomas, 1968:104.

The examination of the oral cavity should address those problems for which the patient is at a relatively high risk. These are listed as follows:

- Tobacco products. Especially in conjunction with heavy alcohol consumption, the smoker is at greatly increased risk for the subsequent development of oral and pharyngeal cancer. Only through early detection, while the lesion is small and asymptomatic, is cure probable.
- Human immunodeficiency virus (HIV) infection. Regular, meticulous examination of the mouth is particularly important in the evaluation and management of the HIV-infected patient in whom oral mucosal lesions abound.
- Periodontal disease. Periodontal disease affects almost all adults at some time and is the most common cause of tooth loss. It is, by and large, preventable and treatable. The primary care physician, with a broad range of patients with diverse medical problems, has a somewhat unique opportunity to impact the course of this disease through early recognition and intervention in conjunction with the patient's dentist.

TECHNIQUE

Equipment necessary for an adequate examination of the oral cavity includes a tongue blade, finger cot or examining glove, portable light source (e.g., penlight), dental mirror, and gauge sponges. The patient should wash off any lipstick or lip balm and always remove their dentures.

Inspection of the mouth is accomplished in three stages. First, the patient is asked to open the mouth widely, and the tongue is depressed to visualize the dorsum of the tongue, hard and soft palate, and pharynx. Rather than request the patient to "stick out your tongue and say ah," this part of the examination may be more satisfactorily accomplished by instructing the patient to retract the tongue into the mouth and take deep breaths. Pressing the tongue blade against the mid-dorsum of the tongue will produce gagging in many patients. This bothersome reflex can sometimes be overcome by having the patient sing "ah" in a high-pitched falsetto voice (1). Next, the patient is asked to open the mouth and to press the tip of the tongue against the palate. This allows for visualization of the floor of the mouth and the ventral aspect of the tongue. Finally, the tongue is grasped with a gauze sponge, then withdrawn as far as possible from the mouth and pulled laterally while the ipsilateral cheek is retracted with the tongue blade. In this position, the posterolateral borders of the tongue may be inspected and palpated. In general, palpation of the dorsum of the tongue is best accomplished by allowing the tongue to relax comfortably within the confines of the mouth.

TABLE 1. *Diseases and ingestions associated with unusual breath odors.*

General category of odor	Further description of odor	Disease or offending substance
Sweet	Fruity, acetonelike, like decomposing apples	Ketoacidosis (e.g., diabetes or starvation), lacquer, chloroform, salicylates
	Fruity, alcoholic	Alcohol, phenol
	Fruity, pearlike, acrid, penetrating	Chloral hydrate, paraldehyde
	Wintergreen	Methyl salicylate
	Aromatic, pungent	Ethchlorvynol
Fishy	Flshy	Uremia (trimethylamine)
	Fishy, rancid butter, boiled cabbage	Hypermethioninemla
Musty	Musty fish, raw liver, feculent, new-mown clover (fetor hepaticus)	Hepatic failure (mercaptans, dimethyl sulfide)
Feculent	Feculent, foul	Intestinal obstruction, esophageal diverticulum
Urinelike	Ammoniacal, urinelike	Uremia (ammonia)
Foul	Foul, putrid	Lung abscess, empyema (especially anaerobic), intranasal foreign body
Halitosis	Severe "bad breath"	Trench mouth (Vincent's angina), amphetamines
Other	Sweaty feet, cheesy	Isovaleric acidemia (odor-of-sweaty-feet syndrome)
	Bitter almond	Cyanide (e.g., apricot pits), jetberry bush
	Burned rope	Marijuana
	Camphor	Naphthalene (mothball pica)
	Coal gas (stove gas)	Carbon monoxide (odorless but associated with coal gas)
	Disinfectant	Phenol, creosote
	Garlic	Phosphorus, arsenic, tellurium, parathion, malathion

From Hayden GF. Olfactory diagnosis in medicine. *Postgrad Med* 1980;67:110–8. Reprinted with permission of McGraw-Hill, Inc.

Direct visualization is the primary modality used in assessing the oral cavity. It can often yield findings that are diagnostic of specific diseases, obviating the need for further laboratory studies. Palpation of the contents of the mouth, on the other hand, is generally reserved for special situations. It is a crucial part of the examination of the patient at high risk for oral malignancies or in the patient with unexplained cervical lymphadenopathy. A number of infectious diseases involving the oral cavity are associated with a foul odor detected on the patient's breath but, by and large, the sense of smell has been relegated to a minor role in physical diagnosis. However, recognition of distinctive odors can provide valuable clues to the presence of many diseases or intoxications in that critical period while awaiting laboratory results. Many metabolic disturbances, biochemical abnormalities, and ingested toxins produce characteristic breath odors available to the astute clinician with a "nose" for this neglected clinical skill (Table 1).

NORMAL FINDINGS

The oral cavity includes the mouth, teeth, tongue, hard and soft palate, region of the palatine tonsils, and pharynx. The mouth consists of two parts: the vestibule and the mouth proper. The vestibule is the narrow space bordered by the lips, buccal mucosa of the cheeks, teeth, and alveolar ridges. The lips consist of skin on the outside, mucous membranes on the inside, and the orbicularis oris muscle in between. The upper and lower lips meet at the commissures and are connected to the contiguous gingiva of the alveolar ridge by a midline fold of mucous membrane, the frenulum. The mucous membranes of the cheeks reflect onto the gingiva and are generally pale coral pink in color. In dark-skinned races, it may be dappled with small patches of pigment. The orifice to the parotid gland (Stensen's duct) can be visualized posteriorly opposite the second maxillary molar. The gingiva (or gums) consists of dense fibrous tissue firmly adherent to the underlying alveolar bone. Its free margins surround the neck of the teeth and are covered by pale red mucous membranes. In adults, there are 32 permanent teeth consisting of two incisors, one cuspid (canine), two bicuspids (premolars), and three molars in each half of both the upper and lower jaw. That part of each tooth that projects above the gingiva is referred to as the crown and is covered by white enamel. Devitalized teeth will appear dark or grayish.

The dorsum of the tongue is divided into lateral halves by the median sulcus. The anterior two-thirds of the tongue is separated from the posterior one-third by a V-shaped groove, the terminal sulcus (the apex of which is directed posteriorly to the foramen cecum, the site of closure of the embryonic thyroglossal duct). Occasionally, this area may be the site of lingual thyroid tissue. The dorsum of the tongue is covered with minute projections or papillae. There are three types. Circumvallate papillae are the largest and are generally eight to 12 in number and located just anteriorly to the V-shaped terminal sulcus. Filiform papillae are the smallest and most numerous and impart a velvety texture to the anterior two-thirds of the tongue. Fungiform papillae are most numerous over the apex and lateral margins of the tongue and may occasionally appear pigmented in dark-skinned races.

The posterior third of the tongue has a somewhat nodular, warty appearance, secondary to scattered lymphoid tissue—the lingual tonsils. Under the tongue, a median fold of mucous membrane, the lingual frenulum, anchors the tongue to the floor of the mouth. Prominent lingual veins are noted on either side of this midline fold. At the base of the tongue, on either side of the frenulum, arise the sublingual caruncles, which house the orifices of the submaxillary glands (Wharton's duct). Running posteriorly and laterally to the root of the tongue on the floor of the mouth are prominent ridges of mucosa, the sublingual folds, which contain the orifices of the ducts of the minor sublingual glands.

The roof of the mouth is formed by the hard palate, which separates the nasal and oral cavities, and the soft palate. The uvula hangs from the free posterior border of the soft palate in the midline.

The mouth unites with the pharynx at the faucial isthmus, which is marked by a pair of prominent arches. The palatoglossal arch (also called the anterior pillars of fauces) extends from the anterior soft palate to the dorsolateral tongue. The palatopharyngeal arch (also called the posterior pillar of fauces) arises at the posterior edge of the soft palate and inserts into the side wall of the pharynx. Within the triangular depression bounded by these prominent arches lies the palatine tonsils. Their color usually matches that of the surrounding mucosa. Their size may vary, but hyperplasia is common in childhood and obesity. The surface is frequently marked with deep clefts and crypts which may contain debris, a finding often mistaken as a sign of infection.

ABNORMAL FINDINGS

Lips

Generalized *enlargement of the lips* may be seen in a number of endocrinopathies, including hypothyroidism and acromegaly.

Mucoceles are localized swellings that most commonly involve the lower lip but may be found anywhere in the oral cavity where mucous glands are plentiful. Typically, these lesions are nontender, fluctuant to palpation, with a bluish tinge. They rarely reach dimensions greater than 1 cm in diameter. They are the result of obstructed or traumatized excretory ducts.

Actinic cheilitis, a condition caused by chronic sun exposure, involves predominantly the lower lip. Initially, there is a subtle obscuring of the normally sharp vermilion border of the lip. In its chronic form, the lip becomes firm and scaly with occasional ulcerations and crusting. This is felt to be a precancerous lesion and warrants close follow-up. Any ulceration persisting beyond 2 weeks should raise suspicion of a squamous cell carcinoma and be examined via biopsy.

Angular cheilitis may accompany excessive pooling of saliva in those who are edentulous or have poorly fitting dentures. It is also seen as a result of a deficiency of the B group of vitamins. Fissures, which frequently become inflamed, extend from the corners of the mouth. In time, these crevices may deepen, erode, and crust. Secondary infection with candida or staphylococcus is frequent.

Multiple punctate lip telangiectasias may be seen in *hereditary hemorrhagic telangiectasia (Rendu-Osler-Weber disease)*, an autosomal dominant disease characterized by similar lesions in the gastrointestinal tract. This disorder may be complicated by recurrent episodes of bleeding and by the presence of pulmonary arteriovenous (AV) fistulas.

Multiple brown macules may be seen on the lips and buccal mucosa in *Peutz-Jeghers syndrome* (hereditary intestinal polyposis). This autosomal-dominant condition is characterized by gastrointestinal polyposis, especially involving the ileum. Gastrointestinal bleeding is common, and there exists an increased risk for development of cancers of the gastrointestinal tract, requiring regular surveillance.

The chancre is the oral hallmark of *syphilis*. It is seen as a painless nodule that subsequently ulcerates. The ulcer crater is covered by a serous exudate teeming with spirochetes and is highly infectious. Healing occurs spontaneously in 2 to 4 weeks.

Oral Vestibule

Inspection of the buccal mucosa of the cheeks may reveal brown streaking or stippling in *adrenocortical insufficiency (Addison's disease)*. The pigmentary changes may extend onto the tongue and lips and gradually recede with adequate replacement therapy with corticosteroids.

Clusters of small (less than 1 mm in diameter) yellowish papules, termed *Fordyce's granules*, may be found on the buccal mucosa, lips, tongue, and gingiva. Painless and harmless, they are indicative of increased sebaceous activity. Small amounts of whitish sebum can be expressed from the individual papules.

Koplik's spots are small white spots with a surrounding red areola generally found on the buccal mucosa opposite the molars. They herald the exanthema of measles, which generally follows in 1 or 2 days.

The *linea albus* is a white, slightly raised, somewhat wavy line located on the buccal mucosa opposite the site of contact of the upper and lower teeth, occurring as a result of chronic friction.

Lichen planus is a common skin disorder that frequently has oral cavity manifestations. The buccal mucosa of the cheeks is most commonly affected, although lesions also may be seen on the tongue, lips, gingiva, and floor of the mouth. The eruption tends to be bilateral and symmetrical. A white, lacy, weblike pattern, termed Wickham's striae, is characteristic.

Irritation fibromas typically appear as well-defined, round, sessile, slowly enlarging papules arising from any soft tissue area of the mouth. Individual lesions seldom exceed 1 cm in diameter and have no malignant potential.

Epulis fissuratum is a fibrous, hyperplastic response of the vestibular mucosa resulting from chronic irritation from the flange of a poorly fitting denture.

Gingiva

Inflammation of the gums (*gingivitis*) is caused by microorganisms residing in supragingival plaques. The free margins of the gingiva and the interdental papillae appear red and swollen. If this process is left unchecked, the infection may spread to the soft tissues and bones surrounding the teeth (*periodontitis*). *Pericoronitis* (operculitis) is a localized gingivitis in the tissues surrounding a partially erupted or impacted wisdom tooth. *Hormone gingivitis* (pregnancy gingivitis) affects females at the time of puberty, pregnancy, and menopause. Persistent gingivitis may be seen as a complication of poorly controlled diabetes mellitus (*diabetic gingivitis*). In acute leukemia, the gingival tissue may become red, tender, and boggy as a result of leukemic infiltration with white blood cells (*leukemic gingivitis*).

Generalized *hyperplasia* of the gums is commonly seen in patients taking diphenylhydantoin or calcium channel blocking drugs (2). In time, growth may become so exuberant that the teeth are completely engulfed.

Chronic ingestion of heavy metals taken either medicinally (e.g., bismuth in antidiarrheal agents) or from occupational exposure (e.g., lead used in paints and plumbing) may produce a linear, blue-black pigmentary deposition within a millimeter of the free margins of the gums. This finding occurs only in the presence of supragingival bacteria and will not occur when the teeth are absent.

Palate

In about 20% of the adult population, a non-neoplastic, slowly enlarging, bony protuberance—the *torus palatinus*—involves the hard palate. It is generally of no clinical significance other than interfering with the fitting of dentures. Less commonly, multiple smaller exostoses—*mandibular tori*—may be found on the floor of the mouth adjacent to the maxillary alveolar ridge.

Papillomas are the most common benign epithelial neoplasm involving the oral cavity. Generally solitary and pedunculated, these lesions rarely reach dimensions greater than a centimeter in diameter. The surface appears pink and may be smooth or verrucous. There is a predilection for the hard and soft palate, uvula, and tongue.

Kaposi's sarcoma is the most frequent oral malignancy in the HIV-infected patient. Most commonly, it is located on the hard palate but it may involve the buccal mucosa or gingiva. Initially, the lesion appears as a rather innocuous red macule that, in time, enlarges into a bluish nodule that may be lobulated. The tumor may ulcerate and be quite painful. Oral Kaposi's sarcoma may precede skin and visceral lesions. It may be the first manifestation of AIDS in an otherwise apparently normal individual.

Floor of the Mouth

Obstruction of the excretory duct from sublingual or submaxillary salivary glands produces a translucent, mucin-filled, domed retention cyst—a *ranula*—located on the floor of the mouth. The lesion is unilateral and fluctuant when palpated.

A *dermoid cyst* also may present as a localized swelling on the floor of the mouth but can be distinguished from a ranula in that it arises in the midline, is opaque, and has a doughy consistency.

Salivary calculi (*sialoliths*) are concretions within the salivary gland duct and also may produce transient swelling in the floor of the mouth. These lesions are firm and may be quite tender.

Tongue

Generalized enlargement of the tongue may be seen in a number of systemic illnesses, including acromegaly, infantile hypothyroidism, amyloidosis, and Down syndrome.

Asymmetric swelling of the tongue can be caused by lymphangiomas, neurofibromas, or hemangiomas. Hemangiomas are benign vascular hamartomas that usually develop about the first year of life. There is a slight predilection for females. Its color will depend on its depth below the mucosal surface and may vary from red to blue or even purple when quite superficial.

Dilated tortuous veins, or varices, are frequently found in the oral cavity, especially in the elderly. These lesions are benign and exhibit a predilection for the lips and ventral surface of the tongue. Varices feel fluctuant to palpation, and applied pressure will disperse blood from the vein.

Geographic tongue is a common, benign, inflammatory condition of unknown etiology. The eruption usually involves the dorsal and lateral borders of the tongue and is characterized by periodic desquamation of the superficial keratin and filiform papillae. Single or multiple denuded patches may be bordered by a raised white serpiginous rim. The pattern changes constantly and may migrate from site to site.

Atrophy of the filiform papillae of the tongue, producing a smooth balding appearance, is a nonspecific response to a number of nutritional deficiencies and anemias (including iron, B12, and folic acid deficiencies). In advanced cases, the surface of the tongue may appear fiery red. This condition is frequently symptomatic, producing pain (glossodynia) and burning (glossopyrosis).

A *hairy tongue* results from elongation of the filiform papillae and is associated with a variety of conditions, including cancer chemotherapy and irradiation, poor oral hygiene, smoking, and prior antibiotic use. The abnormal color of the tongue is caused by overgrowth of mycelial threads of chromogenic organisms, e.g., *Aspergillus niger* and *Candida albicans*. Extrinsic factors, including food and tobacco stain, also may play a role. Changes begin posteriorly near the foramen cecum and spread anteriorly and laterally. This condition is usually asymptomatic and is generally only of cosmetic concern.

Hairy leukoplakia presents as a somewhat vague, poorly demarcated, white lesion with a corrugated or "hairy" surface occurring on the lateral surface of the tongue of HIV-infected patients. It is generally asymptomatic. Biopsy confirmation of this lesion is important and predicts the subsequent development of AIDS, usually within 1 to 3 years.

EVALUATION OF THE SORE THROAT

Sore throat is one of the most common patient complaints encountered in ambulatory medicine. Although these patients are rarely seriously ill, reports of resurgence in the incidence of acute rheumatic fever have imparted a new urgency to the recognition of streptococcal pharyngitis (3). Examination of the pharynx typically shows erythema and swelling involving the tonsils and pillars, often extending onto the contiguous soft palate and uvula. Frequently, an associated exudate appears as a white or grayish scum that can easily be wiped away from the underlying mucosa. The overall prevalence of streptococcal infection in the adult population presenting with sore throats is surprisingly low (approximately 10%). Komaroff et al. have demonstrated that the individual signs and symptoms of streptococcal infection are of insufficient sensitivity and specificity to be of much value in establishing this diagnosis (4). However, combinations of findings may substantially increase the likelihood of this disease. The presence of exudative pharyngitis, fever, and tender anterior cervical lymphadenopathy inflates the postexamination probability of streptococcal disease to approximately 50%. In the absence of any of these findings, there is only a 3.4% likelihood of disease. Streptococcal pharyngitis is generally recognized as a self-limited disease resolving, on average, in 5 days. Trismus, inability to handle one's own secretions, dysphonia, and dysphagia should alert the clinician to the possibility of peritonsillar abscess (*quinsy*). This complication is seen as a bulging of the peritonsillar space, often with displacement of the soft palate and uvula to the contralateral side. Palpation of this area shows a fluctuance. If unrecognized, this suppurative process can progress to produce upper airway obstruction or extend into contiguous structures of the neck, including the great vessels.

Acute *infectious mononucleosis* is caused by the Epstein-Barr virus and is typically seen in teenagers and young adults. It is an uncommon (approximately 2%) cause of acute pharyngitis in adults (5). The diagnosis is suggested by a foul-smelling tonsillar exudate (fetor oris) and bilateral posterior cervical and/or postauricular lymphadenopathy. The tonsillar hypertrophy may be prominent, even to the point of pharyngeal obstruction (kissing tonsils syndrome). Early in the course, there may be palatal petechiae, which generally fades over the ensuing 7 to 10 days.

Oral *candidiasis* is the most common form of oral fungal infection. It is an opportunistic infection caused by *Candida albicans,* a normal inhabitant of the oral cavity, gastrointestinal tract, and vagina. A white, curdlike membrane with an erythematous border occurs commonly over the buccal mucosa, palate, or tongue. Attempts to scrape away the membrane usually produce superficial bleeding. Occasionally occurring de novo, it is more frequently associated with conditions that alter the normal intraoral bacterial ecosystem or compromise immunity, including recent use of systemic antibiotics, corticosteroids (either systemic or inhaled), diabetes mellitus, HIV disease, or chemotherapy. Chronic atrophic candidiasis (denture sore mouth) is the most common form of chronic candidiasis. It is seen as a localized, erythematous eruption involving that part of the hard palate directly in contact with a maxillary denture, especially when the appliance is worn throughout the night.

Oral ulcerations discovered in the patient complaining of sore mouth or throat can be caused by a diverse group of diseases. *Primary herpes gingivostomatitis* is a vesicular eruption caused by the herpes simplex type 1 virus. Typically, this infection occurs in children and, less commonly, in young adults. The infection is frequently subclinical but may occasionally be so severe as to interfere with mastication and swallowing. Initially, an intense inflammation is noted at the gingival margins with subsequent formation of yellowish vesicles, which may occur on mucosal surfaces throughout the oral cavity. After several days, these vesicles rupture, leaving painful ulcerations. The individual ulcers are small, seldom reaching diameters greater than 3 mm, and are surrounded by an inflammatory halo. Lesions frequently coalesce, forming larger, irregular ulcerations. Hemorrhagic crustations involving the lips are also characteristic.

Approximately one-third of these individuals will subsequently experience recurrent eruptions (*secondary herpes simplex*) (6). Lesions most commonly involve the vermilion border of the lip (herpes labialis, or cold sores) and are frequently preceded by several days of localized burning, soreness, or swelling at the site of the impending eruption. Clusters of small vesicles appear, which ulcerate and coalesce to form a large crusted ulcer. Less commonly, recurrences may involve the oral mucosa with vesicles generally limited to "attached" mucosa bound to the alveolar ridges and hard palate.

Herpangina is another vesicular eruption of the oral cavity that affects children primarily. It is caused by the coxsackie virus and generally occurs during the summer months. Vesicles appear over the soft palate, uvula, and tonsils, then rupture, leaving multiple shallow ulcerations that have an intense inflammatory border.

The coxsackie virus is also the causative organism in *hand, foot, and mouth disease*. Outbreaks are seen during the warmer months of the year. Vesicles tend to involve the anterior oral cavity, including the tongue, lips, and hard palate. The lesions ulcerate and may coalesce to form larger erosions. A similar eruption may be seen to involve the hands and soles of the feet.

Recurrent *aphthous stomatitis* (canker sores) is a common malady affecting 20% to 60% of the population (7,8). It can be distinguished from herpes simplex infection in that there is no prodrome of fever, headache, or malaise; there is no vesicular phase; and lesions tend to occur on freely movable (unbound) mucosa (i.e., buccal mucosa, tonsillar pillars, soft palate, tongue, and floor of the mouth). The ulcer is shallow with a fibrinous, yellowish base and erythematous rim. Individual lesions are generally larger than those seen with herpes simplex—frequently greater than 5 mm in diameter. The ulcers are painful and tend to be solitary.

Acute necrotizing ulcerative gingivostomatitis (ANUG; Vincent's angina or trench mouth) is an infection caused by fusobacterium nucleatum or the spirochete, borrelia vincenti, and usually affects teenagers and young adults. The illness begins as an intense, painful inflammation of the gingiva with subsequent formation of a foul-smelling gray slough. Flattening of the interdental papillae is characteristic. Ulcers form and may spread to involve the mucosa of the entire oral cavity and pharynx.

In addition to the above diseases, oral ulcerations may occur in association with a number of systemic illnesses, including systemic lupus erythematosus, Behcet's disease (oculo-oral-genital syndrome), erythema multiforme, pemphigus, pemphigoid, Crohn's disease, sprue, cyclic neutropenia, allergic reactions, and a number of nutritional deficiencies. Such a diverse list of illnesses compels the physician to consider the total patient when evaluating the finding of oral ulcerations.

EARLY DETECTION OF ORAL AND OROPHARYNGEAL CANCERS

Leukoplakia is a term used to describe nonspecific white patches occurring over the oral mucosa that cannot be rubbed off or explained by any other clinically diagnosable disease. It represents a mucosal response to chronic irritation and does not correlate with any specific microscopic finding. Preferential sites include the ventral and lateral portion of the tongue, floor of the mouth, alveolar ridge, lower lip, soft palate, and the area immediately posterior to the lower molars. The majority are benign, but 2% to 4% of these white patches will be found to have invasive cancer or carcinoma in situ if examined via biopsy at the time of their discovery. An additional 4% to 6% will transform into malignancies if observed over a prolonged period of time (9).

Erythroplasia, a much more ominous finding, is any persistent red patch of the oral mucosa that cannot be attributed to any other diagnosable condition. The lesion may appear completely red or may be interspersed or speckled with white patches or granules. Lesions may be formed anywhere in the oral cavity but have a predilection for the lateral border of the tongue, soft palate, and floor of the mouth. Despite their rather innocuous appearance, these lesions are the most common early presentation of squamous cell cancer of the oral cavity. Eighty percent of erythroplasias occurring in high-risk areas will be found to have invasive cancer at the time of biopsy.

Squamous cell cancer is the most common type of oral malignancy. Three sites appear to be predisposed: the floor of the mouth (50%), especially at the base of the tongue in the vicinity of Wharton's duct; the ventral lateral portion of the tongue (17%); and the soft palate complex (including the soft palate, anterior tonsillar pillars and retromolar trigone) (9). The appearance of this cancer is highly variable, with both red and white components, but in the majority of instances, the erythroplakic quality predominates. In time, mucosal changes occur with induration and ulceration.

REFERENCES

1. Friedman IH. Say 'ah!' [Letter]. *JAMA* 1984;251:2086.
2. Steele RM, Schuna AA, Schreiber RT. Calcium antagonist-induced gingival hyperplasia. *Ann Intern Med* 1994;120:663–4.
3. Veasy LG, Wiedmeier SE, Orsmond GS, et al. Resurgence of acute rheumatic fever in the intermountainous area of the United States. *N Engl J Med* 1987;316:421–7.
4. Komaroff AL, Pass TM, Aronson MD, et al. The prediction of streptococcal pharyngitis in adults. *J Gen Intern Med* 1986;1:1–7.
5. Aronson MD, Komaroff AL, Pass TM, et al. Heterophile antibody in adults with sore throat. *Ann Intern Med* 1982;96:505–8.
6. Balciunas BA, Overholser CD. Diagnosis and treatment of common oral lesions. *Am Fam Physicians* 1987;35:206–20.
7. Bell GF, Rogers RS. Observations on the diagnosis of recurrent aphthous stomatitis. *Mayo Clin Proc* 1982;57:297–302.
8. Burns RA, Davis WJ. Recurrent aphthous stomatitis. *Am Fam Physicians* 1985;32:99–104.
9. Mashberg A, Samet AM. Early detection, diagnosis, and management of oral and oropharyngeal cancer. *CA Cancer J Clin* 1989;39:67–88.

SUGGESTED READING

Greene JC, Louie R, Wycoff SJ. Preventive dentistry II. Periodontal diseases, malocclusion, trauma, and oral cancer. *JAMA* 1990;263:421–5.
Krull EA, Fabian LA, Fellman AC. White lesions of the mouth. *CIBA Clin Symp* 1973;25:1–32.
Langlars RP, Miller CS. *Color atlas of common oral diseases.* Philadelphia: Lea & Febiger, 1992.
Schleupner CJ, Overall JC. Infectious mononucleosis and Epstein-Barr virus. 1. Epidemiology, pathogenesis, immune response. 2. Clinical picture, diagnosis, management. *Postgrad Med* 1979;65:83–7,95–105.
Yeatts D, Burns JC. Common oral mucosal lesions in adults. *Am Fam Physicians* 1991;44:2043–50.

Clinical Skills for Adult Primary Care
edited by M. E. Silverman and J. W. Hurst.
Lippincott-Raven Publishers, Philadelphia © 1996.

9

Examination of the Ear, Nose, and Paranasal Sinuses

Mark E. Silverman, M.D.

*Emory University School of Medicine, Atlanta, Georgia 30322
and Piedmont Hospital, Atlanta, Georgia 30309*

"Let not your ear hear the sound of your voice raised in unkind criticism or ridicule or condemnation of a brother physician."

William Osler, quoted in Bean WB. *Sir William Osler: Aphorisms.*
Springfield, IL: Charles C Thomas, 1968:89.

EXAMINATION OF THE EAR

During the routine examination, the ear is usually examined for gross findings and hearing. When a problem-focused examination requires a detailed examination, the primary care physician must be conversant with the many problems—infections, growths, and so forth—that may cause drainage, pain, bleeding, obstruction, or impaired hearing.

Technique

An otoscope with a strong light and a 256- and 512-Hz tuning fork are required. A pneumatic apparatus to pneumomassage the tympanic membrane can be useful. The examination begins with external inspection of the auricle, helical folds, tragus, the lobule of the ear, and the mastoid region (Fig. 1). Next, an otoscopic examination is conducted using the fingers of the free hand to retract the auricle backward and upward to straighten the canal so that the entire passageway and tympanic membranes are fully in view. Care is taken to insert the otoscope short of the tender bony canal. The fourth and fifth digits of the examiner can be propped against the temporal area of the patient's head in order to maintain position and avoid pain in case the patient suddenly turns his or her head. The auditory canal is then inspected for skin disease and color, infection, masses or foreign objects, and the presence of cerumen. Obstructive cerumen

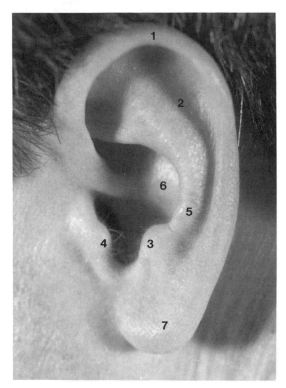

FIG. 1. Anatomy of the auricle. 1, helix; 2, scaphoid fossa; 3, antitragus; 4, tragus; 5, antihelix; 6, concha; 7, lobule.

can be removed through the otoscope, if necessary. Auditory function is grossly evaluated by whispering numbers in each ear while occluding the opposite ear and by performing the Rinne and Weber tests.

The *Rinne test* is performed by holding a gently tapped, 256-Hz tuning fork against the mastoid bone, then in front of the external ear, and asking the patient to decide which location seems louder. Each side is tested. In the *Weber test*, a vibrating (512 Hz) tuning fork is placed on the middle of the frontal bone just below the hairline while the patient is asked if he or she hears better in one ear compared with the other. These tests are inexact screening tests.

Normal Findings

The external ear includes the auricle (pinna), auditory meatus, and the auditory canal up to the tympanic membrane. The normal external ear displays smooth, tight skin over well-formed helical folds, tragus, and concha, and a patent external auditory meatus (Fig. 1). There should be no discharge, tenderness, or erythema. The auditory canal easily admits the speculum. A small amount of cerumen is common. The bony portion has thinner skin that may be pale in appearance. The auditory canal is about 2.5 to 3 cm in length in the adult and takes an upward course. At its far end, the canal is separated from the middle ear by the tympanic membrane, which slants obliquely facing slightly downward (Fig. 2). The tympanic membrane has a slight conical configuration with the center, or apex, concave to the examiner. The umbo of the malleal manubrium attaches at the apex. The tympanic membrane can be conveniently divided into four quadrants with a line through the malleus representing the vertical axis and a transverse line through the umbo at the center as the horizontal axis. The normal tympanic membrane is thin, semitransparent, and has a pearly grey appearance with a sharp light reflex extending from the center to the anterior-inferior quadrant. Blood vessels may be seen coursing on the drumhead. Above the umbo, the handle of the malleus is visible as it extends upward at a 12:00 position considering the drumhead as a clock face. Sometimes the long process of the incus is seen behind the tympanic membrane (Fig. 2).

The tympanic membrane should move in and out as the pneumatic otoscope bulb is squeezed and released. Normal findings for the Rinne test are air con-

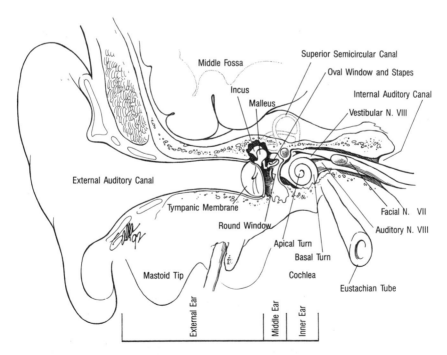

FIG. 2. Schematic drawing of the components of the ear. Reprinted by permission of the *New England Journal of Medicine.* From Nadol JB. Hearing loss. *N Engl J Med* 1993;329:1093. Copyright 1993, Massachusetts Medical Society. All rights reserved.

duction better than bone conduction bilaterally. Generally, air conduction is heard twice as long as bone conduction. The Weber test should be midline (heard equally well by both ears).

Abnormal Findings

Abnormal findings can be anatomically divided into the external ear, auditory canal, middle ear, and inner ear.

External Ear

Exposure

The salient position of the external ear and its exposure to the elements makes it susceptible to *trauma, sun damage,* and *frostbite.*

Skin Diseases

Any skin disease, from *eczema* to *lupus erythematosus*, can involve the auricle and may extend into the auditory canal.

Inflammation

A red-hot ear, very tender and sometimes edematous, is a sign of *perichondritis. Pseudomonas aeruginosa* is the most common infecting organism. An infection or abscess of the lobule or helix can occur, particularly related to piercing of the ear for jewelry. With *polychondritis*, an inflammatory disorder of collagen, the ear may become inflamed, then collapse, forming a "cauliflower" ear. Acute *mastoiditis* causes painful swelling and erythema posterior to the auricle. Healing may leave a depressed scar.

Tumors

Squamous cell carcinoma is the most common histologic type of malignancy involving the ear, occurring five times more frequently than *basal cell carcinoma*. These lesions are recognized as indurated, ulcerated, or crusted lesions that may erode, enlarge, and sometimes fungate. *Melanomas* can present on the auricle (see description in Chapter 6). Benign tumors include *lipomas, cysts, hemangiomas,* and *papillomas* (including warts).

Inherited Problems

The ear may be grossly deformed or missing in inherited diseases such as the *Goldenhar syndrome, trisomy 13-15 syndrome, Klippel-Feil syndrome, Turner's syndrome,* and *chromosome 9 and 22* abnormalities. *Low-set ears* are common to syndromes that have a high cranial vault, a short mandibular ramus, a short neck, or a hyperextended head. These include *Down syndrome, Noonan syndrome, Cornelia de Lange, Turner syndrome, Pierre Robin syndrome, Rubinstein-Taybi syndrome,* and others. A *protruding ear* (lop ear) is an inherited anomaly caused by maldevelopment of the antihelix. A tiny dimple in front of the helix indicates a *congenital preauricular fistula.* These are usually bilateral and may become infected.

Coronary Disease

Coronary artery disease and stroke have been linked to a diagonal earlobe crease.

Metabolic/Endocrine Disease

Ochronosis (alkaptonuria) and *Addison's disease* may cause hardening of the auricle, and ochronosis may produce a bluish discoloration. A tophus is an uncommon manifestation of *gout*, appearing as an inflamed nodule on the helix.

Auditory Canal

Trauma

The auditory canal is subject to traumatic injury from inserted objects or finger nails. Foreign bodies of various sorts may be encountered.

Cerumen

Impacted cerumen may partially or completely obstruct the canal, impairing hearing. The cerumen can become tenacious and induce a bony erosion (*keratosis obturans*).

Infection

External otitis begins in the auditory canal and can extend to the external ear. It may be acute, chronic, or recurrent and caused by bacteria, viruses, fungi, seborrheic dermatitis, allergic reactions to topical medicines, nearby chemicals or metals, or for systemic reasons. Vesicles are due to herpes zoster. A *swimmer's ear* is a particular type of acute external otitis, occurring in the summer from swimming or bathing and due most commonly to *Pseudomonas aeruginosa* infection. The findings of external otitis are inflammation, watery or purulent discharge, odor, edema, and crusting. Tugging the ear may elicit pain. The external ear may become tender and inflamed. *Necrotizing (malignant) external otitis* is a particularly dangerous form that may extend into the soft tissues of the base of the skull in diabetes and immunocompromised patients. A localized infection may be due to *staphylococcal folliculitis* developing into a *furuncle*.

Growths

Exostoses, sometimes multiple, occur in the external canal, usually near the drum. They appear as smooth, hard, white masses. An *aural polyp* is a serious manifestation of deeper disease such as a cholesteatoma or malignancy. They may be infected or bleed easily.

Middle Ear

Perforation of the Tympanic Membrane

Perforation of the tympanic membrane is common from external or internal injury or infection. An acute perforation has a slitlike appearance with a ragged edge. When the perforation is related to chronic otitis media or a cholesteatoma, the appearance is more rounded and the location on the margin of the membrane.

Infection

Acute otitis media is common, especially in children or following colds. Most cases are secondary to viral or bacterial infection from the nasopharynx, complicated by blockage and impaired drainage of the eustachian tube. The otoscopic findings include a change in the surface of the drumhead from shiny and white to dull, red, or blue. Outward bulging of the drumhead and a loss of landmarks is ominous. A bleb on the tympanic membrane may be a sign of impending perforation. Layering of fluid and/or pus may be observed behind the membrane. *Serous otitis media* may follow in the wake of acute otitis media or from blockage of the eustachian tube. The major finding is a nonpurulent amber-colored fluid collection behind the tympanic membrane. The membrane may be normal, scarred, or retracted and fail to move with pneumomassage. A retracted membrane brings the malleus into sharp outline. A collection of thick mucoid fluid may impart a dark appearance and is sometimes called a *glue ear*. *Chronic otitis media* may develop because of infection or for other reasons. In chronic otitis media, the drum may appear bluish and a fluid level can be seen. Chalky white plaques on the drumhead (*tympanosclerosis*) are sequelae of chronic otitis media. Perforation of the membrane and chronic discharge are frequently present.

Cholesteatoma

A *cholesteatoma* is a cyst lined with squamous epithelium and filled with keratin debris. It may be congenital or acquired. As it develops, it may expand, causing bony destruction of nearby structures. Clues to the presence of a cholesteatoma include squamous epithelium in the middle ear, debris behind the tympanic membrane, evidence for bony destruction, polypoid granulation, and perforation in the attic area.

Trauma

Fractures of the temporal bone or barotrauma may cause hemorrhage into the middle ear that is visible behind the tympanic membrane. It may be blue-black in color.

Otosclerosis

Otosclerosis and other diseases involving the ossicles present with conductive hearing loss. The Weber test will lateralize to the affected ear, and bone conduction will be greater than air conduction by a Rinne test. The eardrum will appear normal; however, a pinkish area may be seen due to increased vascularity behind the drumhead.

Sensorineural Hearing Loss

This is due to damage of the cochlea or eighth nerve. The Weber test will lateralize to the good or better ear; the Rinne test will remain normal (air conduction longer than bone conduction).

Inner Ear

Inner ear disease affects hearing and vestibular function. Patients present because of a hearing loss, tinnitus, vertigo, or gait imbalance. Audiometric studies and electronystagmography are important tests used in the evaluation and differentiation of disorders affecting this region. An acute loss of hearing with an otherwise normal examination is an emergency that should be referred to a specialist.

EXAMINATION OF THE NOSE AND PARANASAL SINUSES

A history of mouth breathing, snoring, nasal obstruction, epistaxis, postnasal discharge, eustachian dysfunction, facial pain, anosmia or dysosmia usually alerts the primary care physician to do a problem-focused nasal and paranasal sinus examination.

Technique

The examination of the external nose includes inspection of the skin and configuration and symmetry of the osteocartilaginous vault and nares. Optimally, a nasal speculum is used for examining the nasal passages. The speculum is widely opened in a superior-inferior orientation to avoid traumatizing the tender septal area while the other hand is placed firmly on top of the head to turn the head as necessary. The nasal turbinates are then checked for congestion, color, mucus, and for infection, polyps, masses, septal deviation or perforation, or other problems on each side. About one-third to one-half of the distal nasal passage is routinely visualized. Vasoconstriction is useful and may be therapeutic. Effective solutions include 2% ephedrine, 0.05% oxymetazoline hydrochloride, and 0.25% phenylephrine hydrochloride instilled via an atomizer in each nostril while the patient sniffs. The maxillary and frontal sinuses can be palpated and tapped for tenderness and transilluminated in a dark room to see if a normal dim red glow is transmitted. The frontal sinuses are probed with a finger pushing upward from within the superior portion of the orbit. The maxillary sinuses are palpated over each cheek bone. The frontal sinuses are transilluminated by placing a penlight inside the orbit against the thin floor of the frontal sinus. The maxillary sinuses require a light positioned against the roof of the mouth with the lips closed around the instrument.

Normal Findings

The external nose consists of a bony, arched upper portion and a flexible cartilaginous distal end. Each side is normally symmetric and the tip of the nose should be midline. The nostrils consist of the alar cartilages and muscles, which maintain the patency of the nares during inspiration. The inside of the nostrils is lined by nasal hair. Internally, there are two paired nasal passages or chambers that widen and become triangular in configuration, sharing a vertically oriented nasal septum. The turbinates—inferior, middle, and occasionally a small anterior—are positioned on the lateral aspect of each chamber. The anterior aspect of the inferior turbinate and sometimes the smaller middle turbinate can be visualized by the examiner. The turbinates are covered by deep pink mucosa and a thin secretion. The projection of the turbinates creates a cleftlike space—a meatus—where the sinuses and ducts can drain. The anteriorly placed frontal, maxillary, and anterior ethmoidal sinuses drain into the middle meatus. The nasal septum rarely remains straight in the adult.

Abnormal Findings

The nose is susceptible to infections, allergies, trauma, polyps, bleeding, rare tumors, and rare forms of systemic diseases.

Infections

Viral infections, especially due to rhinovirus, are common. The nose is often the focus of the attack and appears red around the nasal alae and congested inside. A clear or mucus type of secretion is present and the turbinates are boggy and glistening, sometimes obstructing the nasal passages. *Influenza*, other viruses, *staphylococcus*, *measles*, *rubella*, and *chicken pox* also may inflame the nose. *Furuncles* just inside the nares are common. *Acne rosacea*, consisting of pustules, telangiectasia, and an erythematous swelling, is particularly prone to involve the nose and may develop into rhinophyma.

Rhinophyma

In this disorder of men, the distal half of the nose enlarges, sometimes grotesquely, because of overgrowth of sebaceous glands and connective tissue.

Chronic Rhinitis

Patients may have chronic nasal inflammation with enlarged, wet, pale, or inflamed turbinates. Possible contributing causes include *allergy*, *dry air*, *environmental factors*, *cigarette smoke*, *hormones*, *medicines*, and *abnormal ciliary action*. The term *vasomotor rhinitis* is often used to describe a hyperreaction to stimuli such as cold air or emotion.

Trauma

The nose and maxillary area are extremely vulnerable to trauma, which can produce swelling, ecchymoses, displacement, and epistaxis.

Perforation of the Nasal Septum

Perforation of the nasal septum results most commonly from a surgical procedure, but also because of *infection*, *vasculitis*, or *tumor*, or an exposure to an *inhaled irritant*.

Tumors

Polyps appear as a pale, pedunculated mass projecting from the maxillary or ethmoid sinus. They may herniate forward and obstruct the nasal passage. Chronic inflammation, allergy, and aspirin sensitivity are associations. *Mucoceles, osteomas, papillomas, granulomas*, and *carcinoma* are rare occurrences. Basal cell and squamous cell cancers can present on the external nose.

Foreign Bodies

Objects of all sorts can be lodged within the nasal passage and cause bleeding and obstruction.

Epistaxis

The superficial location of the vascular supply of the nasal septum makes it particularly prone to bleed from *trauma, inflammation, infection, hypertension, coagulation disorders, local tumors, foreign bodies*, or for no apparent reason. Bleeding most commonly stems from the anterior nose from Kiesselbach's vascular plexus. A rare but well-known cause of bleeding is *hereditary hemorrhagic telangiectasia* (Rendu-Osler-Weber disease), in which abnormal fragile blood vessels are present and recurrent epistaxis is frequent.

Deviation of the Nasal Septum and Spurs

This may be on a congenital or traumatic basis and is recognized by simple inspection. The septum is usually deviated somewhat in an adult. Septal spurs or humps may be seen.

Cerebrospinal Rhinorrhea

The finding of a clear fluid drainage should raise the question of a communication between the nose and the central nervous system.

Acute Sinusitis

Acute pain in the area of the sinus after a respiratory infection is the usual presentation. The pain is worse with bending or straining. On examination, there may be detectable erythema and swelling overlying the affected sinus. Tapping the sinus aggravates the pain. Transillumination may be poor. The nasal mucosa may be inflamed, boggy, and covered by purulent bloody drainage.

Chronic Sinusitis

The findings can vary according to the location, type of infection, and possible extension into neighboring structures. Mucoceles and polyps may develop and cause obstruction. The diagnosis is suspected from the history, location of the pain, loss of transillumination of the affected sinus, and X-ray/computerized tomography studies.

SUGGESTED READING

Ballenger JJ. *Diseases of the nose, throat, ear, head, and neck.* Philadelphia: Lea & Febiger, 1991.
Chole RA. *Color atlas of ear disease.* New York: Appleton-Century-Crofts, 1982.
DeWeese DD, Saunders WH. *Textbook of otolaryngology.* St. Louis: C.V. Mosby, 1982.
Goldman JL. *The principles and practice of rhinology.* New York: Wiley, 1987.
Goodhill V. *Ear: diseases, deafness, and dizziness.* Hagerstown, MD: Harper & Row, 1979.
Mawson SR. *Diseases of the ear.* Baltimore: Williams & Wilkins, 1963.
Schuknecht HF. *Pathology of the ear.* Cambridge, MA: Harvard University Press, 1974.

Clinical Skills for Adult Primary Care
edited by M. E. Silverman and J. W. Hurst.
Lippincott-Raven Publishers, Philadelphia © 1996.

10

Examination of the Thyroid Gland

N. Spencer Welch, M.D.

Piedmont Hospital, Atlanta, Georgia 30309

"Absolute diagnoses are unsafe, and are made at the expense of the conscience."
William Osler, quoted in Bean WB. *Sir William Osler: Aphorisms.*
Springfield, IL: Charles C Thomas, 1968:129.

The thyroid gland is the dynamo that drives cellular metabolism. Because it is located low in the anterior neck, it is readily accessible to examination. A multitude of systemic complaints can be attributable to malfunction of the thyroid. Because of these two factors, the thyroid should be examined regularly. It is important to examine the thyroid gland expertly and to recognize external manifestations of thyroid disease.

TECHNIQUE

The examination of the normal thyroid gland is difficult because the normal gland is wafer thin and difficult to differentiate from surrounding cartilage and muscle. The examination of the anterior portion of the neck should be done with the patient seated comfortably in a well-lit room, preferably in front of a window. The examiner should face the patient and visually inspect the anterior portion of the neck. After inspection, the patient should be asked to swallow and then protrude the tongue to check the motion of the thyroid and larynx. Palpation of the thyroid gland may be performed by either an anterior or posterior approach. In the anterior approach, each lobe of the thyroid is felt individually (Fig. 1). With the examiner standing slightly to the right of the patient, the right hand is placed in the midline of the neck in order to palpate the thyroid and cricoid cartilage. The right hand is then moved downward and laterally, until the left lobe of the thyroid is palpated completely. Standing on the patient's left, the same procedure is used with the left hand now palpating the right lobe. In the posterior approach, the examiner stands behind the patient, places the fingertips of both hands on the midline of the neck, and palpates the thyroid and cricoid cartilage (Fig. 2). The fingertips then sweep inferiorly and laterally, palpating both lobes of the thyroid

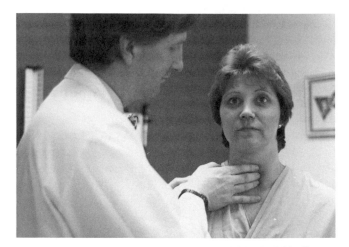

FIG. 1. Anterior approach, palpating each lobe individually.

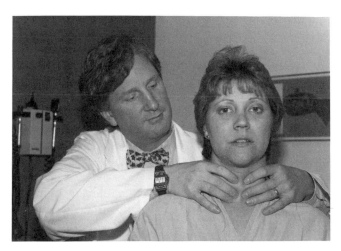

FIG. 2. Posterior approach, palpating both lobes at once.

simultaneously. The patient should be asked to swallow to elevate the gland so that all aspects of the thyroid may be felt. Sipping water greatly aids the patient when repetitive swallows are requested.

NORMAL FINDINGS

The usual dimensions of the thyroid are 2.5 to 3.0 cm in length, 1.5 to 2.0 cm in width, and 0.2 to 0.3 cm in depth. This translates to each lobe being about the size of the thumbnail and the thickness of a quarter. The texture of the gland is smooth to slightly gritty. It is not unusual for one lobe, especially the right, to be slightly larger than the other. On occasion, a third lobe, the pyramidal lobe, arises from the mid-portion or isthmus of the thyroid and may be palpated.

ABNORMAL FINDINGS

Seven percent of the population has either enlargement or nodular disease of the thyroid. At times, it may seem that the examination of the abnormal thyroid may be accomplished with only visual inspection. However, careful palpation of the thyroid to assess for overall size, texture (smooth or nodular), consistency (firm or soft), and tenderness is necessary if a proper diagnosis is to be made. Enlargement of the thyroid, whether it is unilateral or diffuse, is referred to as a *goiter*. A diffuse goiter can be either nodular or smooth in texture. A diffusely nodular goiter is almost always benign and is due to disordered growth of normally functioning thyroid follicles. A smoothly diffuse goiter is most often associated with global hyperfunctioning of the thyroid, hence it is called a diffuse *toxic goiter*. If a goiter and exophthalmos are both present, *Grave's disease* is the diagnosis. At times, some parts of the multinodular goiter may begin to hyperfunction. This is known as a toxic multinodular goiter or *Plummer's syndrome*.

Unilateral enlargement, a single nodule, or a dominant nodule in a diffusely multinodular goiter have a 20% chance of harboring a malignancy. Therefore, careful assessment of these findings is mandatory. If the contralateral lobe of a unilaterally enlarged thyroid cannot be palpated, either congenital absence or suppression of this lobe by a hyperfunctioning nodule is suggested. However, if the contralateral lobe is normal to palpation, the nodule in the enlarged lobe must be carefully examined for consistency. A firm nodule may hide a malignancy, whereas a soft or fleshy nodule is most likely cystic and usually benign. A solitary nodule, whether firm or soft, should be assessed via fine-needle aspiration so that cytology can yield the proper diagnosis. If the nodule is purely cystic, it may disappear totally after aspiration.

Pain and tenderness in the thyroid may be caused by either benign or malignant conditions. If pain and tenderness present acutely in a young woman with a small diffuse goiter, the diagnosis is most likely to be *subacute thyroiditis*. If the onset of pain is insidious and progressive in an older patient and the skin above a rock-hard goiter is red and indurated, the diagnosis of *anaplastic carcinoma* must be considered.

It must be emphasized that thyroid abnormalities cannot be assessed solely by examination of the thyroid gland itself. Unilateral or diffuse enlargement can occur in hyperthyroid, hypothyroid, or euthyroid states. Patients must be carefully assessed for signs and symptoms of thyroid dysfunction because this may further help delineate the underlying cause for the thyroid enlargement.

HYPERTHYROIDISM

Hyperthyroid patients present complaining of fatigue, weight loss, irritability, tremors, and palpitations. They have decreased stamina, perspire with minimal effort, and suffer heat intolerance. Female patients may have scant menses or no menses at all. On physical examination, the hyperthyroid patient may appear gaunt and nervous. They have a staring gaze. Their skin is warm and moist. They may have tachycardia and hyperreflexia.

HYPOTHYROIDISM

Patients with hypothyroidism may be asymptomatic or complain of fatigue, sluggishness, constipation, weight gain, sleepiness, or edema. Depression occurs. Female patients may have menorrhagia and painful menses. Cold intolerance is a specific clue. The hypothyroid patient is usually overweight and plethoric. They may have periorbital or peripheral edema. Their skin is cool and dry and the hair brittle and sparse, especially the outer eyebrows. They may have bradycardia and their reflexes are slowed.

SUGGESTED READING

Bates B. *A guide to physical examination and history taking.* Philadelphia: J.B. Lippincott, 1991:167–71.
Braverman LE, Utiger RD. *Werner and Ingbar's, the thyroid.* 6th ed. Philadelphia: J.B. Lippincott, 1991:572–7.
Sapira JD. The art and science of bedside diagnosis. Baltimore: Urban & Schwarzenburg, 1990:231–5.
Slater S. Palpation of the thyroid gland. *South Med J* 1993;86:1001–3.

Clinical Skills for Adult Primary Care
edited by M. E. Silverman and J. W. Hurst.
Lippincott-Raven Publishers, Philadelphia © 1996.

11

Examination of the Chest

Jonne B. Walter, M.D.

Piedmont Hospital, Atlanta, Georgia 30309

"But it is by your eyes, and your ears and your own mind and (I may add) your own heart that you must observe and learn and profit."
William Osler, quoted in Bean WB. *Sir William Osler: Aphorisms.*
Springfield, IL: Charles C Thomas, 1968:121.

The seasoned clinician may tailor the chest examination to the patient's symptoms, being careful to palpate any painful places, inspect for breathing pattern and anxiety in patients with lung disease, and auscultate for subtle findings. The examination is done in an orderly fashion with the patient undressed to the waist and adequately draped. It is useful to follow Osler's traditional sequence: inspection, palpation, percussion, and auscultation. What you do not see, hear, or feel may be just as important as the more obvious findings.

INSPECTION

Breathing Pattern

Normal Findings

The normal breathing frequency is 12 to 18 breaths per minute and is linked to the metabolic rate. Normal breathing does not cause visible intercostal, neck, or abdominal muscle use or produce audible noise at the mouth. Chest wall motion should be symmetric with lateral chest wall expansion occurring as the ribs move upward and outward in a "bucket handle" fashion. Each side of the chest is symmetric with the expected contour of the chest wall and spine. When the normal patient is recumbent, the chest and abdomen move upward and outward with inspiration.

Abnormal Findings

Abnormal breathing may be described as tachypnea (more than 24 breaths/ minute), hyperpnea (increased rate and depth of breathing), hypopnea (reduced depth of breathing), or apnea (transient cessation of breathing). Dyspnea is the patient's subjective perception of being short of breath. Specific abnormal patterns of breathing have been identified:

- Cheyne-Stokes respirations are characterized by progressive hyperpnea in a crescendo followed by apnea before the cycle is repeated. This is a type of periodic breathing seen in severe heart failure, uremia, and at high altitudes.
- Kussmaul breathing is a form of hyperpnea seen in metabolic acidosis.
- Anxiety and hyperventilation. Unexplained dyspnea due to anxiety is a common clinical condition. The patient may present with unexplained shortness of breath, usually in the absence of cough or wheeze. Such patients may appear depressed or anxious and sigh frequently throughout the interview. Some may have symptoms of flatus or belching due to air swallowing and may complain of an inability to get a satisfactory inspiratory breath to "catch." A timed 2-minute period of voluntary hyperventilation may reproduce the patient's own familiar symptoms of chest heaviness, tightness, dyspnea, and dizziness and associated digital or perioral numbness (typical of hyperventilation). Often the patient requires considerable coaching to continue the full 2-minute hyperventilation, but sometimes individuals seem to become engaged and hyperventilate almost uncontrollably even if asked to stop. When this exercise reproduces the patient's symptoms completely, the patient gains insight and can be taught to control the symptoms.
- Pursed lips breathing. Patients with severe obstructive lung disease (COPD) often exhale through pursed lips, a technique which appears to delay airway closure and reduce air trapping. Obstructive lung patients may contract their neck accessory muscles to assist tidal breathing, using the upper intercostals and the supraclavicular neck accessory muscles to pull upward on the clavicle to expand the chest. Fixation of the clavicle by leaning forward with the elbows bent improves the effectiveness of this accessory muscle action. The chest may be hyperexpanded (barrel chest) with diminished lateral chest wall motion due to the disadvantaged and flattened position of the diaphragm. In such patients, the chest may appear to be moving in an upward, en bloc fashion (pump handle), and lower intercostal retractions are apparent. Flaring of the nostrils may be seen when the work of breathing is increased for any reason.
- Paradoxical abdominal breathing. Paradoxical inward abdominal motion on inspiration (Hoover's sign) indicates that the expected intraabdominal positive pressure is not occurring due to weakness or paralysis of the diaphragm. Hoover's sign may be seen in patients with severe obstructive lung disease who are using neck accessory muscles and have a low-lying diaphragm. It also may be pre-

sent in patients with bilateral or unilateral diaphragm paralysis due to neuro-muscular disease or trauma. Inspiratory retractions between the ribs in the lateral lower chest indicate contraction of the lower intercostal muscles and occurs in COPD patients with hyperinflated lungs.

Chest Wall Deformities

Patients with kyphoscoliosis have one side that is relatively hyperexpanded and one side in which the ribs are collapsed downward. Kyphoscoliosis may progress to produce a severe restrictive ventilatory defect, particularly when the scoliotic curve angle is greater than 100 degrees (Fig. 1). Pigeon breast (pectus carinatum) and pectus excavatum sternal deformities rarely, if ever, alter chest wall motion (Fig. 2). Asymmetric or abnormal motion is perhaps best appreciated on palpation but also can be seen.

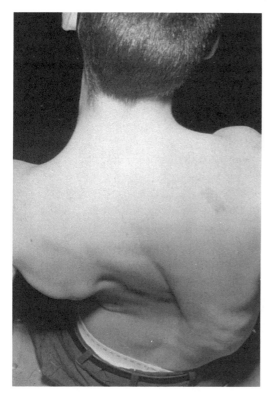

FIG. 1. Pectus excavatum. From Silverman ME, Hurst JW. Inspection of the patient. In: Hurst JW, ed. *The heart*. 4th ed. New York: McGraw-Hill, 1978. Used by permission of McGraw-Hill.

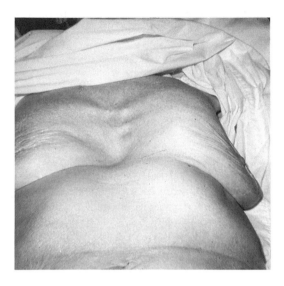

FIG. 2. Kyphoscoliosis. From Silverman ME, Hurst JW. Inspection of the patient. In: Hurst JW, ed. *The heart.* 4th ed. New York: McGraw-Hill, 1978. Used by permission of McGraw-Hill.

Other Organs Significant to the Chest Examination

Digital clubbing and cyanosis should be noted. Digital clubbing is usually bilateral and often develops initially in the thumb and first finger. The fingers are examined in profile for the angle between the root of the nail plate and the distal phalanges. Pressure on the root of the normal nail produces no movement; however, the clubbed digit is spongy when pressure is applied because the nail root is

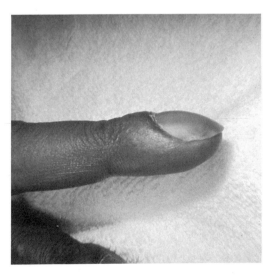

FIG. 3. Clubbing of the fingers.

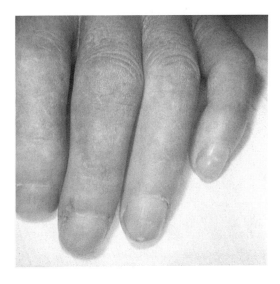

FIG. 4. Scleroderma.

separated from the bone by edema and additional soft tissue. Pressure on the soft nail plate depresses it toward the bone. The normal angle is approximately 160 degrees between the bone and the nail. In clubbing, the angle is obliterated and exceeds 180 degrees (Fig. 3). The pathogenesis of clubbing is not known but it is associated with hypoxic lung disease, especially in children with cystic fibrosis, cyanotic congenital heart disease, pulmonary neoplasm, chronic infection, and subacute bacterial endocarditis. There are many other diseases occasionally associated with digital clubbing, including the hypertrophic osteoarthropathy associated with cancer.

Examinations of the digits for pruning from arthritis, skin tightness, and Raynaud's phenomenon may offer clues to collagen vascular disease that may involve the lungs (Fig. 4).

PALPATION

Technique

The cervical trachea is palpated to determine its midline position. The cricohyoid membrane should be identified by a fingertip placed beneath the thyroid cartilage, normally several centimeters above the clavicle. Chest wall motion is observed by placing the thumbs together over the posterior spine while the fingers are fanned laterally over the posterior lung bases to feel the chest as it expands laterally with inspiration (Fig. 5). The abdominal rectus sheath is palpated to determine whether active abdominal wall expansion is assisting tidal exhalation. Tactile fremitus is appreciated by placing the palmar surface of both hands

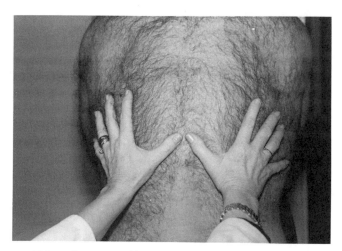

FIG. 5. Technique of feeling the chest for lateral expansion.

on the chest wall, moving from apex to base, while the patient is asked to breathe deeply or speak (vocal fremitus). The patient is asked to repeat the word "ninety-nine" or to count "1-2-3" while the examiner feels for vibration as the sound is transmitted through the chest. One side is compared with the other. The anterior chest wall, especially the costochondral junctions, should be palpated for tenderness. The heel of the hand or loose fist can be used to lightly tap the spine for tenderness.

Normal Findings

The cervical trachea should be in the midline. The lungs normally expand laterally and upward with inspiration, causing the examiner's fingers to move outward and the angle between the thumbs to widen. The accessory respiratory muscles—the sternocleidomastoid, scalenus anticus, and rectus abdominalis—are not recruited in normal breathing except during vigorous exercise (note that as you feel your own neck muscles and take a slow, deep inhalation your neck muscles are recruited at a point 75% of maximal lung capacity). The chest wall and spine are not normally tender to palpation.

Abnormal Findings

In patients with very severe airway obstruction, the cricohyoid membrane may descend beneath the sternum during tidal inspiration instead of maintaining its normal position in the mid-neck. This sign has been called a tracheal tug. The entire chest is palpated carefully in patients receiving mechanical ventilation or in patients with chest tubes or central venous catheters in place to feel for subcutaneous air crepitations indicative of subcutaneous emphysema.

Patients with hyperinflated lungs display decreased lateral chest movement as the chest is moved upward by the accessory neck muscles (pump handle). The use of neck accessory muscles may be appreciated best only by palpation, particularly in an obese patient. Inspiratory contraction of the sternocleidomastoid or scalenus anticus muscles is an important clinical sign that the respiratory system ventilatory reserve is lost.

Contraction of the rectus muscles to assist expiration is seen in patients with severe obstructive lung disease or increased airway resistance, even when no audible wheezing is present. It indicates increased work of breathing because exhalation is normally a relatively passive phenomenon. Often, but not always, this accompanies accessory neck muscle use.

Differences in fremitus between the two sides of the chest suggest an abnormality that should be pursued more carefully during the remainder of the physical examination. Absent vocal fremitus suggests severe airway obstruction, a fluid-filled pleural space blocking vibration, or a pneumothorax. Tactile fremitus is increased in conditions that increase the density of the lung, such as consolidation pneumonia. In this circumstance, the consolidated lung acts as an amplifier to increase the vibrations of the chest as long as airways are patent. Vocal fremitus is also amplified.

If the patient complains of chest pain, it is extremely important for the examiner to touch the painful area and to palpate carefully over the ribs to determine the source of the pain. Careful examination, even if unrevealing, may reassure patients that their symptoms have been addressed. Patients with pleurisy may rarely demonstrate palpable friction rubs. With rib fractures, localized rib tenderness and possible crepitus may be found. These are important signs that may confirm a clinical suspicion of rib fracture, especially in the lateral portion of the ribs, which can be missed on X-ray films of the chest. The examiner should make a special effort to apply pressure to the costochondral junctions above the lateral sternal borders because this is a common area for costochondral arthritis or "costochondritis."

Costochondral pain is a frequent cause of elusive chest pain that may simulate coronary disease. It is easy to miss unless firm pressure along the sternal border reproduces the pain. Palpation below the xiphoid for the point of the maximal cardiac impulse is useful in patients with severe COPD. Sometimes the thrust of a hypertrophied right ventricle can only be felt by pressing upward from underneath the xiphoid.

PERCUSSION

Percussion of the chest wall was introduced by Auenbrugger in a 1761 Latin treatise published in Vienna. The idea of identifying thoracic structures during life was startling and not well accepted until the 19th century. Today, percussion has been mostly replaced by radiography but is still a valuable way to identify lung size, diaphragm mobility, and the approximate density of the underlying lung.

Technique

Percussion is performed by placing the distal phalanx of the middle finger of one hand firmly against the chest wall, parallel to the ribs, in the intercostal space (Fig. 6A). The finger is struck with a quick, sharp tap using the tip of the middle finger of the other hand (Fig. 6B). The nails should be trimmed short and the wrist kept loosely flexible. First one side is percussed and then the corresponding level on the other side, starting at the top of the lung posteriorly and going from side to side down to the diaphragm. To determine the position of the diaphragm and its mobility, the patient is asked to take a maximal deep breath and hold it in while the examiner quickly percusses to the low point of the diaphragmatic dullness, first on one side and then the other. The patient is allowed to breathe normally for several breaths to recover, then asked to take a deep breath and blow out completely, holding the breath out while the percussion is then repeated to find the highest expiratory position of the diaphragm. The level of dullness can be noted with an ink mark on the skin or with a mental note of the maximal inspiratory and expiratory position.

Normal Findings

Percussion notes are described as dull, resonant, and hyperresonant (or tympanic). The air-filled lung is resonant, the gastric air bubble is tympanitic, and bone or solid organs (e.g., liver) are dull on percussion. The normally resonant, hollow percussion note of the lung is related to its air-filled state. The diaphragm should move 2 to 4 cm by percussion when the patient takes a full inspiration.

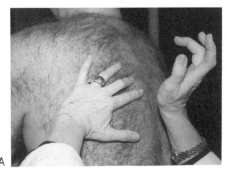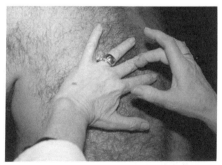

A   B

FIG. 6. Technique of percussion. **A:** Position of fingers. **B:** Striking the knuckle.

Abnormal Findings

Hyperexpansion of the lung, as in COPD, produces hyperresonance. A dull percussion note is appreciated when air is replaced by fluid in the alveoli or compressed by overlying pleural effusion or atelectasis. The keen observer will look for diminished chest wall motion over the area of dullness along with the abnormal breath sounds. Diaphragm mobility is decreased in severe COPD because the diaphragms are fixed in a relatively low position. Patients with severe restrictive lung diseases will also have poor diaphragmatic mobility, although the diaphragms will be elevated in a relatively high position by percussion.

AUSCULTATION OF THE CHEST

When Laennec introduced the stethoscope in 1816, he changed medicine forever (1). At that time, diagnoses were made primarily from the patient's symptoms along with observation and palpation of the pulse. The stethoscope enabled the physician to listen directly to the underlying organs. The information made available was so revolutionary that it was not quickly accepted. Laennec used Auenbreugger's percussion techniques along with his auscultation. He published thorough accounts of his patient's histories, clinical course, and auscultatory data and correlated these with subsequent autopsy examinations, most of which he performed himself (1). He described categories of lung sounds using terminology based on familiar sounds of his day. A later English translation of Laennec's work changed his terminology. Subsequent modifications have led to further confusion in the description of lung sounds that persist to this day. Laennec, for example, used the terms "rale" and "rhonchus" interchangeably to describe the same sound, but also added qualifiers (humide, sibilant, sonore) which have passed down through time and been variously interpreted. Laennec noted that the sounds were easier to recognize than to describe. Interest in auscultation waned after X-ray films of the chest proved superior in establishing anatomic diagnoses, but recently has been rekindled by studies into the mechanisms of breath sound production (2–5).

Technique

The patient should fully undress before auscultation. Auscultation should never be performed over the patient's gown or drape. Patients with excessive chest hair are difficult to auscultate. The hair can be moistened with water before auscultation is attempted. Auscultation is performed anteriorly and posteriorly over the apex, middle, and lower chest wall. The stethoscope filters out extraneous noises if the ear pieces fit snugly. The bell is best for hearing lower pitched sounds and the diaphragm better suited for higher pitched sounds, including most breath sounds. The patient is instructed to breathe in and out with the mouth open as the stethoscope is moved from side to side, up and down both sides of the chest. Because sounds are proportional to flow, the patient should then be asked to pant with the mouth open to increase air flow and bring out latent abnormal breath sounds. Normal individuals are able to produce polyphonic wheezing on a forced expiratory maneuver so breathing must not be overly forced (6,7). It is useful to check for normal airway resistance by asking the patient to inhale as fully as possible and then exhale as rapidly as possible through an open mouth (8).

Normal Breath Sounds

Normal breath sounds are described as tracheal, bronchial, bronchovesicular, and vesicular (or normal). These sounds can be diagrammed (Fig. 7). Tracheal and bronchial sounds are so similar that separating them may not be helpful.

- Tracheal breath sounds are audible over the trachea. The sound is loud, high pitched, and is clearly audible all the way through to the end of expiration. A pause is noted between the inspiratory and expiratory components. The expiratory phase is slightly longer.
- Bronchial breath sounds are similar to tracheal breath sounds, also harsh and high-pitched, with approximately equal inspiratory and expiratory duration. This breath sound also may be heard just over the surface projection of the major bronchi during normal breathing.
- Bronchovesicular breath sounds are heard just distal to the central airways. They are somewhat lower pitched but also have an equal inspiratory and expiratory component.

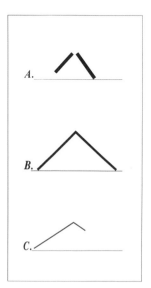

FIG. 7. Diagram of normal breath sounds. A: Tracheobronchial. B: Bronchovesicular. C: Vesicular. The ascending limb represents inspiration and descending limb represents expiration. Line thickness is proportional to sound intensity. Redrawn from Wilkins RL, Hodgkin JE, Lope B. Lung sounds, a practical guide. St. Louis: Mosby, 1988. Reproduced by permission of Mosby Publishers.

- Normal breath sounds, called by Laennec vesicular but by Forgacs normal, are lower pitched, less intense sounds primarily audible during inspiration. It is not clear how these sounds are generated, although they probably are not generated from the "vesicles" (alveoli) as Laennec thought because there is insufficient flow in the alveoli to induce sound. These sounds may reflect regional ventilation and be generated by turbulent airflow in larger airways (9). The expiratory component of the normal breath sounds is audible only in the first third of the expiratory phase. It is heard throughout all areas of the chest beyond the central airways and is characterized by silence in the latter two-thirds of the expiratory cycle.

Abnormal Breath Sounds

Forgacs introduced an entirely new terminology for abnormal or "adventitious" sounds based on an acoustic analysis of lung sounds and interpreted in the light of new developments in pulmonary physiology (2). His acoustic classification separated adventitious sounds into continuous (wheezes) and discontinuous (crackles) and eliminated the term *rale* (Table 1). Later, objective data were found for using the qualifiers "fine" and "coarse" for crackles. The American Thoracic Society largely adopted the Forgacs classification system in 1980 (10), preserving the old term *rhonchus* for a low-pitched wheeze (Table 1). In the future, the information attainable at the bedside with a stethoscope may well be more precise as pathophysiologic correlations between breath sounds and regional pulmonary function are further refined using acoustic techniques.

Tracheal and Bronchial Breath Sounds

Tracheal and bronchial breath sounds are similar and considered abnormal if heard over the periphery of the lung, implying lung compression or consolidation (Table 2). When the air-filled lung is replaced by exudates or tissue consolidation in the presence of a patent airway, a loud amplified bronchial breath sound results. The air-filled lung normally filters out these high-frequency sounds; consolidation of the lung amplifies them.

TABLE 1. *Recommended terminology for adventitious lung sounds* (10)

Classification	Recommended term	Old term (discarded)
Discontinuous	Crackles	Rales, crepitations, creps
Continuous	Wheezes, high-pitched	Musical rales, sibilant rhonchi, sibilant rales
	Wheezes, low-pitched (rhonchi)	Sonorous rales

TABLE 2. *Abnormal breath sounds*

Egophony over consolidated or compressed lung
Bronchial breath sounds over consolidated lung
Coin sign (pneumothorax)
Absent breath sounds: pneumothorax,
    pneumonectomy, atelectasis, hemothorax,
    pleural effusion, immobile chest wall

Adventitious Sounds

Adventitious sounds have been divided into two categories: continuous (wheezes) and discontinuous (crackles) (Tables 3 and 4). Continuous lung sounds are musical sounds with a constant pitch. They are longer than 250 ms in duration, are more frequently heard during exhalation, and are often associated with airway obstruction. Forgacs used the term *wheeze* for these sounds and further defined them as high pitched or low pitched, then timed them within the respiratory cycle (Table 3).

Often wheezes of various pitches are audible simultaneously, designated by the term *polyphonic*. Wheezing is thought to be produced by rapid airflow through an obstructed bronchus, creating vibration of the bronchus and resulting in an asthmatic sound. The pitch of the wheeze is related both to the degree of obstruction in the bronchus and the flow rate of air traversing the obstruction. High-pitched sounds result from more rapid flow or more narrowed airways. Because airways narrow during exhalation as lung volume decreases, wheezes are most often heard during exhalation. Wheezing audible on inspiration reflects more severe obstruction and demands urgent therapeutic action. Each wheeze represents airflow traversing one bronchus. Polyphonic wheezing in an asthmatic sounds different from monophonic expiratory wheezing related to obstruction of a main stem bronchus by mucus or tumor. A monophonic inspiratory wheeze (termed *stridor*) is characteristic of upper airway obstruction in the larynx during epiglottitis or after tracheal extubation.

Wheezing heard during leisurely deep breathing implies diffuse airway obstruction. Obstructed patients may have noisy breathing at the mouth audible with the unaided ear during tidal breathing but diminished breath sounds with the stethoscope over the chest wall. Forced expiratory wheezing is not indicative of disease

TABLE 3. *Wheezes*

Timing	Inspiratory or expiratory
Pitch	High, low
Number	Monophonic (one pitch, one airway)
Stridor	Inspiratory, lower pitched, related to upper airway obstruction
Diseases	Asthma, chronic bronchitis, airway edema in severe heart failure, fixed obstruction due to tumor, stridor heard in epiglottitis, laryngeal edema

TABLE 4. *Crackles: timing and clinical diagnoses*

Early	Late
Chronic bronchitis	Interstitial fibrosis (all causes)
Asthma	Pneumonia
Emphysema	Congestive heart failure, restrictive lung disease

because it can be heard in normal subjects making a great expiratory effort (6,7,11). In respiratory failure, there may be inadequate flow to produce wheezing in compressed central bronchi and exhalation may be silent. Breath sound intensity has been quantitated using both acoustic and subjective measurements (2,4). A decrease in breath sound intensity heard over the chest wall is a useful sign in predicting the presence of obstructive lung disease and correlates better with reduced airflow than any other auscultatory finding, including forced expiratory wheezing (11,12).

Discontinuous adventitious sounds are intermittent, crackling, and of short duration, acoustically distinguished from wheezes by lasting less than 20 ms. These brief bursts of sound are heard most commonly during inspiration in any portion of the inspiratory cycle. They may be present in both restrictive and obstructive diseases (11) (Table 4). Early inspiratory crackles are associated with severe airway obstruction and are usually low pitched and few in number (13). Late inspiratory crackles suggest restrictive defects and loss of lung volume (13,14). Crackles are thought to be caused by the sudden opening of small airways during inspiration or by bubbling of air through secretions. Each crackle represents one airway opening. Crackles from large airways are coarse and may occur during both inspiration and expiration. A cough or airway suctioning may cause them to clear. As collapsed regions of the lung are inflated, peripheral airways may be heard to pop open, producing crackles. Atelectasis due to a shallow breathing pattern also may produce crackles; however, these disappear after a few deep breaths or change in position. In patients with pulmonary fibrosis, the crackles will persist and will not be altered by coughing. Whenever crackles or wheezes are heard over the lung field, the patient should be coached to cough, which may propel secretions through the airways, resolving the sound. The terminology for lung sounds is more logical when based on adjectives that can be acoustically characterized. Therefore, terms such as "wet," "sonorous," "sibilant," and so forth, which have no acoustic basis, should be replaced with more accurate terms, such as *high pitched* and *low pitched,* fine, and coarse, when describing wheezes or crackles. A popular exception is the descriptive term *"Velcro" crackles.* Velcro crackles have not yet been acoustically defined, but sound like two pieces of Velcro fastener being pulled apart. These crackles are fine, high-pitched, multiple, and are typical of interstitial pulmonary fibrosis. In addition, adventitious sounds should be described according to their occurrence in the appropriate respiratory phase: inspiratory, expiratory, or both. Timing and pitch may be described or diagrammed.

Pleural Friction Rub

The pleural friction rub is a low-pitched sound, of longer duration than crackles, and commonly present during both inspiration and expiration. Rubs are caused by fibrin deposits or pleural inflammation causing friction between the pleural layers. To distinguish between a monophonic low-pitched wheeze and a friction rub, the patient again should be asked to cough. Friction rubs are unaltered by coughing and are often compared with creaking leather.

Abnormal Sounds Related to Voice

Vocal resonance is created by the vibration of the bronchial tubes in response to sound energy. Normal vocal resonance is low pitched and is not transmitted well. The normal lung acts as a low-pass filter. The consolidated lung no longer acts as a low-pass filter; instead, sound is amplified, producing high-pitched bronchial breath sounds. Bronchial breath sounds may be easy to detect over an area of consolidation; they may be so augmented and amplified that they induce a nasal, tubular, bleating sound called "egophony" by Laennec (Table 2). Egophony is audible throughout expiration and sometimes is likened to sounds echoing in a wind tunnel or tube and heard as an "AA" when the patient says the letter "E." It is characteristic of consolidation pneumonia and heard also over lungs compressed by pleural effusions. Similar physiologic circumstances of consolidation with sound amplification also account for the phenomenon of whispered pectoriloquy. The patient is asked to whisper the numbers "1-2-3." This would not be audible over normal lung, but through a consolidated area the sounds are amplified and transmitted with greater clarity to the chest wall.

The Coin Sign of Pneumothorax

Pneumothorax is characterized by loss of lung parenchyma adjacent to the chest wall. The coin sound is characteristic of pneumothorax (Table 2). A coin is placed flat on the chest. The listener puts the stethoscope on the opposite side of the chest, then strikes the coin with the edge of a similar coin. The high-pitched sound so produced would be absorbed by normal lung, but when a pneumothorax exists, a high-pitched clink is heard. Breath sounds are absent or diminished, the percussion note hyperresonant, and, in tension pneumothorax, other signs such as respiratory distress and jugular venous distension may be present.

Mediastinal Crunch

Patients who have undergone chest or heart surgery will frequently have a perioperative pneumomediastinum. A crunching or crackling sound, often quite loud, may be heard with each heart beat. This is referred to as a systolic crunch. This same sound of air in the pleural space is also heard in spontaneous or traumatic pneumothorax.

SUMMARY OF ABNORMAL FINDINGS FOR SPECIFIC DISEASES

- Chronic obstructive lung disease: flat diaphragms, poor chest wall expansion, hyperresonant percussion note, decreased breath sounds, noisy breathing at the mouth, early and late soft and low-pitched inspiratory crackles, expiratory wheezing (polyphonic or monophonic), pursed lips breathing, contraction of neck muscles with inspiration, and contraction of abdominal wall musculature with expiration.
- Asthma: polyphonic, variably pitched expiratory wheezing, inspiratory high-pitched wheezing if severe. In glottic closure, wheeze may be loudest over anterior neck, mimicking asthma.
- Pleural effusion: decreased chest expansion, dull percussion note, decreased breath sounds or bronchial breath sounds over top of effusion. Signs depend on degree of underlying lung compression and extent of disease.
- Atelectasis: decreased chest expansion, dull percussion note, decreased breath sounds, coarse inspiratory crackles.
- Pneumothorax: decreased chest expansion on the side of the pneumothorax, decreased or absent breath sounds, coin sign, jugular venous distention on the side of the pneumothorax, respiratory distress, and agitation.
- Interstitial pneumonia: decreased chest wall mobility and diaphragm excursions, normal to decreased resonance on percussion, pan-inspiratory or late, high-pitched, fine to medium inspiratory crackles, often superimposed on loud or bronchial breath sounds.
- Pneumonia without consolidation: dull percussion note, if extensive; coarse or fine pan-inspiratory crackles; wheezes may be present.
- Pneumonia with consolidation: normal or decreased chest wall motion, depending on extent of involvement; dull percussion note, diminished breath sounds, abnormally loud, tubular breath sounds, egophony and whispered pectoriloquy, early or late inspiratory crackles; wheezes may be present.
- Congestive failure: normal chest wall motion, normal percussion note, fine, late, high-pitched peak inspiratory crackles; wheezing may be present; signs of large pleural effusion may also be present.

REFERENCES

1. Laennec RTH. *A treatise on the diseases of the chest* [Translated by John Forbes, 1821]. Special ed. Classics of Medicine Library. Birmingham, AL: Gryphon, 1979.
2. Forgacs P. *Lung sounds.* London: Bailliere, Tindall, 1978.
3. Forgacs P. Breath sounds. *Thorax* 1978;33:681–3.
4. Forgacs P, Nathoo AR, Richardson HD. Breath sounds. *Thorax* 1971;26:288–95.

5. Forgacs P. The functional basis of pulmonary sounds. *Chest* 1978;73:399–405.
6. Beck R, Gavriely N. The reproducibility of forced expiratory wheezes. *Am Rev Resp Dis* 1990;141: 1418–22.
7. Kraman SS. The forced expiratory wheeze. Its site of origin and possible association with lung compliance. *Respiration* 1983;44:189–96.
8. Kory RC. Clinical spirometry: recommendation of the section on pulmonary function testing. *Dis Chest* 1963;43:214.
9. Kraman SS. Vesicular (normal) lung sounds: how are they made,where do they come from, and what do they mean? *Semin Resp Med* 1985;6:183–91.
10. Report of the ATS/ACCP Ad Hoc Subcommittee on Pulmonary Nomenclature. *ATS News* 1977;3:5–6.
11. Bohadana AB, Peslin R, Uffholtz H. Breath sounds in the clinical assessment of airflow obstruction. *Thorax* 1978;33:345–51.
12. Badgett RG, Tanaka DJ, Hung DK, et al. Can moderate chronic pulmonary disease be diagnosed by historical and physical findings alone? *Am J Med* 1993;94:188–96.
13. Nath AR, Capel LH. Inspiratory crackles—early and late. *Thorax* 1974;29:223.
14. Earis JE, Marsh K, Pearson MG, et al. The inspiratory "squawk" in extrinsic allergic alveolitis and other pulmonary fibroses. *Thorax* 1982;37:923–6.

SUGGESTED READING

Loudon R, Murphy RLH. Lung sounds. *Am Rev Respir Dis* 1984;130:663–73.
Robertson AJ. Rales, rhonchi, and Laennec. *Lancet* 1957;1:417–23.
Wilkins RL, Hodgkin JE, Lope B. *Lung sounds, a practical guide.* St. Louis: Mosby, 1988.

Clinical Skills for Adult Primary Care
edited by M. E. Silverman and J. W. Hurst.
Lippincott-Raven Publishers, Philadelphia © 1996.

12

Examination of the Heart

Mark E. Silverman, M.D.

*Emory University School of Medicine, Atlanta, Georgia 30322
and Piedmont Hospital, Atlanta, Georgia 30309*

> *"The four points of a medical student's compass are: Inspection, Palpation, Percussion, and Auscultation."*
>
> William Osler, quoted in Bean WB. *Sir William Osler: Aphorisms.*
> Springfield, IL: Charles C Thomas, 1968:103.

A cardiac examination is regularly performed to check the heart rhythm and rate, to listen for a murmur(s), gallop(s), or click(s), and to detect evidence for heart failure. The components of a thorough cardiac examination include inspection of the jugular veins, palpation of the carotid artery and precordium, and auscultation with the diaphragm and bell. These are often performed simultaneously for purposes of timing and enhancing the diagnostic findings.

EXAMINATION OF THE JUGULAR VEINS

The jugular veins offer valuable visual clues to right heart physiology and several cardiac disorders (1–3). The estimation of venous pressure and the analysis of the various venous waves should be done on all patients with suspected heart disease. Proficiency develops when this is incorporated into the routine examination of all patients.

Venous Pressure

Thomas Lewis, in 1930, suggested the use of the external jugular veins to measure venous pressure (1):

> Of paramount importance, however, are the signs in the veins; that is so because they are usually amongst the earliest that can be detected; for that reason every medical student should make a full study of them. . . . Thus, normally, all veins which lie higher than the manubrial point are collapsed, all which lie below it are distended. If, therefore, we can gauge the precise level at which the veins collapse we have a gauge of the filling of the

venous reservoir and of general, or to be more exact, of right auricular venous pressure. Another and better gauge is to place the subject upon his back, the head resting upon pillows. The external jugular veins are then usually to be seen as swollen vessels in the neck, but, as they are traced upwards, the swelling ends; it ends at a point that represents atmospheric pressure in the veins, and in normal people this is at a point of the neck that is level with the sternum, or a little higher or a little lower.

Technique

The upper body is elevated or lowered (preferably on a slant) until the external jugular vein, as it crosses the sternocleidomastoid muscle, is seen to remain distended up to a point, then collapse forming a meniscus (Fig. 1). A tangential light forming highlights and shadows across the neck is a great aid in visualizing the meniscus as well as the internal jugular venous pulsations (3).

The venous pressure is then estimated by measuring the vertical difference in centimeters from the sternal angle of Louis to the upper level of the external jugular meniscus. With very high venous pressure, the external jugular meniscus may not be seen even with the patient upright.

Normal Findings

The external jugular veins are often normally distended when the patient is lying flat. When the trunk is elevated to 30 degrees, flickers of venous pulsations may be seen; however, the external jugular veins will not be engorged unless ve-

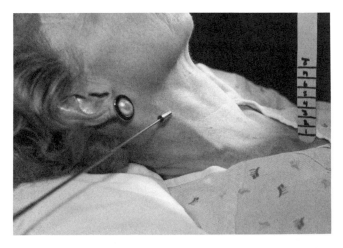

FIG. 1. Examination of the jugular veins. The external jugular vein is highlighted by tangential light. The pointer marks the meniscus, which is sighted across to a level of 4 cm above the sternal angle.

nous pressure is increased. A semiquantitative estimate of venous pressure can be made by measuring the vertical distance between the meniscus and the sternal angle (Fig. 1). The sternal angle is approximately 5 cm above the mid-right atrium. The measured height of the venous pressure can be added to 5 cm to express the total central venous pressure as centimeters of H_2O above the sternal angle (Example: 3 cm + 5 cm = 8 cm H_2O).

Abnormal Findings

The jugular venous pressure is an indirect measure of central venous pressure. An elevated jugular venous pressure is an indication of volume overload, right ventricular dysfunction or noncompliance, or tricuspid regurgitation. Rarely, it may be caused by a right atrial tumor or tricuspid stenosis. The most common cause of elevated venous pressure is heart failure due to left ventricular dysfunction. There is a good correlation of estimated jugular venous pressure with an elevation of pulmonary capillary wedge pressure (18 mm Hg) in patients with chronic congestive heart failure (2). In acute left heart failure and many cases of chronic left heart failure, right atrial pressure remains normal. Therefore, a normal jugular venous pressure does not exclude significant left ventricular failure. Serial measurements are particularly helpful in following the status of a volume-overloaded patient (4,5).

Abdominojugular Reflux

Technique

The patient is positioned with the head and trunk elevated about 30 degress (4). The external jugular venous pressure is estimated. Firm pressure is then maintained over a nontender area of the abdomen for 30 to 60 seconds while observing for an increase in the venous pressure (Fig. 2). The patient must not strain or resist pressure during the test.

Normal Response

The venous pressure stays the same or transiently increases, then decreases while pressure is maintained.

Abnormal Response

The venous pressure increases 4.0 cm or more and persists (4).

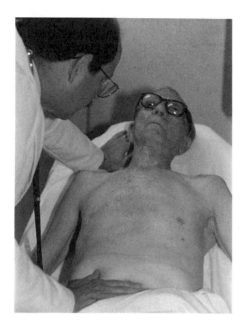

FIG. 2. Abdominojugular reflux. Pressure is exerted with the hand on the abdomen while observing for an increase in external jugular venous distention.

Alternative Test

The abdominojugular test uses the same technique but pressure is applied for only 10 seconds, then removed (5).

Normal Response

A normal response consists of no increase or a quick increase, then rapid decrease of venous pressure.

Abnormal Response

Patients with a sustained increase whose venous pressure decreases by 4 cm of H_2O or more upon pressure release are likely to have a pulmonary wedge pressure of 15 mm Hg or more. A positive test is strong supportive evidence for left ventricular dysfunction (in the absence of right ventricular failure).

The Jugular Venous Pulsations

We come now to the study of a subject which gives us far more information of what is actually going on within the chambers of the heart. In the study of the venous pulse we have often the direct means of observing the effects of the systole and diastole of the right auricle, and of the systole and diastole of the right ventricle. The venous pulse represents therefore a greater variety of features, and is subject to influence so subtle that it may manifest variations due to the changing conditions of the patient, during which the arterial pulse reveals no appreciable alteration. (5a)

Technique

The individual jugular venous waves and their descents can be evaluated best by observing the right internal jugular venous movement seen beneath the sternocleidomastoid muscle. The level of the trunk must be adjusted and tangential light used to find just the right level for optimal pulsations. The head is turned slightly to the left. A pillow under the shoulders may be helpful. With practice, the jugular movements are easily separated from the carotid arterial pulse by observing the following:

- Venous pulsation is slower and multiple waves occur.
- Venous waves are altered by position, respiration, abdominal compression, and a Valsalva maneuver.
- Venous pulsation can be easily blocked by compressing the vein.
- Venous pulsations are usually not palpable.

The individual venous waves are timed by simultaneously listening to the heart sounds and feeling the carotid arterial pulse. The A wave is normally seen when the first heart sound is heard and just before the carotid pulse is felt (unless the PR interval is long). Sometimes the X descent is well seen and can be used to time the A wave that precedes it.

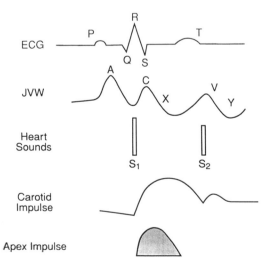

FIG. 3. The three normal internal jugular venous waves (A,C,V) and their descents (X,Y) are illustrated. Simultaneous electrocardiograms (ECG), jugular venous waves (JVW), heart sounds, carotid impulse, and apex impulse.

Normal Findings

Normally, there are three positive jugular venous waves (Fig. 3). The first, and usually the most prominent, is the A wave, which is due to right atrial contraction. The C wave closely follows the A wave and interrupts the X descent. It is due to bulging of the tricuspid valve into the right atrium from right ventricular contraction. The A and C waves are visualized as two quick fluttering movements before the second heart sound. The A wave is usually larger and seen at the time of the first heart sound. The C wave may not be seen. The V wave, caused by overflow of venous return to the right atrium during ventricular systole, is small and may or may not be seen at the time the second heart sound is heard. The Y descent follows the V wave and is very shallow and difficult to appreciate.

Abnormal Findings

A Wave

The amplitude of the A wave is heightened when the right atrium contracts against resistance, as seen with any cause of right ventricular hypertrophy, a stenotic or closed tricuspid valve, or right atrial tumor or clot. It also is augmented by tricuspid regurgitation. When the right atrium contracts against a closed tricuspid valve, as occurs with complete atrioventricular block or accelerated junctional rhythm, a large retrograde wave, called a cannon wave, is produced. The A wave is absent with atrial fibrillation; however, irregular flickering movements may be seen. Rapid regular flickering waves at a rate of 280 to 300/min are visible in atrial flutter and are best seen just above the clavicle while the patient inspires slowly.

C Wave

There are no abnormalities of the C wave. It is not often seen. Sometimes the C wave is prominent and can be mistaken for an A wave.

V Wave

The V wave is higher with atrial septal defect, reflecting left atrial physiology, and may equal the A wave. The normal V wave can be altered or replaced when tricuspid regurgitation occurs. Because the resultant wave is not normal, it should be called an R wave, although most clinicians refer to it as a CV wave. The greater the degree of tricuspid regurgitation, the earlier the regurgitant wave will appear during ventricular systole until it fuses with the C wave. When moderate to severe tricuspid regurgitation is present, a forceful venous pulse, resembling an arterial pulse, can be seen as a broad retrograde movement under the sternocleido-mastoid muscle. The Y descent that follows is rapid due to the high right atrial pressure. A bounce of the ear lobe from the underlying venous pulse is a good sign of severe tricuspid regurgitation and may be seen when no murmur of tricuspid regurgitation can be heard.

Pericardial Constriction

The external jugular veins are distended, and a rapid, deep Y descent is seen in the internal jugular veins. This is seen best when the patient is in the upright position. The X descent may be prominent when there is constriction plus pericardial effusion.

Right Ventricular Infarction

The internal jugular venous waves may simulate pericardial constriction with a rapid X and Y descent and a high venous pressure. A *Kussmaul's sign* (increase in venous pressure with inspiration) may be present.

CAROTID ARTERIAL EXAMINATION

The carotid arterial examination is a necessary part of the routine cardiac examination for it provides important information about cardiac and valvular function. In addition, the presence or absence of a carotid bruit may become very useful in long-term follow-up.

Technique

The patient is examined while lying flat or with the head and trunk slightly elevated. The chin is tilted slightly upward and to the left to open up the right cervical area, taking care not to stretch the right sternocleidomastoid muscle. The carotid arteries are each auscultated for bruits and felt for symmetry of pulsation. The carotid artery is then palpated with the second and third fingers while analyzing rate, rhythm, rapidity of upstroke, amplitude, and contour (Fig. 4).

Normal Findings

The carotid arterial pulses should be bilaterally symmetric and have a subjective amplitude of 3+. No bruit is heard over normal carotid arteries; however, loud murmurs from the heart, especially when aortic stenosis is present, may be transmitted to the carotid area and may be difficult to impossible to separate

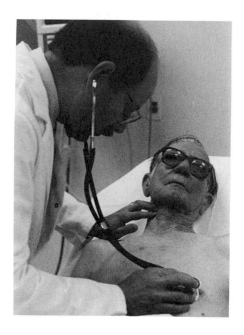

FIG. 4. Examination of the carotid pulse. The second and third fingers of the left hand palpate the pulse while the examiner listens simultaneously.

from a bruit. The normal carotid impulse has a single, brief bump that is easily felt in early systole (Fig. 3).

Abnormal Findings

Weak (Low-Amplitude) Carotid Pulse

A weak carotid pulse may be due to hypovolemia, hypotension, obstruction at the aortic or mitral valve, or a large pericardial effusion. The carotid pulse in patients with severe aortic stenosis classically has a low-amplitude, shuddering, delayed upstroke (anacrotic pulse). However, the elderly and young adults with severe aortic stenosis may have a normal carotid pulse.

Bounding Carotid Pulse

An exaggerated height and brisk upstroke of the arterial pulse may be due to a number of factors:

Increased Stroke Volume

Causes include pregnancy, an early stage of hypertension, athlete's heart, a slow heart rate, patent ductus arteriosus, and an arteriovenous fistula.

Aortic Regurgitation

The large stroke volume, rapid ejection of blood, and low diastolic pressure due to moderately severe or severe aortic regurgitation combine to produce a bounding pulse, sometimes called a *collapsing* or *water-hammer pulse.*

Enhanced Contractility

Examples include anxiety, fever, hyperthyroidism, and postexercise.

Abnormally Stiff Carotid Artery

The elderly artery may stiffen, lose its normal elasticity, and be unable to cushion the force of ventricular systole. This results in a more forceful arterial pulse and a higher systolic pressure.

Hypertrophic Cardiomyopathy

A rapidly rising, slapping arterial pulse, sometimes bifid (pulsus bisferiens), is the clue to hypertrophic subaortic stenosis and may provide an explanation for a harsh systolic murmur at the left sternal border. In this not uncommon condition, the amplitude of the arterial pulse decreases after a premature ventricular contractions (PVC) (the opposite of normal). This phenomenon is called the *Brockenbrough effect* (6).

Alternating Pulse (Pulsus Alternans)

This alternately weak and stronger pulse (in sinus rhythm) is a manifestation of severe heart disease due to a large or multiple infarctions, aortic stenosis, or a cardiomyopathy. It may be appreciated best by palpating the femoral artery. An alternating pulse may be intermittent and apparent only when induced by a premature ventricular contraction. It may be demonstrated by inflating a blood pressure cuff above systolic levels, then slowly deflating the cuff until only every other beat is heard. At a lower cuff pressure, the audible sounds then double.

Paradoxical Pulse (Pulsus Paradoxus)

A paradoxical pulse is defined as a decrease in systolic pressure of 10 mm Hg or more with normal inspiration. Causes include pericardial tamponade, constrictive pericarditis, emphysema, asthma, pulmonary embolus, or superior vena caval obstruction. The patient should be lying flat and breathing normally. The cuff is inflated above systolic pressure, then deflated very slowly until the Korotkoff sounds are first heard. The pulsus paradox is measured from this point to the point where sounds are heard throughout respiration.

PALPATION OF THE PRECORDIUM

The apex impulse should be part of the routine cardiac examination for it can provide useful information about heart size and abnormal physiology without necessarily resorting to chest radiography or echocardiogram.

Technique

With the patient supine and comfortable, the examiner "warms up" the chest with light touches of the fingers. An attempt is made to locate the apical impulse with the second and third fingertips; the distance of the impulse from the midsternal or midclavicular line is then measured. The midclavicular line is less exact but can be used. The intercostal space where the impulse is felt best is also recorded. Other areas of the precordial area are also palpated to check for thrills and abnormal pulsations. The most sensitive technique is to place the fingers of the right hand lightly over the fingers of the left hand while pressing over the selected area (Fig. 5). The patient is then tilted 30 degrees or so to the left to provide a better feel of the apex to seek for the presence of gallops (Fig. 6). Six areas should be carefully palpated (7): (a) adjacent to the upper right sternal border (aortic area),

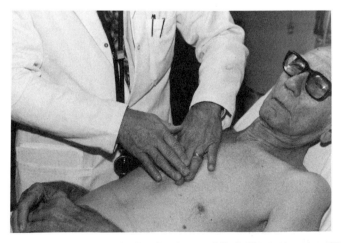

FIG. 5. Two-handed technique for palpating the chest wall for thrills and impulses. The fingers of the right hand press down on the left fingers.

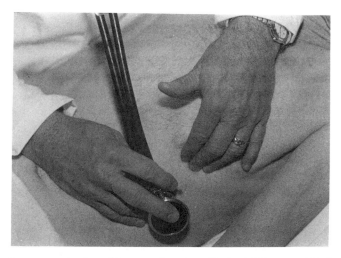

FIG. 6. Simultaneous palpation of the apex impulse with the left fingers while listening to the heart. The patient is turned 30 degrees to the left.

(b) adjacent to the upper left sternal border (pulmonary artery area), (c) midsternum (right ventricular area), (d) apical area, (e) ectopic area, and (f) epigastrium.

Normal Findings

The apex impulse can be palpated in only 40% to 50% of adults when examined in the supine position. The normal apex impulse is found in the fourth or fifth intercostal space within 10 cm from the midsternal line or within the midclavicular line. Heart size cannot be evaluated when the patient has been turned leftward. The normal apex impulse measures less than 3 cm (a quarter is 2.4 cm in diameter) in width and imparts a quick bumping sensation lasting less than one-third that of systole (Fig. 3). No presystolic or early diastolic movements should be felt. The rest of the precordium is motionless, although a slight sternal movement may be felt in young, thin, or anxious individuals. The aorta and pulmonary artery are not normally palpable.

Abnormal Findings

Adjacent to the Upper Right Sternal Border

A dilated aorta or aortic aneurysm may cause a systolic pulsation. A thrill is common in children with valvular aortic stenosis (but best appreciated in the suprasternal notch) although rarely felt in adults.

Adjacent to the Upper Left Sternal Border

A prominent pulmonary artery pulsation can be felt and may also be seen in patients with pulmonary hypertension, especially those with Eisenmenger syndrome, but also with mitral stenosis. An accentuated pulmonic closure sound is often palpable at the end of the impulse. Increased pulmonary flow due to an atrial septal defect may impart a bouncing type of systolic pulsation. A systolic thrill is present in some patients with pulmonic stenosis, whereas a diastolic thrill may be a consequence of pulmonic regurgitation after pulmonic valvotomy or valvuloplasty or tetralogy of Fallot repair.

Midsternal Area

The right ventricle underlies this area. A prominent, relatively slow and sustained pulsation may be felt with conditions that cause right ventricular systolic pressure overload, such as pulmonic outflow obstruction (valvular pulmonic stenosis, tetralogy of Fallot) or pulmonary hypertension (primary pulmonary hypertension, mitral stenosis). A quicker increase and decrease, due to volume overload of the right ventricle, can be felt with atrial septal defect. When severe mitral regurgitation is present, the expansion of the left atrium lifts the right ventricle forward, producing an early systolic pulsation. A systolic thrill along the midsternum is found with ventricular septal defect and subaortic stenosis (idiopathic subaortic stenosis [IHSS] and the membranous type).

Apical Area

The apex impulse is considered displaced when it is found outside the midclavicular line or more than 10 cm from the midsternal line. A slow-onset, sustained, forceful apical impulse, lasting beyond the first half of systole, is a sign of left ventricular systolic overload, as found with aortic stenosis or hypertension. With a volume load on the left ventricle, commonly associated with aortic or mitral regurgitation, the apex impulse is prominently felt and noted to have a brisk onset and offset. A bifid type of apical impulse is a clue to idiopathic hypertrophic subaortic stenosis. A presystolic impulse, occurring just before the first heart sound and sometimes seen as well as felt, indicates a noncompliant ventricle from hypertension, aortic stenosis, or coronary disease. This is always felt best with the patient in a left lateral position while the examiner listens for an atrial gallop and simultaneously feels the apex for two impulses—the atrial gallop followed quickly by the systolic impulse (Figs. 6 and 7). A palpable ventricular gallop may be felt in early diastole with volume overload conditions on the left ventricle, as occurs with heart failure and mitral or aortic regurgitation. Sometimes this can be seen. A ventricular gallop is almost always heard (Fig. 7). For this to be detected, the

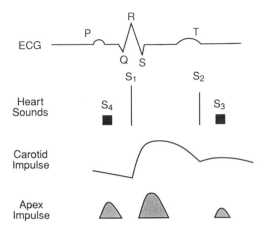

FIG. 7. An audible and palpable left atrial gallop (S_4) and left ventricular gallop (S_3) are shown. Simultaneous electrocardiogram (ECG), heart sounds, carotid impulse, and apex impulse.

patient must be turned to the left. A late systolic outward movement of the apical impulse—a late systolic bulge—indicates an infarction or aneurysm of the left ventricle. A systolic thrill at the apex can be due to severe mitral regurgitation from a ruptured papillary muscle or flail mitral chordae. Mitral stenosis can cause a diastolic apical thrill.

Ectopic Impulse

An ectopic impulse refers to an abnormal systolic movement where none is normally felt. Most commonly this is above the apex and along the left lateral cardiac border due to a myocardial infarct or unusually dilated heart.

Epigastrium

In patients with severe chronic lung disease, the right ventricle may be palpated only in the epigastric region. The abdominal aorta may also be felt in this location.

AUSCULTATION OF THE HEART

The ability to analyze heart sounds and murmurs distinguishes between the serious bedside examiner and someone who resorts to an expensive echocardiogram to sort out their clinical significance. Auscultation should be routinely performed on every patient.

Technique

Using the diaphragm of the stethoscope, the examiner should routinely auscultate at the upper right and upper left sternal border, the mid-left sternal border, and at the apex with the patient in a recumbent position (Fig. 4). Other sites, such as the right sternal border or spine, are occasionally rewarding. Depending on the findings, it may also be important to listen with the patient turned 30 degrees to the left, sitting, standing, squatting, after squatting, and after brief exercise (Fig. 8). The diaphragm is designed to listen to heart sounds and medium- to high-frequency murmurs, such as aortic regurgitation. The bell is used almost solely for gallops or a low-pitched rumble at the apex or left sternal border. A deeply held inspiration is a useful technique to slow a fast heart rate and can provide an easier auscultation for timing and configuration. Inspiration augments or brings forth right-sided gallops and murmurs related to tricuspid valve disease. The ejection sound of congenital pulmonic stenosis decreases with inspiration. Standing may accentuate ejection sounds, mitral valve prolapse clicks, and augment the murmur of IHSS. Squatting decreases the murmur of IHSS, increases the murmurs of mitral stenosis and aortic regurgitation, and may accentuate the late systolic murmur of mitral valve prolapse. During the strain of a Valsalva maneuver, the murmur of IHSS may increase while right-sided murmurs are reduced in intensity. Standing after squatting is an excellent way to bring forth diagnostic changes in the murmur or click of mitral valve prolapse. Isometric handgrip can augment mitral and aortic regurgitation. Bedside exercise, such as situps, then turning the patient to a left lateral position, accentuates the murmur of mitral stenosis. Situps or an isometric handgrip can bring forth an atrial gallop (Table 1). At times, with

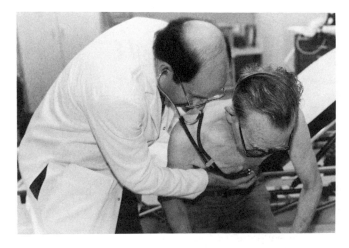

FIG. 8. Listening to the heart while the patient is squatting.

TABLE 1. *Useful bedside maneuvers*

Inspiration
    Slows heart rate to allow better timing
    Changes splitting interval of S_2 and gallops
    Augments right-sided murmurs and gallops
    Decreases innocent murmur and a right atrial gallop
    Decreases pulmonic ejection click
Standing
    Accentuates intensity of aortic ejection sound
    Decreases gallop sounds
    May bring forth click of mitral valve prolapse, especially when preceded by squatting
    Augments murmur of IHSS, mitral valve prolapse, and venous hum
    Decreases murmur of aortic and pulmonic stenosis
Bending over
    Improves ability to hear aortic regurgitation and pericardial rub
Squatting
    Augments murmur of mitral stenosis, aortic regurgitation
    Decreases the murmur of IHSS, mitral valve prolapse (but may bring forth late systolic
        murmur)
Valsalva maneuver
    During the strain, the murmur of IHSS increases and right-sided murmurs decrease
Isometric handgrip
    Augments an atrial gallop and the murmurs of aortic regurgitation and mitral stenosis
Bedside exercise
    Increases gallops and murmur of mitral stenosis

---

fast heart rates, multiple sounds, or more than one murmur, the most expert examiner will find it difficult to time the findings. In this situation, palpation of the carotid impulse to fasten onto systole and simultaneous auscultation is necessary. The technique of "inching" from one secure auscultatory finding to the next or "jumping" from a less-noisy area to the confusing area is most helpful.

Heart Sounds

The First Heart Sound

Normal Findings

The first heart sound relates to closure of the mitral and tricuspid valves. The first heart sound (S_1) should be listened to near the apex with the diaphragm. Normally, there will be a single sound with a fairly solid quality, unlike a click, which is sharper and of briefer duration. There is a wide range of normal intensity. Splitting of S_1 into mitral and tricuspid components may sometimes be heard along the left sternal border, especially in young people. The tricuspid component closely follows the louder mitral component and is sometimes sharp, which may make it difficult to distinguish from an early systolic click (Fig. 9A and C).

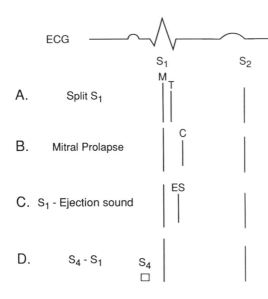

FIG. 9. Sounds that must be differentiated from a split first heart sound (S_1). **A:** Split S_1. **B:** Early systolic click of mitral prolapse. **C:** Ejection sound of a congenital bicuspid aortic valve (S_1). **D:** Atrial gallop (S_4). Reproduced with permission. From Silverman ME. Auscultatory findings in mitral valve prolapse. *Heart Dis Stroke* 1992;1:184–7. Copyright 1992 American Heart Association.

Abnormal Findings

An accentuated S_1 is heard with a short PR interval, mitral stenosis, mitral valve prolapse, a forceful left ventricular contraction (such as seen with exercise, emotion, and hyperthyroidism), and an atrial myxoma. S_2 becomes fainter with a long PR interval, an immobile mitral valve as seen with severe mitral stenosis, feeble left ventricular contraction, severe aortic regurgitation, and with constitutional factors such as obesity and lung disease.

The Second Heart Sound

Normal Findings

The second heart sound (S_2) is due to aortic and pulmonic valve closure. The second heart sound should be listened to at the upper left sternal border because this location is best for hearing both the aortic and pulmonic components. The normal aortic component (A_2) is loud, whereas the pulmonic component (P_2) is much fainter and briefer. The two components are fused into a single sound on expiration and separated by 0.02 to 0.04 seconds with inspiration (Fig. 10A). A normal splitting of 0.02 seconds produces a broadening of the second sound and will not be appreciated as two separate sounds. Wide splitting of S_2 with inspiration is prominent in a young person but not in the middle-aged or older person.

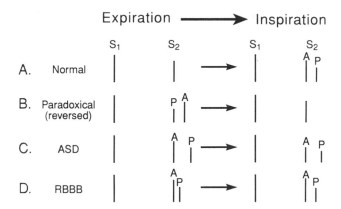

FIG. 10. Normal and abnormal splitting of the second heart sound (S₂).The effects of expiration and inspiration are shown on aortic (A) and pulmonic (P) closure. **A:** Normal splitting. **B:** Paradoxical splitting due to left bundle branch block. **C:** Wide fixed splitting due to an atrial septal defect (ASD) **D:** Splitting with a right bundle branch block (RBBB).

Wide splitting of S₂ may be heard on expiration in some young people in the recumbent position but not when standing.

Abnormal Findings

Aortic valve closure is accentuated by systemic hypertension and may acquire a tambourlike quality. When the aortic valve is heavily calcified and immobile, A₂ becomes faint or inaudible. Pulmonic closure becomes accentuated with pulmonary hypertension, especially in Eisenmenger's syndrome, and can become louder than A₂, in which case P₂ may be heard at the cardiac apex.

Abnormal splitting is of three types (Fig. 10):

Paradoxical Splitting. When the pulmonic valve closure is before the aortic valve closure, the two sounds will come together with inspiration and split apart on expiration—the opposite of normal. This generally occurs when left ventricular systole is longer than normal and aortic closure is delayed. Left bundle branch block or right ventricular pacing are by far the most common causes for paradoxical splitting (Fig. 10B). Severe valvular aortic stenosis and coronary artery disease are less likely considerations.

Fixed Splitting. When the two sounds are widely split (0.04 to 0.06 seconds) and the splitting interval remains fixed throughout respiration, a fixed split due to an atrial septal defect is suggested (Fig. 10C). The patient should then be examined standing because some young people have an apparent fixed split in the recumbent position that will narrow with standing.

Right Bundle Branch Block. With right bundle branch block, the two components of S_2 may not completely fuse on expiration (Fig. 10D). The split still widens with inspiration.

Gallop Sounds

Normal Findings

An apical ventricular gallop (S_3) is a normal finding in a child and it may be quite loud. A normal S_3 may continue to be heard up to age 30 or so but after that age it should be considered to be an abnormal finding. An atrial gallop is rarely, if ever, a normal finding at any age.

Abnormal Findings

Ventricular Gallop. A left ventricular gallop (S_3) is a very important finding for it signifies left heart failure or volume overload with a high degree of specificity. It is a difficult sound to hear because it has a very low frequency and is usually quite faint. The patient should always be turned into a left lateral position and auscultated using the bell applied lightly to the apex. An S_3 has a dull, thudding quality and is heard in early diastole 0.10 to 0.17 seconds after S_2 (Fig. 7). Rarely, it is palpable, in which case it is always loud. Right ventricular gallops also can occur related to right ventricular volume overload or dysfunction. The right ventricular gallop is best heard over the lower sternum, in the epigastrium, and sometimes transmits to the neck where it is heard over the jugular veins. Right-sided gallops are augmented by inspiration.

Atrial Gallop. An atrial gallop (S_4) is common to conditions in which there is an increased wall stiffness. This may be due to hypertrophy, ischemia, or fibrosis of either the left or right ventricle. These conditions cause an elevated diastolic pressure in the ventricle that brings forth a vigorous atrial contraction (Fig. 7). A left ventricular S_4 is dull, low-pitched, and heard best at the apex with the bell of the stethoscope. It may be simultaneously seen and/or felt. Often the left ventricular atrial gallop will be indistinct or not heard with the patient lying flat but will be easily appreciated with the patient in a left lateral position. Its intensity is enhanced by exercise, ischemia, or hand grip. It may be difficult to separate an atrial gallop from a split first heart sound (Fig. 9A and D). The simultaneous pressure of a presystolic impulse is helpful in deciding whether the sound is a left atrial gallop (Fig. 7). An atrial gallop is best heard with the bell because it is a low-frequency sound, whereas both components of a split first heart sound are heard best with the diaphragm of the stethoscope. A right ventricular S_4 is heard closer to the lower sternal edge and is louder during inspiration.

Summation Gallop. With rapid heart rates or long PR intervals, the third and fourth heart sounds may superimpose. This can produce a loud mid-diastolic gallop sound known as a summation gallop. This sound may be as loud as or louder than the first or second heart sounds and, if so, should suggest a summation gallop.

Systolic and Diastolic Sounds, Clicks, and Snaps

Normal Findings

A click should always be considered to be an abnormal sound. On occasion a split S_1 may simulate an early click while a widely split S_2 may raise the misleading possibility of an opening snap (Figs. 9B, 9C, and 11).

Abnormal Findings

A click is a high-frequency sound that is sharper and briefer in duration than a normal sound.

Ejection Sounds. An ejection sound occurs in early systole, closely following the first heart sound, and is related to opening of a congenitally stenotic aortic or pulmonic valve or to a forceful ejection of blood into a dilated or stiff aorta or pulmonary artery (Fig. 9C). The clicking sound is heard best along the left sternal border or near the apex using the diaphragm. Standing will accentuate the ejection sound and make it easier to hear. Right-sided ejection sounds that occur with pulmonic stenosis tend to decrease with inspiration, whereas left-sided aortic valve sounds remain the same intensity. The ejection sound of a bicuspid aortic valve

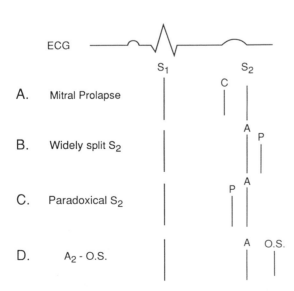

FIG. 11. Sounds that must be differentiated from a split second heart sound (S_2). **A:** Late systolic click of mitral prolapse. **B:** Widely split S_2. **C:** Paradoxically split S_2. **D:** Opening snap of mitral stenosis in early diastole. Reproduced with permission. From Silverman ME. Auscultatory findings in mitral valve prolapse. *Heart Dis Stroke* 1992;1: 184–7. Copyright 1992 American Heart Association.

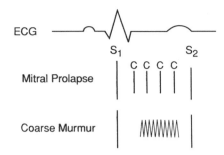

FIG. 12. Multiple systolic clicks at the apex due to mitral prolapse may simulate a coarse systolic murmur. Reproduced with permission. From Silverman ME. Auscultatory findings in mitral valve prolapse. *Heart Dis Stroke* 1992;1:184–7. Copyright 1992 American Heart Association.

is usually loudest near the apex, whereas the pulmonic valve ejection sound is best heard along the left sternal border.

Nonejection Systolic Clicks. Single or multiple clicks may occur in early, mid-, or late systole (Figs. 9B, 11A, and 12). The click(s) is usually due to prolapse of one or both mitral leaflets as they are propelled upward by ventricular contraction. Other rare causes of a systolic click include an aneurysm of the atrial or ventricular septum, IHSS, Ebstein's anomaly (*sail sound*), and tricuspid valve prolapse. The click due to mitral valve prolapse is heard best at the apex and may be a loud, sharp noise or a delicate crisp sound. The timing and intensity may be markedly affected by the position of the patient. At times a click may be absent or heard only in one position (usually standing) while easily heard at other times in multiple positions. Multiple clicks due to mitral prolapse are common (Fig. 12).

Opening Snap. An opening snap is produced by the opening of a stenotic mitral valve. The sound occurs 0.06 to 0.12 seconds after S_2 at the termination of the descent of the thickened mitral valve as it is driven into the ventricular cavity in early diastole by the force of left atrial pressure (Fig. 11D). The sound may be loud or delicate and usually introduces a diastolic rumble. The opening snap is generally best heard along the left lower sternal border while using the diaphragm but may be heard elsewhere, whereas the murmur of mitral stenosis is localized to the apex most of the time. An opening snap along the lower sternal border also can be due to rheumatic tricuspid valve stenosis. An atrial myxoma can simulate an opening snap (*tumor plop*).

Heart Murmurs

Characteristics of Murmurs

If a murmur is detected, it should be described by location, radiation, configuration, pitch, grade, and any alteration that transpires with position, inspiration, or maneuver. Abnormal findings on auscultation are best described by a drawing (Fig. 13). The location of the abnormal sound or murmur is shown by circling the

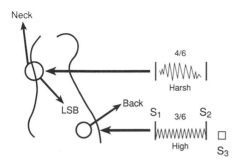

FIG. 13. The technique of diagramming and describing two murmurs. The area of maximal intensity is circled. Arrows show the direction the murmur radiates from the circle. The configuration of the murmur is illustrated with the grade of the murmur placed above and the tonal quality below. In this example, a grade 4/6, harsh crescendo/decrescendo systolic murmur of aortic valve stenosis is illustrated at the right upper sternal border radiating to the neck and to the left sternal border (LSB) and a grade 3/6, high-frequency, holosystolic murmur of mitral regurgitation radiating to the back is shown at the cardiac apex.

area of maximal intensity on the cardiac silhouette. The direction of radiation of a murmur is shown by an arrow(s). The grade of the murmur can be placed above the murmur(s) and the frequency or quality below. The effect of position, respiration, squatting, and so forth should be notated.

Location

The location of the maximum intensity of a murmur is related to the area on the chest wall where the murmur is most intense. This is often closest to the site of origin—valve, septum, great vessel—but also relates to the direction of blood flow and propagation through the chest wall (Fig. 14).

Radiation

The direction of radiation of the murmur from the site of maximal intensity provides some insight into the origin of the murmur. The transmission of sound from the point of origin to the chest wall is complex, depending on the distance from the source and the physical properties of the medium between the source and the stethoscope. Murmurs tend to be transmitted in the downstream direction of the blood flow in the cardiac chambers or blood vessels. Lung and fat tissue dampen the sound considerably, whereas bone may amplify to some extent. Certain frequencies transmit better than others, producing a change in pitch of the

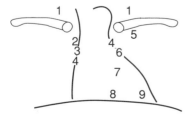

FIG. 14. Diagrammatic sketch of the heart with numbers assigned to locations of greatest intensity of specific murmurs. 1, venous hum, supraclavicular bruits; 2, supravalvular aortic stenosis; 3, valvular aortic stenosis; 4, aortic regurgitation; 5, patent ductus arteriosis; 6, secundum atrial septal defect, pulmonic stenosis; 7, normal murmur, ventricular septal defect, subaortic stenosis; 8, tricuspid regurgitation and stenosis; 9, mitral regurgitation and stenosis.

original sound at different locations. The stethoscope also alters the sound because the diaphragm attenuates low-pitched sounds and accentuates high-pitched sounds, whereas the bell has the opposite effect.

Configuration

A holosystolic murmur can assume one of several configurations: crescendo, decrescendo, and plateau. A crescendo/decrescendo murmur is sometimes called an ejection murmur (a term that should be discarded), a diamond-shaped murmur, a spindle-shaped murmur, or a kite-shaped murmur and may be further characterized as peaking in early, mid-, or late systole (Fig. 15A and B). The configuration of a murmur offers considerable information about the changing pressure difference (gradient) that exists between the two chambers. Systolic murmurs are generated by the ejection of blood from the ventricle into a lower pressure chamber or vessel. When the ventricular pressure is significantly higher then the receiving chamber at the onset of ejection, the systolic murmur begins immediately and continues until the pressures equalize or the second heart sound occurs. For example, the murmur of mitral regurgitation is usually holosystolic because left ventricular pressure greatly exceeds left atrial pressure beginning with the first heart sound and extending throughout systole to the second heart sound. A crescendo/decrescendo configuration occurs when there is an increased volume of blood being ejected or an obstruction to ventricular ejection. In this situation, the intensity of the systolic murmur builds up as the ventricular pressure rapidly climbs and overcomes the resistance to flow. The murmur declines in intensity as ventricular pressure decreases in late systole.

Diastolic murmurs occur during the period of ventricular relaxation when there is an obstruction or increased flow across an atrioventricular valve or if the aor-

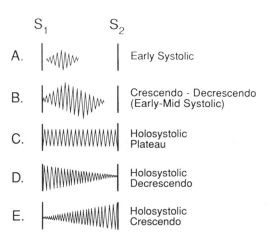

FIG. 15. Configurations of systolic murmurs. **A:** Early systolic. **B:** Crescendo/decrescendo. **C:** Holosystolic/plateau. **D:** Holosystolic/decrescendo. **E:** Holosystolic/crescendo.

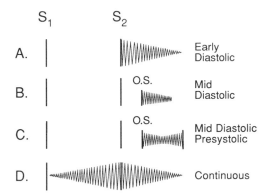

FIG. 16. Configuration of diastolic and continuous murmurs. **A:** Early diastolic. **B:** Opening snap (OS) and mid-diastolic. **C:** Opening snap and mid-diastolic–presystolic murmur. **D:** Continuous murmur.

tic or pulmonic valve is incompetent. Diastolic murmurs are generally timed as early, mid-, or late (presystolic) (Fig. 16A–C). The exact configuration and timing depends on the dynamic pressure gradient existing between two chambers or vessel and chamber. For example, the murmur of aortic regurgitation begins with the aortic component of the second heart sound because aortic root pressure immediately exceeds left ventricular pressure at the onset of diastole. The murmur then has a decrescendo configuration as aortic pressure declines (Fig. 16A). The murmur of mitral stenosis is mid-diastolic because it cannot begin until the mitral valve opens in early diastole. If diastole is sufficiently long, the murmur will decrescendo or disappear as the left atrial–left ventricular pressure gradient rapidly decreases. In presystole, when atrial contraction elevates atrial pressure, the murmur is accentuated (Fig. 16C).

A continuous murmur is generated when a pressure gradient continues from systole into diastole. This usually occurs because of an arteriovenous (AV) communication such as a patent ductus arteriosus or an AV fistula. Because the pressure difference is greatest in systole, the continuous murmur, with the exception of the venous hum, is always loudest in systole with a decrescendo component into part or all of diastole (Fig. 16D). A wind-tunnel type of roaring noise is generated. By definition, a continuous murmur has to continue through the second heart sound but does not necessarily span the entirety of systole and diastole.

Loudness

Cardiac murmurs are graded according to the loudness as perceived by the listener. This is a highly subjective estimate and is based on the following guidelines by Samuel Levine (8):

Grade 1/6   Faint and heard only after several seconds of "tuning in"
Grade 2/6   Slight murmur heard immediately
Grade 3/6   Moderately loud

Grade 4/6   Louder than a grade 3 murmur but not heard when only a portion
             of the rim of the stethoscope touches the chest wall
Grade 5/6   Very loud; can be heard when a portion of the stethoscope is
             touching the skin but not when the stethoscope is just lifted from
             the chest wall
Grade 6/6   Extremely loud; heard with the stethoscope just removed from the
             chest wall

Diastolic murmurs are rarely as loud as systolic murmurs. Generally the same scale is used, however. The presence or absence of a thrill is not used to grade murmurs using the Levine classification.

Pitch and Quality

The pitch of the murmur refers to the frequency range (number of Herz/second) of the murmur. Murmurs are described as low, medium, or high-pitched. A low-pitched murmur has a rumbling, somewhat rough quality (rrr). A high-pitched murmur has a blowing quality (shhh). Medium-pitched murmurs are in between and may have components of both. Most murmurs are noise (mixed frequencies) and can be described as harsh, coarse, blowing, musical, rumbling, and so forth; some may have overtones that impart characteristic musical tones such as cooing, whistling, honking, or whooping.

Normal Murmurs

A normal systolic murmur (formerly called innocent or functional) is common in children and adolescents. The examiner must reach a firm diagnostic decision to avoid alarming the patient and family and thereby producing insurance and antibiotic implications attendant to the diagnosis of a heart murmur. The typical normal murmur is heard in early mid-systole and is often maximally located along the mid-left sternal border (Fig. 15A). The intensity is usually grade 1 to 2, rarely grade 3, and has a coarse or slightly musical (vibratory) quality (*Still's murmur*). The second heart sound should split normally (not fixed), and there is no ejection sound or click. A normal third heart sound is often present in this age group. The murmur will usually disappear with Valsalva maneuver and standing, especially when standing is combined with deep inspiration. An early systolic coarse murmur at the upper left sternal border, due to normal or increased flow or rapid ejection, is not unusual in children or young adults. A similar murmur can be heard over the aortic valve area in adults, especially with anemia, fever, or high cardiac output. A supraclavicular bruit is a brief, sometimes intense systolic murmur loudest above the clavicle in children. It is accentuated by sitting and decreased when the folded arms are extended backwards. During and after pregnancy, a continuous murmur, the *mammary souffle*, may be heard along the sternal border. A normal *cervical venous hum* is present in many children below the age of 10. The murmur is continuous, roaring, and heard best over the neck with radiation down into the upper chest where the diastolic (loudest) component may be the only component heard. The venous hum is only heard when the patient is sitting and the head turned to the side. It can be obliterated by firm finger pressure across the sternocleidomastoid muscle and is inaudible in the recumbent position. It sounds like the "roar" of a large sea shell.

Abnormal Murmurs

Aortic Valve

Aortic Valve Stenosis. The murmur of aortic stenosis is always harsh and diamond shaped, and is usually most intense at the upper right sternal border (Fig. 15B). Occasionally, in the elderly, it is loudest at the mid-left sternal border. It radiates well to the right clavicle and both sides of the neck as well as downward to the left sternal border and apex, where it becomes higher pitched. A thrill at the area of maximal intensity and in the suprasternal notch is common in children but rare in adults. An early systolic ejection sound, best heard at the apex and with standing, indicates a congenital bicuspid aortic valve but is rarely heard after age 40 because of valvular calcification and immobility. A short, coarse systolic murmur at the upper right sternal border due to aortic valve sclerosis without stenosis is a frequent finding in the elderly. The greater the severity of the aortic stenosis, the lengthier the systolic murmur and the later the peak until the murmur may sound holosystolic. With severe left ventricular dysfunction or critical aortic stenosis, the flow across the valve may be so reduced that the murmur is unimpressive or even absent. A palpable or audible left atrial gallop in individuals under age 65, a low amplitude, slowly increasing carotid arterial pulse, and a reduced or absent A_2 are key findings of severe aortic stenosis. In the elderly and the young, the carotid pulse may be surprisingly normal despite severe aortic stenosis. A systolic pressure of 180 or even 200 mm Hg due to a stiff aorta is not inconsistent with severe aortic stenosis in the elderly.

Aortic Valve Regurgitation. Aortic valve regurgitation may be present with or without aortic stenosis and is usually loudest at the upper and mid-left sternal border. With aortic root disease, such as aortic dissection or dilation, the murmur may be loudest along the right sternal border. In the elderly, a "whiff" of aortic regurgitation may only be heard at the apex. The typical diastolic murmur is high frequency and does not radiate widely (Fig. 16B). In general, a short and soft early diastolic murmur indicates mild aortic regurgitation. A longer diastolic murmur may be due to mild, moderate, or severe aortic regurgitation. When the diastolic pressure of the left ventricle becomes severely elevated in long-standing, severe aortic regurgitation, the diastolic murmur shortens and may even temporarily disappear. A cooing or groaning (musical) diastolic murmur is evidence for a flail or retroverted aortic cusp. Signs of severe aortic regurgitation include a forceful, steeply rising arterial pulse, a wide pulse pressure with low diastolic pressure, a left ventricular gallop, a laterally displaced and quickly rising apex impulse, and an Austin Flint murmur. The *Austin Flint murmur* is a mid- or late diastolic rumble simulating mitral stenosis and heard at the cardiac apex. With severe aortic valve regurgitation, a harsh systolic murmur suggesting coexisting aortic stenosis is also present, giving a to and fro or sawing noise to the two murmurs. This systolic murmur is due to increased systolic flow across the abnormal aortic valve. The bounding carotid pulse shows that there is no significant aortic stenosis.

Mitral Valve

Mitral Valve Stenosis. The diastolic rumble of mitral stenosis may be difficult to detect, and technique often makes the difference in picking up a subtle murmur. The examiner is tipped off by an accentuated first heart sound, which may be louder than S_2 even over the base of the heart. The next step is to listen with the bell of the stethoscope applied lightly over the cardiac apex with the patient slanted leftward. Hand grip, situps, and listening while the patient is squatting may be rewarding. An introductory opening snap, best heard along the lower left sternal border but sometimes widely transmitted, follows aortic closure by 0.06 to 0.14 seconds. It may be absent when the mitral valve is immobile. After the opening snap, a diastolic murmur of mitral stenosis may be heard in mid- or late diastole (Fig. 16B and C). The timing and duration of the murmur depends on the gradient across the mitral valve, which in turn is a result of left atrial pressure, left ventricular diastolic pressure, and heart rate.

Mitral Valve Regurgitation. Mitral regurgitation is almost always loudest at or near the apex. The classic murmur is holosystolic and highpitched (blowing); however, the configuration and pitch may vary according to the etiology of the mitral regurgitation and its severity. The murmur radiates laterally from the apex to the axilla.

With mitral valve prolapse, the most common etiology of mitral regurgitation, the murmur may be holosystolic, mid–late systolic, or limited to a brief presystolic period (Fig. 17A–D). A crescendo configuration into the second heart sound is characteristic due to an increasing degree of mitral regurgitation as the mismatch of the two mitral leaflets becomes more pronounced in late systole. A late systolic murmur always means mild mitral regurgitation, whereas a holosystolic murmur may indicate mild, moderate, or severe regurgitation. The presence and length of the murmur is strongly position related; standing and sometimes squatting, then standing, bring forth or augment the murmur. An unusual musical systolic murmur—honking or whooping in tone—may be intermittent or heard only with standing (Fig. 17E). It is always a mild form of mitral regurgitation. Systolic clicks are an important diagnostic feature of mitral valve prolapse and may be single or multiple, early, mid, or late, present intermittently, or not at all (Figs. 9B, 11, and 12).

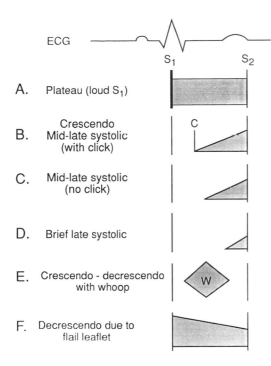

ECG

S₁   S₂

A.   Plateau (loud S₁)

B.   Crescendo
      Mid-late systolic
      (with click)

C.   Mid-late systolic
      (no click)

D.   Brief late systolic

E.   Crescendo - decrescendo
      with whoop

F.   Decrescendo due to
      flail leaflet

FIG. 17. Different configurations of murmurs heard with mitral prolapse. **A:** Plateau with loud first heart sound (S₁). **B:** Mid- to late crescendo systolic murmur introduced by click (c). **C:** Mid- to late systolic crescendo murmur without click. **D:** Brief late systolic murmur. **E:** Musical whooping murmur. **F:** Decrescendo/holosystolic murmur due to a flail mitral leaflet. Reproduced with permission. From Silverman ME. Auscultatory findings in mitral valve prolapse. *Heart Dis Stroke* 1992;1:184–7. Copyright 1992 American Heart Association.

Chordal rupture, usually related to long-standing mitral valve prolapse but also from endocarditis or trauma, causes an intense, harsh, decrescendo holosystolic murmur at the apex (Fig. 15D). The murmur may radiate to the spine and be heard as far as the head or sacrum and occasionally to the base of the heart, where the harsh murmur may simulate aortic stenosis. The murmur has a decrescendo configuration because the severe, acute mitral regurgitation causes the left atrial pressure to increase steeply, thereby decreasing late systolic regurgitation and the intensity of the murmur. An apical thrill and left atrial gallop may be felt at the apex. The apical impulse is thrusting and the carotid arterial pulse brisk but of low amplitude. The combination of these findings, especially the decrescendo configuration, alerts the physician to the presence of acute mitral regurgitation and the possible need for urgent surgery.

Papillary muscle dysfunction, due to myocardial infarction, acute ischemia, or sometimes aortic stenosis, may allow mitral regurgitation. The murmur is heard in a limited area at the apex and is usually of low intensity and slightly coarse. It is often short and may be early, early–mid, or late systolic with a crescendo/decrescendo configuration. Occasionally, the murmur is high frequency and holosystolic. A left atrial and/or left ventricular gallop sound may be present. Listening during acute ischemic pain or while the patient is performing isometric handgrip may be rewarding.

When mitral regurgitation is *rheumatic* in origin, the murmur is usually holosystolic, blowing in quality, and radiates to the left. When the mitral regurgitation is severe, a left ventricular gallop followed by a short diastolic murmur—a *flow rumble*—may be heard (Fig. 15C). If mitral stenosis is also present, the blowing systolic murmur may be short and difficult to appreciate. A cleft mitral valve associated with *ostium primum defect* is a congenital cause of mitral regurgitation.

Tricuspid Valve

The murmur of tricuspid regurgitation and/or stenosis is usually well localized along the lower sternal border. It may be augmented by or only heard with inspiration (*Carvallo's sign*).

Tricuspid Valve Regurgitation. The murmur of tricuspid regurgitation is rarely audible but occasionally can be found with tricuspid valve prolapse, a cleft tricuspid valve, rheumatic tricuspid involvement, pulmonary hypertension, acute pulmonary embolism, severe mitral valve disease, carcinoid syndrome, and right-sided endocarditis. The murmur is heard in a limited area along the lower sternal border or xiphoid area and is low intensity, medium (coarse) frequency, and often not quite holosystolic. It increases with inspiration unless right atrial pressure is extremely high. When there is obvious tricuspid regurgitation seen in the jugular venous inspection, sometimes no murmur is audible. Standing the patient will decrease right atrial pressure and may allow better appreciation of a regurgitant venous wave and inspiratory increase in the murmur.

Tricuspid Stenosis. Although some minor degree of tricuspid stenosis is not uncommon at autopsy in patients with rheumatic heart disease, auscultatory evidence is rare. The diagnosis is established by hearing an opening snap followed by a diastolic rumble, increasing in intensity with inspiration and best heard along the lower left sternal border.

Selected Common Congenital Heart Murmurs

Ventricular Septal Defect. The usual *membranous ventricular septal defect* (VSD) is easily diagnosed by the finding of a typical harsh, holosystolic murmur at the mid-left sternal border with a thrill felt at the same location. However, there are variations. The murmur is sometimes high pitched and soft. With a small VSD, the murmur is sometimes high pitched and brief, ending by mid-systole. Muscular VSDs may be heard along the lower sternal border, whereas membranous septal aneurysms can be heard best at the second and third left sternal border. A supracristal type of VSD may undermine the aortic valve, causing a diastolic murmur of aortic regurgitation. A flow (mid-diastolic) rumble heard at the cardiac apex indicates that the left-to-right shunt is large. Postoperatively, the systolic murmur should be eliminated; however, a small residual VSD may remain and be heard as a soft, high-frequency systolic murmur.

Atrial Septal Defect. An *atrial septal defect* can be easily missed. The murmur, due to increased flow across the pulmonic valve, is short, coarse, rarely loud, and sometimes not present. The most important clue is a widely split second heart sound that does not vary with respiration. This is heard in 90% of patients with an atrial septal defect. Care must be taken to be sure the split is truly fixed by listening to the patient in the upright position. An apical murmur of mitral regurgitation is found in some cases of ostium primum defect. Rarely, tricuspid regurgitation is present. A tricuspid valve rumble in mid-diastole indicates a sizeable shunt. In some patients, the widely split second heart sound and diastolic rumble will closely simulate the opening snap and murmur of mitral stenosis. An ostium primum type of atrial septal defect may have two systolic murmurs—one due to increased flow across the pulmonic valve and the other from a cleft mitral valve and mitral regurgitation. After atrial septal defect repair, a short, early systolic murmur at the upper left sternal border and a widely split but no longer fixed second heart sound may still be present due to the persisting right ventricular conduction delay.

Pulmonic Stenosis. *Valvular pulmonic stenosis* produces a harsh, crescendo/decrescendo systolic murmur that is always heard best at the upper left sternal border. A sharp ejection sound, typically fading with inspiration, is commonly present although sometimes difficult to hear because of the noisy murmur. If the pulmonic valve is dysplastic, as in Noonan's syndrome, no ejection sound will be heard. The second heart sound splits widely and the pulmonic closure sound is faint.

Coarctation of the Aorta. With *coarctation of the aorta*, an early systolic harsh murmur is heard along the mid-sternal border and also in the back. Asymmetric arm blood pressure readings and a diminished or absent femoral pulse are diagnostic features. A systolic ejection sound with or without a harsh systolic murmur at the upper right sternal border indicates a coexisting bicuspid aortic valve. The ejection sound is commonly loudest at the cardiac apex. Occasionally, a murmur of mitral regurgitation or mitral stenosis is associated. Systolic bruits or even a continuous murmur may be heard in the back. After surgery or balloon valvuloplasty, the systolic murmur is usually no longer heard. The associated defects remain audible.

Tetralogy of Fallot. *Tetralogy of Fallot* is the most common form of cyanotic congenital heart disease that may present to the primary care physician. The cyanosis may be obvious, subtle, or absent (acyanotic tet). Clubbing correlates with the presence of cyanosis. The unoperated patient has a loud, harsh early mid-systolic murmur at the upper and mid-left sternal border due largely to flow across the right ventricular outflow narrowing. If the ventricular septal defect is large and the infundibular stenosis mild, the longer, higher frequency murmur of the ventricular septal defect may predominate. The pulmonic valve closure sound is often inaudible. The adult patient will mostly be postoperative total repair. The harsh systolic murmur at the upper left sternal border persists. Almost always there is a low-frequency, short diastolic murmur beginning a short space after A_2.

This murmur is found lateral to the upper left sternal border and is due to surgically created pulmonic regurgitation. The second heart sound is widely split because a right bundle branch block almost inevitably results from the surgical closure of the ventricular septal defect because the right bundle courses along the rim of the defect.

Coronary Artery Disease

The major finding is the presence of an audible and palpable left atrial gallop, which may become louder during an ischemic episode. A systolic murmur, due to papillary muscle dysfunction (see earlier description), is occasionally present. A late systolic impulse along the left lateral cardiac border or apex indicates infarction has occurred.

Cardiomyopathy

Dilated Cardiomyopathy. Soft heart sounds and prominent left atrial and left ventricular gallops are the features. A murmur of mitral and occasionally tricuspid regurgitation may be heard. Signs of volume overload—pulmonary crackles, external jugular venous distention, hepatomegaly, and peripheral edema—are common in advanced stages. A pulsus alternans may be noted on palpation of a peripheral artery.

Hypertrophic Cardiomyopathy. The physical findings associated with *hypertrophic aortic stenosis* are often distinctive. An intense decrescendo, lengthy but not quite holosystolic, along the lower sternal border or near the apex is the classic murmur of idiopathic hypertrophic cardiomyopathy. Additional findings may include a loud S_1, a rapidly increasing (slapping) and sometimes bifid carotid arterial pulse (pulsus bisferiens), and a palpable and/or audible left atrial gallop. With squatting, the murmur usually softens and with standing and Valsalva it becomes louder. After a premature ventricular contraction, the murmur may increase while the peripheral pulse simultaneously diminishes. The presence of IHSS should be strongly suspected if the examiner hears a murmur at the left sternal border and has trouble deciding whether it is due to aortic stenosis or mitral regurgitation. Hypertensive heart disease is a common cause of a hypertrophic cardiomyopathy. An accentuated aortic closure sound, palpable and audible atrial gallop, and sustained apical impulse are supportive evidence.

Restrictive Cardiomyopathy. In this type of cardiomyopathy, diastolic dysfunction predominates. Causes include *amyloidosis, hemochromatosis, scleroderma, sarcoidosis,* and *carcinoid syndrome.* Signs of these diseases may be apparent on general inspection (see Chapter 5). On examination, the external jugular veins are often distended and the internal jugular veins may display a rapid Y and sometimes rapid X descent. Prominent left ventricular third and fourth heart sounds may be heard. Occasionally, mitral and/or tricuspid regurgitation are present. Mixed tricuspid stenosis and regurgitation suggest carcinoid syndrome.

Pericardial Disease

Acute Pericarditis. The cardinal sign is a friction rub usually heard best along the left sternal border. The sound may be squeaky or creaky. Sometimes it sounds smoother, like playing the drum with a brush. It may be very loud or very soft and heard only on expiration, only with deep inspiration, or only with the patient sitting and leaning forward. Classically, three components—presystolic, early systolic, and early diastolic—are present, but not infrequently only one or two components may be heard. The intensity of the rub can vary considerably during the day.

Recurrent Pericarditis. Pleuritic pain is present; however, a friction rub may or may not be heard.

Constrictive Pericarditis. The diagnosis is often appreciated from examination of the neck veins. Venous pressure is very high and the Y descent is rapid. An early diastolic sound—a *pericardial knock*—is sometimes heard and felt. Pulsus paradox may be found.

Pericardial Effusion Causing Cardiac Tamponade. The chief findings include external jugular venous engorgement, a rapid X descent, pulsus paradoxus, a rapid heart rate, low blood pressure, soft heart sounds, and often a friction rub.

REFERENCES

1. Lewis T. Remarks on early signs of cardiac failure of the congestive type. *Br Med J* 1930;1:849.
2. Butman SM, Ewy GA, Standen JR, et al. Bedside cardiovascular examination in patients with severe chronic heart failure: importance of rest or inducible jugular venous distention. *J Am Coll Cardiol* 1993;22:968–74.
3. Benchemol A, Tippit HC. The clinical value of the jugular and hepatic pulses. *Prog Cardiovasc Dis* 1967;10:159–85.
4. Ducas J, Magder S, McGregor M. Validity of the hepato-jugular reflux as a clinical test for congestive heart failure. *Am J Cardiol* 1983;52:1299–1303.
5. Ewy GA. The abdomino-jugular test: technique and hemodynamic correlates. *Ann Intern Med* 1988; 109:456–60.
5a. James Mackenzie. *The study of the pulse, arterial, venous and hepatic, and the movements of the heart.* Edinburgh: Pentland, 1902.
6. Brockenbrough EC, Braunwald E, Morrow AG. A hemodynamic technique for the detection of hypertrophic subaortic stenosis. *Circulation* 1961;23:189–94.
7. Hurst JW. The physical examination, in cardiovascular diagnosis: the initial examination. St. Louis: Mosby, 1993:141–6.
8. Levine SA, Harvey WP. *Clinical auscultation of the heart.* Philadelphia: W.B. Saunders, 1949:145–6.

SUGGESTED READING

Abrams J. *Essentials of cardiac physical diagnosis.* Philadelphia: Lea & Febiger, 1987.
Constant J. *Bedside cardiology.* 2nd ed. Boston: Little, Brown, 1976.

Dalen JE, Alpert JS. *Valvular heart disease.* 2nd ed. Boston/Toronto: Little, Brown, 1987.

Emery RW, Arom KV. *The aortic valve.* Philadelphia: Hanley & Belfus, 1991.

Fye WB. *William Osler's collected papers on the cardiovascular system.* The Classics of Cardiology Library. Birmingham, England: Gryphon, 1985.

Harvey WP. *Cardiac pearls.* Newton, New Jersey: Laennec, 1993.

Hurst JW. *Cardiovascular diagnosis: the initial examination.* St. Louis: Mosby, 1993.

Marriott HJL. *Bedside cardiac diagnosis.* Philadelphia: J.B. Lippincott, 1993.

O'Rourke MF, Kelly RP, Avolio AP. The arterial pulse. Philadelphia: Lea & Febiger, 1992.

Perloff J. *The clinical recognition of congenital heart disease.* 4th ed. Philadelphia: W.B. Saunders, 1994.

Roberts WC. *Adult congenital heart disease.* Philadelphia: F.A. Davis, 1987.

Clinical Skills for Adult Primary Care
edited by M. E. Silverman and J. W. Hurst.
Lippincott-Raven Publishers, Philadelphia © 1996.

13

Examination of the Peripheral Arteries and Veins

*Stephen M. Barnett, M.D., and †Mark E. Silverman, M.D.

*Piedmont Hospital, Atlanta, Georgia 30309; and †Emory University School of Medicine,
Atlanta, Georgia 30322 and Piedmont Hospital, Atlanta, Georgia 30309

"There is no disease more conducive to clinical humility than aneurysm of the aorta."
William Osler, quoted in Bean WB. *Sir William Osler: Aphorisms.*
Springfield, IL: Charles C Thomas, 1968:138.

The evaluation of the peripheral vasculature encompasses an examination of the arteries and veins and an indirect measurement of blood pressure. A normal examination provides an initial data base with which future findings may be compared. Abnormal findings formulate the basis for further investigation, based on symptomatology. The elements of the vascular examination are inspection, palpation, and auscultation. Information from the patient's history helps to focus the examination. Supplementary tools useful to the examiner include the stethoscope, sphygmomanometer, Doppler ultrasound velocity detector, and a tuning fork. Findings should be recorded in an organized format for future use.

TECHNIQUE OF MEASURING ARTERIAL PRESSURE

The arterial blood pressure is indirectly measured using a compression cuff containing an inflatable rubber bag. The bag should have a width that is 20% greater than the diameter of the arm and a length that encircles two-thirds of the arm. Initially, the cuff is inflated to a pressure greater than the systolic pressure as determined by feeling the radial pulse. By measuring the palpable systolic pressure first, an auscultatory gap will not be missed and the true systolic pressure will be correctly estimated by auscultation. The cuff is then inflated above the palpable pressure and slowly deflated at a rate of 3 to 5 mm Hg/second. The diaphragm of the stethoscope is firmly held over the brachial artery with the thumb on top and the fingers behind the arm while the examiner listens for the appearance and disappearance of the Korotkoff sounds. The peak systolic pressure is taken at the point where the first tapping sound is heard for two consecutive beats. The diastolic pressure in adults is recorded as the point where all sounds disappear. In children and in patients with a hyperkinetic circulation, the diastolic pressure is the point where the Korotkoff sounds muffle. A mean pressure can be estimated by adding one-third of the difference between the systolic and diastolic pressure to the diastolic pressure.

The normal middle-aged or younger adult systolic blood pressure can be as high as 140 mm Hg or as low as 100 mm Hg; the normal diastolic pressure is between 60 and 90 mm Hg. The systolic pressure may decrease as much as 10 mm Hg with inspiration. The blood pressure should be taken in at least one arm (and often both) sitting and, if indicated by symptoms or medications, lying down, then standing.

If the blood pressure is elevated, a coarctation of the aorta should be considered. The femoral arterial pulses are felt and compared with the carotid arterial pulses. If the femoral pulse is weak or absent, a blood pressure is determined by auscultating in the popliteal area while slowly deflating a thigh-sized cuff around the proximal leg.

In patients with orthostatic symptoms, the standing blood pressure may be taken repetitively for 5 to 15 minutes to see if a delayed decrease occurs.

Examination of the Arteries

Technique

Inspection of the patient is performed looking for asymmetry, atrophy, absence of digits or extremities, paralysis, surgical scars, and variations in skin color and integrity. The color and thickness of the nails and the presence or absence of digital hair are noted.

Superficial palpation shows information regarding temperature, turgor, tenderness, and thrills. Deeper palpation is performed to assess the status of the arteries. Arterial pulsations should be evaluated with regard to intensity, contour, width, and symmetry. Variations are noteworthy. The magnitude of the pulsation is graded and recorded using a subjective system. Consistency by the individual examiner is most important. A useful and reproducible scale is shown in Table 1.

The superficial temporal artery is palpable anterior to the ear and continues onto the forehead within several millimeters of the hairline. The carotid artery lies

TABLE 1. *Scale assessing magnitude of arterial pulsation*

4+	Increased arterial pulsation
3+	Normal arterial pulsation
2+	Mildly decreased arterial pulsation
1+	Significantly decreased or barely palpable arterial pulsation
0	No palpable arterial pulsation

along the anterior margin of the sternocleidomastoid muscle. Palpation should be performed gently with the patient recumbent. Simultaneous bilateral palpation of the carotids can be performed with a light touch; however, moderate pressure should be avoided. When stimulated, a hypersensitive carotid sinus can, on rare occasions, cause a serious slowing of the heart rate or even a cardiac arrest. The subclavian artery may be felt behind the upper side of the clavicle. Bending the neck toward the side being examined facilitates subclavian artery palpation, especially in muscular people. The arteries of the arm are usually palpated most easily by supporting the patient's arm with one hand while palpating with the fingers of the other hand. The axillary artery is felt best behind the head of the pectoralis muscle while the arm is held out at 90 degrees. The brachial artery may be felt above the antecubital crease, along the bicipital groove just medial to the biceps tendon, while the patient's arm is held with the hand in the thumb-up position. The radial artery is best palpated at the wrist. The patient's hand is held with the palm up, the wrist in a neutral position, and the fingers slightly flexed. The Allen test is used to assess patency of the radial and ulnar arteries and the palmar arch. It is performed by compressing both the radial and ulnar artery at the wrist after the patient makes a tight fist (Fig. 1A–C). The hand is then opened, showing palmar and digital pallor. The examiner then releases one vessel and observes the time for return of normal color throughout the hand and fingers, thus demonstrating patency of the released vessel and adequate collateral flow via the palmar arch. The test is repeated, releasing the other vessel. Normally, the hand and fingers will pink up quickly. With compromised flow, the pallor persists for at least several more seconds.

Examination of the abdominal aorta is performed with the patient recumbent and the legs supported and slightly flexed, thereby relaxing the abdominal muscles. Normally, the aorta is palpable in the midline between the tip of the xiphoid and the umbilicus. The bifurcation of the aorta is usually found at the level of the umbilicus. The fingers of each hand are used to locate the aorta by gently increasing downward pressure until the aortic pulsation is felt with each hand (Fig. 2). The aortic width is estimated by measuring the distance between the fingers. Examination of the abdominal aorta is dependent on the patient's size. In thin people, the iliac arteries may be palpable along the sides of the rectus muscle below the umbilicus.

The femoral artery is most easily palpated just below the inguinal ligament in the medial aspect of each groin. The patient should be recumbent and the foot rotated slightly outward. Palpation of the popliteal artery can be more difficult. The patient should be recumbent with the knees slightly bent. Both thumbs are placed on the patella while the third and fourth fingers of each hand are positioned directly on the popliteal fossa behind the knee (Fig. 3). Anterior-posterior pressure is increased until the pulse is felt. Alternatively, the patient may be sitting with the legs hanging freely and the same maneuver used. Another method is to place the patient face down on the examining surface, flex the knee with one hand, and palpate for the pulse with the thumb of the other hand while the fingers apply

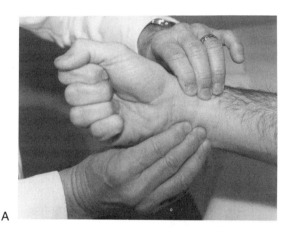

A

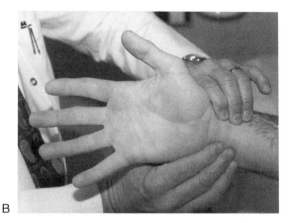

B

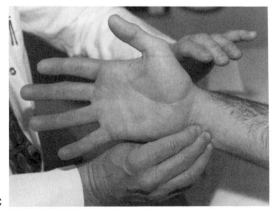

C

FIG. 1. Allen test. **A:** Hand is first clenched, then both radial and ulner arteries are compressed. **B:** Hand is opened while both arteries are still compressed. **C:** One artery is released while rate of return of blood flow is checked.

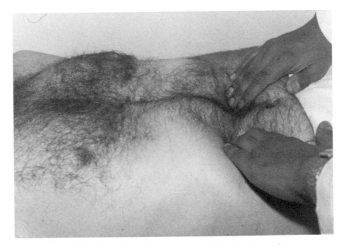

FIG. 2. Technique for palpating abdominal aorta.

counterpressure against the patella. This last position may be uncomfortable or difficult for many patients and should be avoided in frail people.

The pedal vessels may be examined with the patient sitting or supine. The posterior tibial artery is felt best at the ankle by applying gentle pressure to the soft tissue behind the medial malleolus (Fig. 4). Occasionally, the continuation of this artery can be felt on the plantar surface underlying the shaft of the first metatarsal. The dorsalis pedis artery is the continuation of the anterior tibial artery. It may be

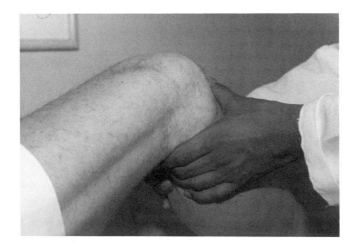

FIG. 3. Technique for palpating popliteal arterial pulsation.

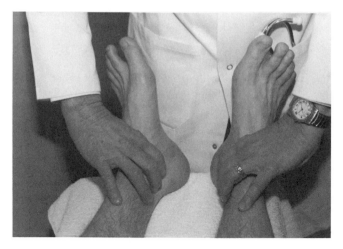

FIG. 4. Technique for palpating posterior tibial arterial pulsations.

absent in up to 10% of normal people. This pulse is generally palpable just below the ankle lateral to the tendon of the extensor hallicus longus (Fig. 5).

Auscultation is generally performed over the carotid artery, the anterior border of the sternocleidomastoid muscle, the superior border of the clavicle, over the abdomen between the xiphoid and umbilicus, between the umbilicus and each groin, and over both flanks and both groins. Bruits are recorded and subjectively graded as soft or harsh. The length of the bruit may be significant.

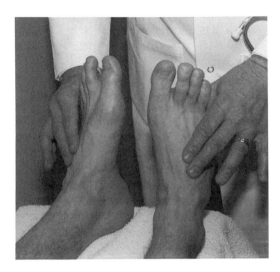

FIG. 5. Technique for palpating dorsalis pedis arterial pulsations.

A Doppler ultrasound probe can be useful to assess arterial flow. Conductive gel is placed over the vessel to be examined, and the probe is then placed at a 45 to 60 degree angle over the vessel. The nature of the signal is recorded as triphasic (three components), biphasic (two components), or monophasic (one component). The intensity of the signal is recorded as weak, moderate, or strong. Using pressure cuffs placed around the thigh or calf and listening with the Doppler probe over the pedal vessels, segmental pressures can be estimated. The ratio of the ankle pressure and brachial pressure is calculated as the ankle/brachial index. Normally, the index is 1 or greater. Vibratory sense can be tested by placing a vibrating tuning fork firmly against the tissues overlying the metatarsal head and recording the duration of the perceived vibration.

Normal Findings

Arteries are normally soft, smooth, and compressible. When arterial flow is occluded by a tourniquet or cuff, the distal vessel cannot be palpated. The arterial pulse rapidly expands the width of the vessel as blood flows through the lumen in systole. As the pressure decreases during diastole, the vessel caliber narrows. The rhythmic ebb and flow of the blood conveys a sense of elasticity. The smooth contour of the artery is free of angulations and bulbous protrusions. The caliber is variable, but should be symmetrical. The abdominal aortic width should not exceed 3 cm in lateral measurement. A prominent aortic pulsation in the anterior-posterior plane is not necessarily aneurysmal but may reflect a tortuous vessel or merely a small body habitus. Arterial pulses may be more prominent in the elderly due to loss of subcutaneous tissues and elongation or ectasia of the vessels. These findings are especially noted in the subclavian and carotid arteries.

Abnormal Findings

Sclerotic Arteries

The elderly artery may stiffen, lose its normal elasticity, and be unable to cushion the force of ventricular systole. This results in a more forceful arterial pulse and a higher systolic blood pressure. This can be recognized by palpating a cord-like radial vessel after occluding proximal flow with a finger or blood pressure cuff and emptying the vessel by pressing it against the bone. If the emptied vessel feels as prominent as when full, the vessel is sclerotic. This is known as *Osler's sign* (1).

Acute Arterial Insufficiency

Etiology includes embolus (clot, myxoma, cholesterol plaque), trauma, and compression. The involved extremity may be pale, mottled, or bluish, and may be asymmetrically cold. Livedo reticularis (reddish blue, netlike mottling) may be seen. Capillary refilling of the compressed skin and nails may be delayed or absent. Pain may be present or may have abated; tenderness may not be elicited, reflecting anesthetic changes. Sensation, especially to light touch, and motor strength may be reduced or absent. Pulses may be reduced or absent. If the etiology is penetrating trauma, the presence of a palpable thrill, a bruit, or a continuous murmur may denote an acute arteriovenous fistula. Doppler signals may be diminished or absent.

Chronic Arterial Insufficiency

The characteristic complaint due to chronic arterial insufficiency, most commonly due to atherosclerosis, is pain with use, relief with rest. The pain is usually burning or cramplike and involves the muscle groups distal to the arterial narrowing. Many patients experience muscle weakness without pain. Occlusive disease of the distal aorta or both iliac arteries provokes weakness and pain in the gluteal region as well as the thighs; when coupled with male impotence, this is known as the *Leriche syndrome.* Isolated iliac occlusion may cause unilateral gluteal or thigh symptoms. Superficial femoral artery disease causes typical symptoms of intermittent claudication in the calf of the affected leg. Popliteal and tibial vessel disease may likewise provoke pain in the calf with activity.

Spinal stenosis often mimics the symptoms of intermittent claudication and is referred to as *pseudoclaudication* or *neurogenic claudication.* Because this disorder is caused by nerve compression, the arterial examination is generally normal. Exercise tolerance should be quantitated in terms of distance walked on flat terrain, elevated terrain, or number of stairs ascended.

Occlusive disease of the upper extremity also may provoke pain with use. Upper extremity ischemia is clinically far less frequent than leg pain because of the rich collaterals in the arm and a lower incidence of significant disease in this vascular distribution. Hemispheric neurologic symptoms provoked by use of the arm—the *subclavian steal syndrome*—is caused by proximal blockage in the subclavian artery with retrograde collateral flow via the ipsilateral carotid and vertebral circulation to the distal subclavian artery. With mild to moderate chronic arterial insufficiency, the skin may become thin or shiny, progressing to rubor, which may be exaggerated with dependency or activity. Hair may disappear over the affected area, and the nails may be thickened. A bruit may be audible over a stenotic vessel proximal to the affected region. Pulses may be diminished or absent and may disappear with exercise. The Doppler signal may be weak or monophasic. Blood pressure in the affected extremity will be decreased with an ankle/brachial index usually less than 0.7, although the recorded pressure may be falsely elevated with calcified or incompressible vessels. The pressure may diminish further with exercise. More severe chronic arterial insufficiency is associated with pain at rest and usually involves the foot (characteristically across the instep). This pain is due to ischemia of the nerves and portends impending tissue loss. It may be absent in patients with peripheral neuropathy. Absence of vibratory sense, elicited by placing a vibrating tuning fork on the skin overlying the metatarsal head, implies peripheral neuropathy. The skin may be thin, tight and shiny, ruborous, pale, or dusky. Ulcers may appear on or between the digits, or over pressure areas such as the malleoli. Pulses are commonly absent, and Doppler signals are usually weak and monophasic or absent. The ankle/brachial index is usually less than 0.5 but may be falsely elevated. These flagrant findings are often the result of occlusion at several arterial sites rather than isolated occlusion. Patients with prior amputations may develop progressive arterial insufficiency; the onset of stump pain (as opposed to phantom pain, in which the patient experiences itching or pain in the amputated tissues) may herald tissue breakdown.

Vasospastic Disorders

Vasospastic disorders, such as Raynaud's phenomenon, generally provoke digital pain during exposure to cold. Rubor of the fingertips may progress to blanching, and peripheral pulses are diminished or absent. Symptoms are usually episodic and reproducible with cold exposure.

Cholesterol Embolization

Cholesterol emboli, flaking off of severe aortic atherosclerosis, may cause diffuse or focal discoloration, gangrene, or the sudden onset of digital pain and ischemia (*blue toe syndrome*). Livedo reticularis is sometimes present. The onset is usually acute and may follow arterial catheterization, cardiac surgery, or be spontaneous. Peripheral and even digital pulses may remain palpable, and tissues proximal to the microemboli are undisturbed. Repeated episodes are common, producing extensive tissue damage.

Buerger's Disease

Buerger's disease (*thromboangiitis obliterans*) is a chronic disorder of uncertain etiology in which inflammatory changes in the arteriolar wall leads to progressive ischemic rest pain in the hands, fingers, feet, and toes. The physical findings include diminished radial, ulnar, and pedal pulses, and skin changes due to chronic arterial insufficiency.

Abdominal Aortic Aneurysm

Abdominal aortic aneurysms may be asymptomatic or present dramatically. A pulsatile mass located above the umbilicus estimated to be greater than 3 cm wide should suggest an aortic aneurysm. Associated back, flank, groin, testicular, or abdominal pain heightens suspicion and requires urgent investigation. Plain abdominal X-ray films, abdominal ultrasound, and computerized axial tomography are useful tests to define the problem. Aneurysms that have lost their integrity may leak slowly or rapidly, the latter provoking more intense pain. With significant blood loss, mottling of the abdominal wall and/or extremities may be noted; pulses may become thready or absent; and the blood pressure may decrease to hypotensive levels, indicating an emergency situation. Although the peripheral pulses may be abnormal because of associated atherosclerotic vascular disease, the aneurysm itself does not compromise the peripheral circulation and the status of the distal arterial pulses is not useful.

Aortic Dissection

Aortic dissection develops from an intimal tear of the aorta or, rarely, without a tear. Blood driving between the intima and adventitial layers creates a false lumen and a double-barrelled aorta. A significant widening of the aorta gives rise to the term *dissecting aortic aneurysm*. Aortic dissections often occur in association with hypertension. The proximal aorta just above the aortic valve and the descending aorta at the origin of the left subclavian artery are the most frequent starting sites. The sudden onset of severe, ripping, midline chest pain is characteristic. Major findings relate to which vessels are occluded by the dissection. A stroke is common when the dissection involves the aortic arch. Often the false channel provides adequate arterial flow and no ischemic findings develop. If flow through the false channel is inadequate, ischemia or infarction in the unperfused tissue occurs. Depending on the level and extent of the dissection, arterial pulses may be diminished in one or both arms, in one or both carotid arteries, in visceral vessels, in one or both legs, or in any combination. In a proximal (type A) aortic dissection, the normal suspension of the aortic valve may be altered and an acute murmur of aortic regurgitation can be heard.

Arteriovenous Fistula

An arteriovenous fistula may be congenital or acquired. Acquired causes include penetrating trauma, biopsies, catheter insertions, surgery, aneurysms, cancer, and atherosclerosis. A communication between a large artery and vein is detected by listening for a continuous, roaring noise over the area. Listening over scars, biopsy sites, and insertions of catheters may be rewarding. A rapid resting heart rate, increased stroke volume, and low diastolic pressure are signs of a large arteriovenous fistula. Over time, heart failure may develop. When the artery leading to a large arteriovenous fistula is occluded by sudden compression, the heart rate slows. This is known as *Branham's sign*.

EXAMINATION OF THE VEINS

Technique and Anatomy

Inspection should be performed in a well-lit room. The legs are inspected with the patient standing. The greater saphenous vein may be seen just anterior to the medial malleolus. It continues upward along the medial aspect of the calf, across the knee joint on its medial surface, along the medial aspect of the thigh, and enters the deep venous system several centimeters below the inguinal ligament. The lesser saphenous vein originates near the lateral side of the Achilles tendon and continues up the posterolateral calf, terminating in the popliteal fossa. When these veins are visible, they are normally straight and of relatively constant size. The skin overlying the course of these veins is carefully inspected for variation in color, thickness, or signs of healed scars or ulcers. The presence and distribution of secondary venous networks and capillary beds are noted.

The legs should also be palpated while the patient is standing. Superficial palpation along the course of the greater and lesser saphenous veins shows information regarding tenderness, thickness, and compressibility. The presence, extent, and anatomic distribution of edema are noted. Deep palpation is performed and tenderness noted.

Normal Findings

When superficial veins are visible, they are of uniform caliber and contour. There should be no variation in skin consistency or color. When palpable, the veins are soft, supple, and not tender. The walls are thin and the blood can be evacuated by gentle digital compression.

Abnormal Findings

Varicose Veins

The most common disorder of the venous system is varicose veins. Afflicted patients may have no symptoms or may complain of burning or aching pain, itching, or swelling. The pain is often relieved by leg elevation. A hereditary tendency is common. Other etiologic factors relate to pregnancy, obesity, prolonged standing, and a past history of thrombophlebitis. Primary varicosities involve the greater and lesser saphenous veins, and afflicted veins are dilated and tortuous. The overlying skin may be coarse, and dermatitis may be present. Venous insufficiency occurs due to dilatation of the vessel and associated venous valvular incompetence. The insufficiency may be limited to the superficial venous system, the perforating veins communicating between the superficial and deep system, or the deep venous system. When perforating veins are affected, they are often visible as focal dilatations and can be palpable as they exit through the fascia. Deep venous insufficiency is often accompanied by significant edema, more advanced stasis dermatitis characterized by red-blue discoloration, or brown discoloration due to hemosiderin deposition. Venous ulcers are more likely to occur when deep venous insufficiency is present. The *Trendelenburg test* is useful in demonstrating incompetence. The patient is placed in the recumbent position and the legs are elevated to empty the veins. The saphenous vein is compressed with a tourniquet or finger, and the patient then stands. The compression is released and the recurrence of venous dilatation is observed. If incompetent perforating veins are present, the superficial veins will dilate before the release of superficial compression.

Thrombophlebitis

The characteristic findings in acute thrombophlebitis are pain and swelling of the involved vein. The surrounding area may be red and tender. Findings are quite varied, however, and patients may experience only tightness or even no symptoms at all. Superficial phlebitis may be manifest by a tender, firm, red cutaneous vein. The acute onset of edema and thigh pain implies the presence of ileofemoral thrombosis. Few findings may accompany deep venous thrombophlebitis, and noninvasive Doppler studies, including ultrasound imaging (duplex scan), are most useful when this diagnosis is suspected. *Phlegmasia cerulea dolens* is the most severe and dramatic presentation of acute venous thrombosis. It is characterized by the rapid onset of leg edema accompanied by blue or violet discoloration of the skin. Diffuse cyanosis and bullae supervene, accompanied by a decrease in arterial pulsation. Unchecked, this disorder commonly eventuates in massive tissue loss and even death.

REFERENCE

1. Osler W, McCrae T. *Diseases of the arteries. Modern medicine, its theory and practice.* Philadelphia: Lea & Febiger, 1908:426–47.

SUGGESTED READING

Crawford ES, Crawford JL. *Diseases of the aorta.* Baltimore: Williams & Williams, 1984.

Haimovici H. *Vascular surgery.* 3rd ed. Norwalk: Appleton & Lange, 1989.

Joyce JW. Examination of the patient with vascular disease. In: Loscalzo J, Creager MA, Dzau VJ, eds. *Vascular medicine.* Boston: Little, Brown, 1992:401–18.

Lindsay J Jr. Aortic dissection. In: Lindsay J Jr., ed. *Diseases of the aorta.* Philadelphia: Lea & Febiger, 1994:127–43.

Miller DC, Roon AJ. *Diagnosis and management of peripheral vascular disease.* Menlo Park: Addison-Wesley, 1982.

Pousti TJ, Wilson SE, Williams RA. Clinical examination of the vascular system. In: Veith FJ, Hobson RW, Williams RA, Wilson SE, eds. *Vascular surgery.* 2nd ed. New York: McGraw-Hill, 1994:74–89.

Clinical Skills for Adult Primary Care
edited by M. E. Silverman and J. W. Hurst.
Lippincott-Raven Publishers, Philadelphia © 1996.

14

Examination of the Abdomen and Rectum

Valerie J. Jagiella, M.D.

Piedmont Hospital, Atlanta, Georgia 30309

"The chief function of the consultant is to make a rectal examination that you have omitted."

William Osler, quoted in Bean WB. *Sir William Osler: Aphorisms.*
Springfield, IL: Charles C Thomas, 1968:104.

The history of gastroenterology and liver disease dates back to antiquity. In the third century B.C., Praxagoras performed surgery for a strangulated hernia and seems to have made an artificial anus. Traditional Japanese medicine emphasized the abdominal examination because of the belief that most illnesses declare themselves by abdominal symptoms categorized in 16 forms. Presently, the examination of the abdomen and rectum play an important part in evaluating a patient. The history is extremely useful in directing attention to specific areas of the abdomen. Inspection, palpation, percussion, and auscultation are the primary elements of physical diagnosis. It is generally recommended that the same sequence be followed each time to avoid overlooking anything of importance. With the abdominal examination, the sequence is usually auscultation before palpation and percussion (1). This can directly follow cardiovascular auscultation.

TECHNIQUE

Abdominal Topography

When examining the abdomen, the location of the findings must be evaluated in a systematic and descriptive way using specific terminology. There are basically two ways to map the abdominal surface (1). The most commonly used map divides the abdomen into four quadrants: the right and left upper quadrants and the right and left lower quadrants. This map divides the organs according to location (Fig. 1A). Less commonly in the United States, but frequently elsewhere, the abdominal area is divided into nine sections. With this division, there are two imaginary parallel, horizontal lines crossing the lower border of the costal mar-

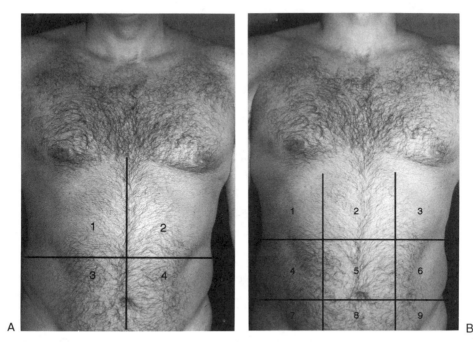

A   B

FIG. 1. Map of abdominal surface. **A:** Four-quadrant map: 1, right upper quadrant; 2, left upper quadrant; 3, right lower quadrant; 4, left lower quadrant. **B:** Nine-area map: 1, right hypochondriac; 2, epigastric; 3, left hypochondriac; 4, right lumbar; 5, umbilical; 6, left lumbar; 7, right inguinal; 8, hypogastric; 9, left inguinal.

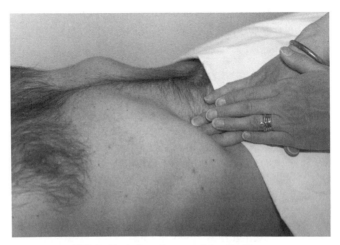

FIG. 2. Technique for examining the liver.

gins and at the level of the anterior-superior aspects of the iliac crests. There are two vertical lines descending from the midclavicular line approximately aligned with the lateral border of the abdominal recti muscles. With this system, the surface of the abdomen is divided into nine areas: the right hypochondriac, epigastric, left hypochondriac, right lumbar, umbilical, left lumbar, right inguinal, hypogastric, and left inguinal quadrants (Fig. 2B).

There are other anatomic landmarks that are useful in the description of pain, tenderness, and other abnormal findings. These basic landmarks include the xiphoid process, the costal margin, the epigastric area, the umbilicus, the anterior-superior iliac spine, Poupart's ligament (which is in the lower abdomen), and the superior margin of the os pubis. The back forms the posterior wall of the abdomen and should not be overlooked. This part of the examination is more easily performed when examining the lungs and spine with the patient sitting.

INSPECTION

The patient should be suitably draped for the examination. Observation should be accomplished first, and can be done while auscultating the area. One approach is to ask the patient to point to the area(s) of pain and then to place the stethoscope over that area. The patient then understands that the physician is listening to their complaints and is paying attention to the area involved. This does not imply that palpation is done with a stethoscope at that moment. Inspection includes the overall appearance of the patient, including the skin color, and findings such as the stigmata of liver disease. The patient's breath should be sniffed at the same time.

Normal Findings

The contour of the abdomen can be flat, rounded, or scaphoid. No asymmetry or localized bulges should be visible. In women, respiratory movement is mainly costal and little abdominal wall movement is seen. In men, respiration is predominately abdominal. Normally, the veins coursing in the abdominal wall are barely visible or not seen. When present, the venous flow is cephalad for those veins above the umbilicus and caudad for those veins below.

Abnormal Findings

The side profile of the abdomen can help distinguish the underlying area of pathology. Distention of the lower half or third is more consistent with ovarian tumors, pregnancy, bladder distention, or uterine fibroids. If the distention is in the upper half, gastric distention, a pancreatic cyst, or carcinomatosis should be considered. Generalized distention with an inverted umbilicus is often due to obesity or abdominal gas; if the umbilicus is everted, ascites and/or an umbilical hernia should be considered. Respiratory movement should be noted. Compromise in the abdominal respiratory movement can be due to disease below the diaphragm, especially peritonitis. Markings, such as stretch marks and ecchymoses, may be seen on the abdomen. Striae are usually red, but sometimes purple as in idiopathic Cushing's syndrome or postpregnancy. Cullen's or Turner's signs, a hemorrhagic discoloration of the abdominal wall, are the same entity. Unfortunately, this sign is not sensitive for intraabdominal hemorrhage from pancreatitis or a ruptured ectopic pregnancy. Moreover, the sign usually becomes visible late, around the second to sixth hospital day. Venous markings should be looked for. A reversal in the direction of venous blood flow is seen with obstruction of the inferior vena cava and in portal hypertension. Unfortunately, the direction of venous flow can be difficult to ascertain. Compressing, then decompressing the vein and watching for the direction of venous flow may be nondiagnostic. Nevertheless, it should be attempted when indicated. Characteristic odors that can be identified include acetone (diabetic ketoacidosis), fetor (liver failure), fetid (esophageal diverticulum or lung abscess), or feculent (bowel obstruction) (1). Physicians with a genetic ability to identify the aroma of bitter almond may be able to diagnose cyanide poisoning as well.

AUSCULTATION

Auscultation of the abdomen can be useful to identify the presence or absence of bowel sounds, bruits, or rubs. The diaphragm of the stethoscope is used to auscultate the abdomen because it accentuates the high-pitched sounds. Faint peristaltic sounds can be missed with the bell; however, the bell is often preferred when listening for arterial bruits and venous hums. Proficiency occurs with time and practice (1). Auscultatory sounds can be classified by their source, i.e., visceral, arterial, muscular activity sounds, venous hums, and parietal friction rubs.

Normal Findings

In the normal abdomen, bowel sounds caused by interfaced fluid and air are always present but vary in frequency, intensity, and pitch, depending primarily on the phase of digestion. Due to the complexity of the sounds, the examiner must establish a normal basis of comparison after having listened to the peristalsis of numerous healthy patients (1).

Abnormal Findings

The prevalence of an epigastric systolic bruit in normal adults is as high as 16%. The diagnosis of decreased bowel sounds is a difficult one to make because bowel sounds can intermittently be present. Only a complete absence of bowel sounds for several minutes is considered significant. Clinical conditions that may produce changes in peristaltic sounds include a variety of surgical and medical problems. Absent peristalsis occurs with an ileus from peritonitis, advanced intestinal obstruction, mesenteric thrombosis, pneumonia, myxedema, severe electrolyte abnormalities, and spinal cord injury. Increased peristalsis is frequently seen with diarrhea and early pyloric or intestinal obstruction.

Bruits may indicate aortic disease or stenosis of the celiac or superior mesenteric artery. Renal vascular disease can be diagnosed by the finding of a systolic bruit, especially when the bruit is continuous. Massive splenic enlargement can sometimes produce a left upper quadrant systolic bruit. A hepatic venous hum can be present with portal hypertension. It disappears with pressure from the stethoscope. In the right upper quadrant, hepatic bruits have been associated with cirrhosis, Hodgkin's disease, and aortoportal fistulas. Peritoneal friction rubs usually occur over the liver or spleen. These rubs may be heard by having the patient inspire during auscultation over the area. The most common rub is probably due to splenic infarction and is usually best heard at the left lower costal margin along the anterior axillary line. Friction rubs from the liver can be heard in cases of hepatoma, cholangiocarcinoma, and metastatic carcinoma. They are often present the day of a liver biopsy. They are not as frequent in inflammatory conditions but can be heard in cases of pyogenic abscesses; viral, autoimmune, or alcoholic hepatitis; cholecystitis; tuberculosis; peritonitis; and hepatitis due to lupus erythematosus or a gonococcal infection. If a bruit coexists, tumor is the most likely etiology. A rub also can be heard over an inflamed gallbladder, but this is uncommon. Finally, a succussion splash should be considered. A succussion splash may be heard when there is retained fluid in the stomach or other intestinal organs. This can be helpful when evaluating the patient for possible delayed gastric emptying or gastric outlet obstruction. It is also present at times with a dilated small bowel, particularly when the dilation is proximal to a stricture, as in patients with Crohn's disease.

PALPATION

Palpation of the abdomen is probably the most sensitive and fruitful part of the examination. It can confirm findings noted with inspection and auscultation. Palpation is expected by the patient, especially if there is a complaint of abdominal pain. The physician will "feel where it hurts."

Technique

After evaluating the chest wall and back, especially the flank areas, the patient is placed in the supine position with the legs flat on the table or flexed at the knees, the arms at the side, and the head relaxed. The examiner's hands are important. They should be warm without long fingernails, which could hurt the patient. Finger pads are used for tactile discrimination. The dorsal surface of the hands or fingers are helpful for sensing temperature. The palmar aspect is best for vibration. The fingers also can grasp and help the physician determine the consistency of organs and masses. The technique of palpating the abdomen may vary, depending on whether the patient is having abdominal pain. There are different levels of palpation. Light palpation, considered the scouting expedition, is followed by deeper palpation (1). Light palpation warms up the abdomen and scouts the area by feeling superficially, trying to avoid any unnecessary pain, while checking for skin turgor and possible edema. The examiner also can check for areas of cutaneous hypersensitivity.

Deeper palpation is then performed. Resistance to palpation beyond the superficial layers of the abdomen is noted. Voluntary guarding can be diminished by making the patient feel at ease during the scouting phase. The patient can be asked to take deep, slow breaths that may help relax the abdominal muscles. Involuntary muscle rigidity persisting despite maneuvers to try to relax the abdominal wall often indicates peritoneal irritation. Spasticity or tenderness may be localized to one particular area, such as over the right lower abdomen in appendicitis and the left side in diverticulitis. When feeling the abdomen for possible masses, a distinction can be made between an abdominal wall and intraabdominal mass by palpating while the patient raises his or her head. In the case of an intraabdominal mass, the palpating hand cannot feel the mass when the abdominal muscles are tensed; in a patient with an intramural mass, the mass can still be palpated with the patient's head elevated. Deeper palpation is done systematically, usually beginning away from the area of pain. The palpation can be single or double handed. The palmar surface of the hand is placed on the abdominal wall, and the fingers "do the walking," going deeper while trying to delineate the edges of any palpable organ or mass. If a mass is identified, it can sometimes be grasped between the fingers and thumb. Bimanual palpation is sometimes necessary, especially if the mass or organ is large, as with palpation of the kidneys. Ballottement is done using a bimanual technique for the kidneys. With ascites, a single-handed approach is often used. To palpate the liver, the examiner should start by feeling for the lower liver edge. This is accomplished by exerting gentle pressure with the fingertips in the right upper quadrant several centimeters below the right costal margin and asking the patient to breath in gently and slowly to bring the liver edge down (1) (Fig. 2). With each exhalation, the exploring fingers should be moved upward about 2 cm. If the liver edge is not felt, no further palpation is necessary. If, on the other hand, the liver edge is identified, the lower extent of the liver should be followed by palpating medially as far as the left upper quadrant, particularly in the area corresponding to the midclavicular line. The lower edge can be marked and checked with percussion. Palpation may elicit a tender point left of the 12th thoracic vertebra, known as Boas's point, and sometimes found in patients with gastric ulcers. Costovertebral angle tenderness also should be checked.

Three techniques of palpation are useful in identifying splenomegaly; however, percussion is a more sensitive technique and should be used first as a screen.

Two-handed palpation with the patient in the right lateral decubitus position, or supine position, involves placing the left hand around the left lower chest and lifting the lowermost rib cage anteriorly and medially with the right fingertips pressed beneath the left costal margin. While the examiner's hands are held in this position, the patient is asked to take a long, deep breath. A spleen "tip" is felt when the enlarged spleen descends. The one-handed technique is similar, but there is no counterpressure applied by the left hand. If no spleen tip is palpated with the first attempt, the right hand should be placed lower, farther away from the costal margin before the initiation of the examination to avoid missing a large spleen. The hooking maneuver of Middleton requires cooperation from the patient, who places the left fist under the left costovertebral angle while in the supine position. Both hands of the examiner are curled over and under the costal margin, and the patient is asked to take a long, deep breath (2).

Normal Findings

Normal findings on palpation vary according to the patient's size, particularly the degree of obesity and general body build, as well as the ability of the patient to cooperate with the examination (3). Normally palpable abdominal organs may include the epigastric portion of the aorta, the sigmoid colon and cecum, the kidneys, the edge of the liver on inspiration, and occasionally the bladder or uterus (particularly in women). The spleen tip is rarely palpable in a presumed normal population (4). About half the time when a liver edge can be palpated below the costal margin, the actual size of the liver, as determined by scintigraphy or ultrasonography, is within normal limits (3). If the liver edge is palpable, the overall span of the liver must be assessed as discussed under percussion. When the liver is not palpable, the likelihood is that the liver is not enlarged; however, this is not infallible (3).

Abnormal Findings

Hepatomegaly

A palpable liver edge should be traced to feel for increased firmness or lobularity that might indicate cirrhosis or an infiltrative disease. A tumor mass may be palpated along the edge.

Splenomegaly

A palpable spleen should be quantitated by the extent (finger breadths or centimeters below the left costal margin).

Mass

Any mass that is identified should be described by its position, size, contour, consistency, mobility, and in its relation to other abdominal organs and to the abdominal wall. The presence of tenderness should be noted.

Hyperesthesia

Hyperesthesia to light touch in the referred dermatome can occur in patients with an acute abdominal process. *Boas's sign* is hyperesthesia in the right posterior flank area or over the lower right ribs posteriorly and is often related to gallbladder disease and sometimes ulcer disease. In diabetic patients, neuropathy of the thoracoabdominal area can occur and mimic symptoms of intraabdominal pathology, particularly gallbladder disease or appendicitis. Hyperesthesia along a dermatomal distribution should suggest *herpes zoster*. The characteristic skin eruption will often occur several days later.

Hernia of the Abdominal Wall

Any scars should be palpated for a hernia. A hernia of the rectus sheath and umbilicus is common. The patient should be requested to lift his or her head to see if any protrusion occurs through the scar or defect.

Skin Findings

The skin should be felt for turgor, edema, hypersensitivity, subcutaneous crepitus, or a superficial mass. Crepitus is a crackling sound or tactile sensation noted due to air bubbles present under the skin or in underlying structures. While palpating lightly, the consistency of the skin can be felt, especially by grasping some skin between the fingers. Pitting edema, especially of the flanks, should be looked for in patients with possible anasarca or fluid overload.

Abdominal Pain

Palpation in the presence of abdominal pain includes the use of different methods to study for possible rigidity (local guarding), induced guarding, rebound, referred pain, and hyperesthesia.

Abdominal Wall Pain

Carnett described this test in 1926 to differentiate abdominal wall pain from underlying visceral pathology. It also has been called an *abdominal tension test* and consists of two-stage palpation of the tender area of the abdomen (5). The examiner palpates to try to identify the point of maximum tenderness and to ascertain the relationship between the degree of pressure and the degree of discomfort. The patient is asked to rate the abdominal pain. The examiner then asks the patient to tense the abdominal muscles. If the tenderness is within the abdomen itself, the tenderness is reduced or eliminated. If, on the other hand, the tenderness remains at the same intensity or increases with palpation while the abdominal muscles are tense, the source lies in the abdominal wall. Some patients will evince a general pain response by wincing, crying out, or withdrawing when deep pressure identifies the trigger point. A method to induce guarding is to ask patients to cross their arms while supine and then to sit up. The abdomen is palpated as the patient sits up. When the patient reaches halfway between the recumbent and sitting position, the point of maximal abdominal musculature contraction occurs and there is normal guarding. If the tenderness to palpation decreases at this point, the test result is positive and the tenderness is considered intraabdominal. A negative test result is worsening of pain. The predictive value and sensitivity is high for appendiceal abscess, cholecystitis, bowel obstruction, ruptured ovarian cyst, ureteral colic, and urinary tract infection. The predictive value of a negative test result for patients who have no identifiable cause for the pain is close to 100%.

Rebound and Referred Pain Testing

There are several tests for rebound and referred pain (6). *Blumberg's sign* (rebound tenderness) is a pain test for early peritonitis. This is the classic test in which the examiner palpates the tender area as deeply as possible and then abruptly withdraws the palpating hand. If the peritoneum is inflamed, the patient will usually cry out or wince. It is not a helpful test and probably creates unwarranted pain in patients who have unquestionable involuntary rigidity when initially evaluated. After such a maneuver, any further palpation may not be possible due to voluntary guarding from the patient's fear of recurrent pain. There have been some modifications of this test that are useful in patients who are suspected of not being completely cooperative or who are not precise in reporting any sensation. With *referred rebound testing*, abdominal pressure is exerted in an area where there has been no pain. The pressure is again suddenly released, as with the rebound tenderness test. If the patient points to pain in another area of the abdomen while denying pain in the area that was palpated, the test result is considered positive. The test is considered to be useful only if a positive result is obtained.

Abdominal Palpation with a Stethoscope

Abdominal palpation with a stethoscope can be used in patients who are not cooperative or who describe pain with minimal palpation of the abdomen (7). Patients who develop voluntary rigidity with hand palpation can sometimes be palpated with a stethoscope. Auscultation is repeated and the stethoscope is pushed down slowly while listening. If no rigidity occurs, the rigidity with hand palpation is considered voluntary. The stethoscope also can be withdrawn abruptly, as with the rebound test, and the accuracy of the patient's complaints can be confirmed.

PERCUSSION

Percussion of the abdomen can identify bowel or bladder distention, tumors, fluid, free air, and enlarged solid organs.

Technique

The technique involves both hands. Usually the left hand is placed on the abdomen, and the left middle finger is struck with the tip of the right middle finger. Sometimes several of the left fingers will be struck in succession to identify a change in sound in a specific area (such as over the ribs anteriorly when evaluating the liver or spleen) (3). Another technique is fist percussion over the liver, which can produce tenderness in cases of hepatitis, cholecystitis, or liver abscess. The left hand, palm side down, is placed over the area and struck a light blow with the right hand. Percussion seems to be most useful when evaluating the liver span but is also helpful to identify the spleen and possible ascites. The best technique for evaluating the size of the liver appears to be a combination of palpation for the edge and percussion for the span of the liver (3). The scratch test using the stethoscope over the costal margin has been shown to be less accurate than palpation alone to identify the true liver edge. The vertical liver span is measured by

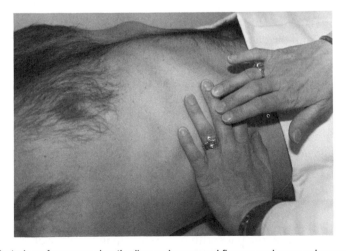

FIG. 3. Technique for percussing the liver using several fingers and percussing each in turn.

percussion at the midclavicular line. However, it is difficult to determine the precise midclavicular line (8). The best way would be to use a tape measure; most examiners palpate the ends of the clavicle and usually estimate the midpoint. Variability seems greatest in obese patients, and clinical estimates are frequently closer to the midsternal line than anticipated. One of the best techniques for percussion of the liver is to percuss down the midclavicular line beginning about the level of the third rib. The pleximeter finger is moved progressively downward. Resonance from the lung will be heard first. As the finger is moved from one rib space to the next, the tone will change at the level of the interposition of the dome of the liver with the air-filled lung. There is usually a gradation of increasing dullness. A good technique to confirm the increased dullness is to lay the entire left hand across several ribs, spreading two or three pleximeter fingers over adjacent rib spaces, then percussing each quickly (back and forth) (3) (Fig. 3). The percussion should go from greater to lesser resonance and vice versa. If the patient is asked to take a deep breath and hold it, percussion will then elicit an unequivocal increase in resonance at one rib space. This will help confirm the upper border of the liver. The examiner should always try to identify the upper and lower borders of the liver in quiet respiration or with deep inspiration. Both borders should be measured at the same phase of respiration. The lower edge of the liver also can be determined by percussion; however, palpation is more reliable because of the thin edge of the liver. Moreover, palpation can help delineate any abnormality in the consistency of the liver or any mass on the liver edge. Studies using ultrasound and scintigraphy have validated that correct liver span can be determined clinically when percussion and palpation are combined and that direct percussion of the liver along the midclavicular line can be accurate (9). Measurement is especially useful when following certain patients in fulminant hepatic failure to document reduction in liver size (3).

The spleen should be percussed before palpation is attempted. If no splenic dullness is elicited by the following approaches, palpation is not necessary (4). Three percussion methods for identifying the spleen have been validated when compared with ultrasonography or scintigraphy (4). These include Nixon's, Castell's, and Traube's methods. Nixon's method, modified by Sullivan and Williams, involves placing the patient in the right lateral decubitus position and percussing the left costal area. The left costal margin is identified, and, at its halfway point, percussion is initiated and extended upward along a perpendicular line from the costal margin. Normally, dullness extends no more than 8 cm above the costal margin (Fig. 4). Using Castell's method, the patient is supine and percussion is done in both expiration and full inspiration. The fingers percuss the area where the lowest intercostal space meets the left anterior axillary line (10) (Fig. 5). This is *Castell's spot*, which should remain resonant throughout the examination. If it becomes dull with inspiration, splenomegaly is considered to be present. Traube's space also can be evaluated (2). This area is defined by the sixth rib superiorly, the midaxillary line laterally, and the left lower costal margin inferiorly. With the patient breathing normally, percussion is considered normal if this area is reso-

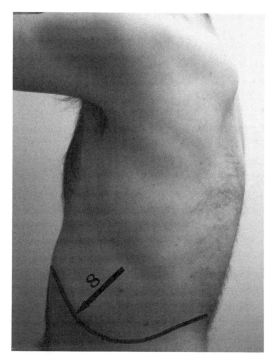

FIG. 4. Nixon's method for determining splenomegaly. Dullness should not extend more than 8 cm above costal margin.

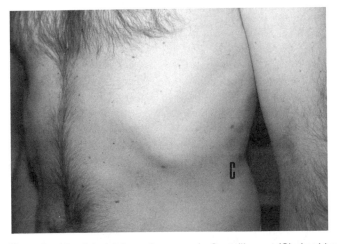

FIG. 5. Castell's method for determining splenomegaly. Castell's spot (C) should remain resonant in inspiration unless splenomegaly is present.

nant. When the area is dull to percussion, splenomegaly is diagnosed. There is a high false-negative rate of identifying splenomegaly; however, the specificity of a positive finding is high when results of both percussion and palpation are positive. Radiologic studies or scintigraphy may be needed to verify the findings.

Normal Findings

The normal size of the liver varies with each individual. There is a correlation between the size of the liver and the estimated total lean body mass, sex, and height of the patient (3). For example, a 10-cm span of liver is considered hepatomegaly in a 5-foot-tall, 100-pound woman, but would be normal for a 6-foot-tall, 200-pound man. The air-filled intestines provide a hollow note to percussion throughout the abdomen.

Abnormal Findings

Hepatomegaly

The liver span, by combined percussion and palpation, can vary depending on body size and sex, being greater in men and in taller people. As a general rule, the vertical span should not exceed 13 cm (3).

Splenomegaly

A spleen that is enlarged by percussion, as described under normal findings, should be considered abnormal and investigated further.

Mass

A lower abdominal midline mass may be a distended bladder or enlarging uterus. Other masses are usually best delineated by palpation; percussion is used to detect air inside the mass.

Ascites

The most sensitive sign for ascites is "shifting dullness" (11). The most specific finding is a prominent fluid wave (11). Unfortunately, the overall predictive value of either of these findings is low. The accurate interpretation for ascites depends on the prevalence of ascites and the type of patient examined. There is no single sign for ascites that is both sensitive and specific. The most sensitive findings are the presence of flank dullness, bulging flanks, or shifting dullness (11,12). In eliciting the *puddle sign*, the patient is placed on his or her hands and knees for several minutes; the diaphragm of the stethoscope is then placed over the most dependent portion and the examiner listens as the abdominal wall is flicked with the finger (13). The stethoscope is then moved laterally. The flicked sound is greatest when the edge of the puddle of ascites is passed. This test has a sensitivity of only 55% (12). The most specific finding for ascites is a fluid wave (12). Overall, the findings of a fluid wave, shifting dullness, and peripheral edema increase the likelihood of ascites. To rule out ascites, a negative history, the absence of bulging or dull flanks, and shifting dullness are useful. The clinical history becomes quite important because it will identify patients with high versus low probability. The probability is low if the patient does not complain of a recent increase in abdominal girth or has no history of recent ankle swelling (12). The maneuvers are easily reproducible, and there is little discrepancy from one examiner to another.

SUMMARY OF ABNORMAL FINDINGS FOR
SPECIFIC DISEASES

Cholecystitis

Constant tenderness is localized behind the inferior margin of the liver. There may be inspiratory arrest when the examiner's fingers are held under the right costal margin and the patient is asked to inspire (*Murphy's sign*). With severe cholecystitis, a tender globular mass may be felt behind the lower border of the liver.

Acute Pancreatitis

Epigastric tenderness is always present. A tender mass may be palpated in the epigastrium. Jaundice may be present. Blue or green ecchymoses may occasionally appear in the flank after 2 to 3 days (*Turner's sign*). Bluish discoloration of the umbilicus (*Cullen's sign*) also may occur.

Splenic Infarction

Tenderness will be present in the left upper quadrant. A splenic friction rub may be present over the infarcted area after a few days.

Acute Abdomen

Diffuse or localized tenderness will be present. Bowel sounds may be present and the abdomen may be distended. There may be boardlike, involuntary rigidity if peritonitis is present.

Appendicitis

Tenderness is usually present in the right lower quadrant. A tender mass may be palpated in the area if an abscess has formed. A palpable tender mass also may be detected on the rectal examination. Suprapubic pain with flexion of the thigh and rotation of the femur internally and externally may be present (*obturator test*).

Diverticulitis

Tenderness is present in the left lower quadrant. A palpable mass may be felt in severe diverticulitis or when an abscess has developed. A fistulous tract may connect to the bladder and air bubbles and/or feces may be seen in the urine.

Irritable Bowel Syndrome

Generally the examination is normal. There may be some mild tenderness over the sigmoid colon area. A mass may be felt in the lower left quadrant from stool in the sigmoid colon if constipation is a problem.

Regional Enteritis

Tenderness in the right lower quadrant is often present if the distal ileum is inflamed. A tender mass also can be palpated if there is extensive inflammation. Arthritis may occur.

Ulcerative Colitis

Tenderness is present over the affected area of the colon. The most common area of tenderness is the left lower quadrant. Abdominal distension and absent bowel sounds may be a clue to the development of a toxic megacolon.

Intestinal Infarction

Diffuse tenderness is present and bowel sounds are usually absent. Abdominal distention may reflect intestinal perforation.

Strangulated Hernia

A tender painful mass is present at the hernia site. Signs of bowel obstruction will eventually be present.

Volvulus

The site of the volvulus most commonly occurs in the sigmoid colon or cecum. Tenderness or a tender mass may be detected over these areas.

Cirrhosis

Signs of hepatic cirrhosis include ascites, pedal edema, jaundice, palmar erythema, vascular spiders, gynecomastia, loss of axillary and pelvic hair, and testicular atrophy. The liver edge may be firm or nodular when palpated.

THE RECTAL EXAMINATION

Regular examination in an adult should include the examination of the anorectal area. Anoscopy, proctosigmoidoscopy, or flexible sigmoidoscopy should be considered in any patient with specific anorectal complaints.

Technique

Preparation is of the utmost importance. The physician should explain each step. The patient needs to be reassured by the physician before the examination. The patient should be draped appropriately so that only the perineum is exposed. The knee-chest or lithotomy position can be used, but generally the left lateral decubitus position is easier because there is no need for a special examining table and it is better tolerated in the elderly and the debilitated patient. Placing the right knee across the left and resting it on the table enables a better examination. Unfortunately, in this position, the contents of the peritoneal cavity are not as readily palpable. The buttocks are spread apart with gloved hands. Inspection is performed of the buttocks, thighs, sacrococcygeal region, vulva, or base of the scrotum. The skin is inspected for signs of inflammation, sinuses, masses, and fistulas. Palpation of these areas also should be performed before the examination of the perianal area. The contour of the anal verge is studied. The mucocutaneous junction is then everted with bilateral traction of the adjacent skin. The lower anal canal can be seen at this time, and any lesions identified should be described. The gloved index finger is used to palpate while also searching for tenderness, fullness, mass, or induration. Sometimes a fistulous tract can be palpated and pus may be expressed. Surgical jelly is applied to lubricate the finger and perianal area, and palpation is repeated. This second palpation is usually the most sensitive for identifying any induration or mass. A subcutaneous cord may be felt when a fistula is present. The digital anorectal examination follows and is generally performed with the index finger; the small finger may be used when anal stenosis or a painful lesion is present. If a painful area is encountered, an anesthetic ointment may be necessary and can be applied before the digital examination using a small cotton-tip swab. If pain occurs during the examination, gentle pressure to overcome the sphincteric contraction should be applied to the opposite side. The caliber of the canal and sphincter tone should be estimated as the finger is inserted. The intersphincteric groove, where an abscess is sometimes located, is then palpated circumferentially. The finger should then sweep the lower anal canal. Bimanual palpation with the index finger inside and the thumb externally will help delineate an abscess. The finger is then inserted its full length and should again sweep the rectal area. The average index finger is 10 cm long; however, the depth of insertion will depend a great deal on the size of the buttocks. The anorectal ring is palpated during this part of the examination. The ring is generally more prominent posteriorly and laterally and can be studied by asking the patient to contract their anus. The strength and tone of the contraction is then noted. By asking the patient to strain, the examiner can palpate more deeply into the rectum. Masses in the anterior peritoneal reflection are often within reach, especially in women. The cervix or a vaginal tampon may be mistaken for a tumor. The prostate examination is discussed in Chapter 18. The coccyx is felt by grasping it with the thumb on the perineum and the index finger in the rectum. The bone is then moved slightly to elicit pain. At the completion of the examination, the examiner's glove should be examined for pus, blood, or mucus. The stool can be stained for the presence of blood (14,15).

Normal Findings

Normal findings include a good sphincter tone with no palpable masses except for stool in the rectal area. Internal hemorrhoids are generally not palpable, but prominent papillae may be felt.

Abnormal Findings

Infections of the perianal and anal areas may show a number of abnormalities (Table 1) that may be associated with cancer, inflammatory bowel disease, AIDS,

TABLE 1. *Detectible abnormalities with inspection*

Perianal	Deformity or asymmetry (tumors, warts, cysts, scars)
	Dermatologic disorders (psoriasis, atopic dermatitis, contact dermatitis, pruritus ani)
	Fistula or sinus (with drainage of pus, feces, or mucus)
Anal	Deformity or asymmetry of anal verge
	Skin tag or hypertrophied anal papilla
	Fissure in ano
	Tumor, abscess
	Anal ulcers, condylomata acuminata
	Hemorrhoids (thrombosed, prolapsing, external)
	Prolapse of an internal hemorrhoid, polyp, or rectal mucosa

TABLE 2. *Causes of abnormal anal sphincter tone*

Tight	Relaxed
Apprehension	Laceration of anal muscles
Fissure in ano	Atony of muscles
Anal stricture	
Fibrosis of the anal muscles	
Anal carcinoma	
Abscess, thrombosed hemorrhoid	

or autoimmune disorders. The anal sphincter tone may be noticeably abnormal, either too tight, tender, or too relaxed, as in cases of incontinence (Table 2).

REFERENCES

1. Judge RD, Zuidema GD. Gastrointestinal system. In: Delp MH, Manning RT, eds. *Major's physical diagnosis.* Philadelphia: W.B. Saunders, 1981:331–61.
2. Barkun AN, Camus M, Green L, et al. The bedside assessment of splenic enlargement. *Am J Med* 1991;91:512–8.
3. Naylor CD. Physical examination of the liver. *JAMA* 1994;271:1859–65.
4. Grover SA, Barkun AN, Sackett DL. Does this patient have splenomegaly? *JAMA* 1993;270:2218–21.
5. Thomson WHF, Daives RFH, Carter S St C. Abdominal wall tenderness, a useful sign in chronic abdominal pain. *Br J Surg* 1991;78:223–5.
6. Liddington MI, Thomson WHF. Rebound tenderness test. *Br J Surg* 1991;78:795–6.
7. Meyerowitz BR. Abdominal palpation by stethoscope. *Arch Surg* 1976;111:831.
8. Naylor CD, McCormack DG, Sullivan SN. The midclavicular line: a wandering landmark. *Can Med Assoc J* 1987;136:48–50.
9. Skrainka B, Stahlhut J, Fulbeck CL, et al. Measuring liver span: bedside examination versus ultrasound and scintiscan. *J Clin Gastroenterol* 1986;8:267–70.
10. Castell DO, Frank BB. Special aspects of primary care: abdominal examination. *Postgrad Med* 1977;62:131–4.
11. Cummings S, Papadakis M, Milnick J, et al. The predictive value of physical examination for ascites. *West J Med* 1985;142:633–6.
12. Williams JW Jr, Simel DL. Does this patient have ascites? *JAMA* 1992;267:2645–8.
13. Sackett DL. A primer on the precision and accuracy of the clinical examination. *JAMA* 1992;267:2638–44.
14. Sapira JD. *The art and science of bedside diagnosis: the rectum.* Baltimore: Urban & Schwarzenberg, 1990.
15. Schrock TR. Examination of the anorectum, rigid sigmoidoscopy, flexible sigmoidoscopy, and diseases of the anorectum. In: Sleisenger MH, Fordtran JS, eds. *Gastrointestinal disease.* 4th ed. Philadelphia: W.B. Saunders, 1989:1570–89.

Clinical Skills for Adult Primary Care
edited by M. E. Silverman and J. W. Hurst.
Lippincott-Raven Publishers, Philadelphia © 1996.

15

Examination of the Musculoskeletal System

Kimberley E. Wilson, M.D., and W. Hayes Wilson, M.D.

Piedmont Hospital, Atlanta, Georgia 30309

"In its more aggravated forms diffuse scleroderma is one of the most terrible of all human ills. Like Tithonus to 'wither slowly' and like him to be 'beaten down and marred and wasted' until one is literally a mummy, encased in an evershrinking, slowly contracting skin of steel, is a fate not pictured in any tragedy, ancient or modern."
William Osler. On diffuse scleroderma. *J Cutan Genitourin Dis* 1898;16:49.

The Centers for Disease Control has predicted that by the year 2020 there will be an estimated 59% increase in arthritic conditions and that one in five Americans will have an arthritic condition as the "baby boomers" continue to age (1). Therefore, a careful joint examination is important and should be part of every physical examination. The frequency with which the musculoskeletal examination should be performed varies with the severity of the arthritic illness. A patient with stable osteoarthritis on nonsteroidal antiinflammatory drugs may routinely be monitored at 6- to 12-month intervals, whereas a patient with an inflammatory arthropathy on second-line antirheumatic drugs may require monitoring at 1- to 3-month intervals.

HISTORICAL FOCUS

Simple questions can help the examiner direct the examination:

- Is the musculoskeletal complaint confined to one area or many?
- Is the problem symmetrical or asymmetrical?
- Is the problem articular, periarticular, or muscular?

Specific characteristics include the following:

- Pain: location, duration, frequency, alleviating or exacerbating factors
- Swelling: articular, periarticular, nodules
- Warmth
- Erythema
- Duration of morning stiffness

- Weakness: functional impairments
- Associated systemic manifestations: fever, weight loss, skin rash, mucosal ulcerations, dry eyes, dry mouth, visual changes, chest pain, diarrhea, etc.

A systematic approach from head to toe is necessary when investigating rheumatologic complaints. Comprehensive discussion of systems other than the musculoskeletal system are found in other chapters; however, there are important clues from these systems that must be considered when performing a musculoskeletal examination.

EXAMINATION OF THE HEAD AND NECK

- Hair pull test: hair is pulled through the examiner's fingers to see if it easily falls out (two or more hairs come out). Alopecia is a significant problem in systemic lupus erythematosus and a positive hair pull test is an important clue.
- Scalp and ears should be diligently inspected for psoriatic plaques that may be associated with psoriatic arthritis. Psoriatic arthritis may involve the spine, as well as the peripheral joints, and at times can be very destructive (e.g., arthritis mutilans). Discoid lesions are associated with lupus and frequently involve the scalp and ears as well.
- Facial skin: a malar rash (sparing the nasolabial fold) is consistent with systemic lupus erythematosus; a discoid rash is characterized by depressed scarring and follicular plugging.
- A careful fundoscopic examination may show papilledema, suggestive of increased intracranial pressure or optic neuritis. Retinal changes may indicate thromboembolic or other systemic diseases (such as diabetes) that have associated musculoskeletal syndromes.
- Inspection of nasal and oral mucosa: mucosal ulcerations are one of the 11 criteria for lupus. These ulcerations typically occur on the nasal septum and at the junction of the hard and soft palate. Check under the tongue to assess salivary pooling. In Sjogren's syndrome, there may be little or no salivary pooling.
- Palpate the parotid and submandibular salivary and lymph glands for enlargement and/or tenderness. These glands may be enlarged as a manifestation of Sjogren's syndrome. In addition, Sjogren's syndrome is associated with an increased incidence of lymphoma. Therefore, lymph node examination should be performed routinely and recorded in patients with Sjogren's disease.
- Palpate the thyroid for enlargement or nodules. Hypothyroidism as well as malignancy can be associated with a symmetrical polyarthritis.

EXAMINATION OF THE LUNGS

Auscultate for evidence of a pleural friction rub, pleural effusion, interstitial lung disease, or fibrosis. These findings are common in systemic collagen vascular diseases, such as rheumatoid arthritis, progressive systemic sclerosis, CREST syndrome, and systemic lupus erythematosus.

EXAMINATION OF THE HEART

Auscultate for pericardial friction rub, heart murmurs, evidence of pulmonary hypertension. Serositis is one of the 11 criteria for the diagnosis of systemic lupus erythematosus. Also important are signs of aortic root dilatation that can be found in the spondyloarthropathies, the Marfan syndrome, Takayasu's arteritis, and giant cell arteritis.

Palpate arterial pulses, particularly when there is evidence of possible peripheral vascular compromise. Rheumatic diseases associated with diminished peripheral circulation include Takayasu's arteritis, extracranial giant cell arteritis, and other forms of vasculitis or vasoocclusive disease. Raynaud's syndrome is present in 3% to 5% of the general population; however, it is also commonly associated with systemic lupus erythematosus, mixed connective tissue disease, CREST, and scleroderma (2).

EXAMINATION OF THE GASTROINTESTINAL SYSTEM

Palpate for hepatosplenomegaly, masses, tenderness/peritoneal signs looking for hepatitis, or intraabdominal neoplasm. Inflammatory arthritis may be the heralding sign of either hepatitis or carcinoma. Abdominal bruits may suggest an intraabdominal vascular abnormality such as vasculitis, e.g., mesenteric or renal.

Rectal sphincter tone and prostate examination are important in evaluating back pain to assess possible neurologic deficit or potential for malignancy, as well as possible referred pain from prostatitis. A positive stool guaiac may be evidence of occult malignancy or side effects from nonsteroidal antiinflammatory therapy.

EXAMINATION OF THE MUSCULOSKELETAL SYSTEM

Examination of the Upper Extremity

Hands and Wrists

Begin by inspecting the hands and wrists for signs of erythema or swelling. The dorsum of the examiner's fingers should be lightly stroked across the dorsum of the patient's hands to feel for increased warmth. Each joint is then palpated at the joint margin, beginning with the metacarpophalangeal joints and progressively moving to the proximal and distal interphalangeal joints. It is important to maintain eye contact with the patient by looking for subtle clues of tenderness such as wincing. Synovial thickening and effusion are looked for as well. Range of mo-

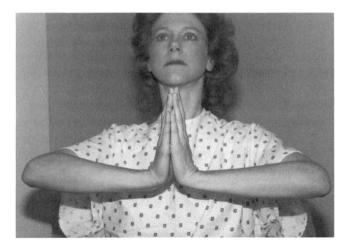

FIG. 1. Wrist extension.

tion is examined by asking the patient to make a tight fist that requires the finger tips to reach the pads at the base of the metacarpophalangeal joints, obliterating any excess space. If there are focal deficits, such as finger locking or loss of range of motion in one or more fingers, the fingers are examined individually for tendon nodules, Dupuytren's contractures, cysts, giant cell tumors, etc. Grip strength may be assessed semiquantitatively using a manometer or qualitatively by having the patient grasp the examiner's index and middle fingers with a maximal effort. The wrists are examined in the same manner for synovial thickening, effusion,

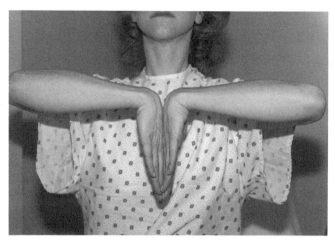

FIG. 2. Wrist flexion.

and tenderness. Range of motion should be near 80 degrees for flexion and 70 degrees for extension and can be checked actively by asking the patient to "say your prayers and raise your elbows parallel to the floor" (Fig. 1). If the patient can accomplish this with the heels of both hands touching, extension is normal. Ask the patient to perform the same type motion with the backs of both hands touching (Fig. 2). Again, if the patient can accomplish this with both wrists touching and elbows near level, there is full range of motion. Any deficit should be investigated by passively flexing and extending the individual wrists and recording any positive findings, including warmth, swelling, lack of normal range of motion, or withdrawal from pain.

Elbows

Inspect the elbows for erythema or swelling. Palpate using the dorsum of the hand to detect warmth. The para-olecranon grooves should be palpated with the elbow in slight flexion to detect joint effusion. The olecranon bursa can be examined with the elbow in extension to detect bursal thickening or fluid accumu-

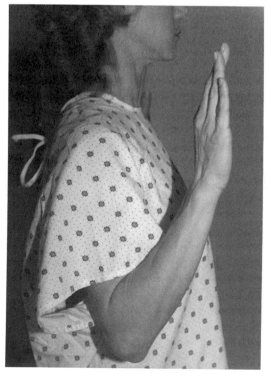

FIG. 3. Elbow flexion.

lation. The surrounding structures of each elbow, including the extensor surface of the forearm, should be palpated for rheumatoid nodules. The lateral and medial epicondyles are palpated to detect tenderness suggestive of epicondylitis. Range of motion is tested by asking the patient to flex and extend the arms. Normal range is from 0 degrees in full extension to 150 degrees in full flexion (Fig. 3); some women are able to extend beyond 0 degrees to –5 degrees; however, hyperflexability is a risk factor for arthritis.

Shoulders

The patient is asked to hold the arms at the side and then abduct them through a complete arch, bringing the outstretched arms together over the head, touching the upper arms to the ears if possible (Fig. 4). Normal shoulder motion ranges from neutral to 180 degrees abduction. The hands are then clasped and placed behind the head. Elbows are brought as far backward as possible and then forward (Fig. 5A and B). Next request that the patient place the hands behind the back, "as if you are scratching your back," and to try to reach up as high as he or she

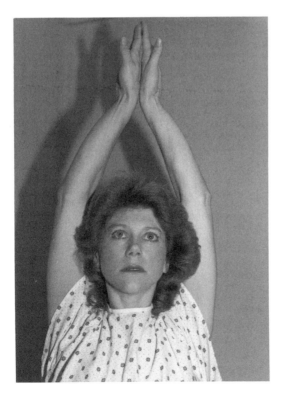

FIG. 4. Shoulder abduction.

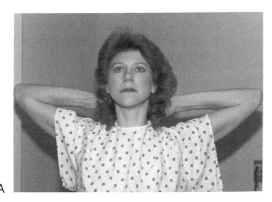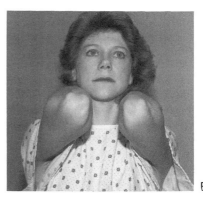

A   B

FIG. 5. A: Shoulder external rotation. **B**: Shoulder forward flexion.

can (Fig. 6). Normally patients can adduct and internally rotate their shoulders so that the hands reach up to T_8 to T_{10}. During these maneuvers, any discomfort or lack of range of motion is noted.

Temporomandibular Joint

The patient is asked to open the mouth as widely as possible. The incisor-to-incisor distance is measured and any discomfort is noted. An oral aperture of less than 4 cm is typically seen in scleroderma. Palpate over the temporomandibular joints as the patient opens and closes the mouth, feeling for crepitation, popping,

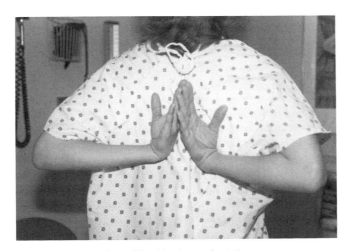

FIG. 6. Shoulder internal rotation.

or malalignment. It is sometimes easier to feel crepitation by placing the tips of the fifth digits into the patient's external ear canals while asking the patient to elevate and depress the mandible.

Examination of the Spine

Cervical Spine

The patient is asked to tip the head back as far as it will go and then to touch the chin to the chest. Next, the patient is asked to touch the chin to the right and then left shoulder. If puzzled, ask the patient to look backward as if looking to see if someone is following. The patient should be able to rotate the neck so that the chin is almost in line with the shoulder. Lastly, the patient is asked to touch the ear to the shoulder to test lateral bending. Normal is about to 45 degrees. It is important to note how comfortably and smoothly the patient accomplishes these tasks. Range of motion may be near normal but is accomplished slowly and painfully when the patient has degenerative arthritis of the spine.

Thoracic and Lumbosacral Spine

The thoracic spine is palpated for excessive kyphosis, as with ankylosing spondylitis or osteoporosis ("dowager's hump"). The lumbar region is palpated for normal lordosis, which is frequently absent in ankylosing spondylitis and low-back syndromes. Alignment is also checked, noting any scoliosis. The paravertebral muscles are palpated for tenderness and spasm. Next, percuss over the spinous processes and sacroiliac areas to detect focal areas of tenderness. Straight leg raise in the sitting position may elicit long tract signs suggestive of sciatic nerve irritation.

Examination of the Lower Extremity

Knees

With the patient recumbent, begin the knee examination with inspection for erythema, swelling, asymmetry, muscle wasting, or malalignment. Common abnormalities include a valgus deformity, with the lower legs making an outward L shape and the knees coming together, also known as "knock knees," and a varus deformity in which the knees are apart and the lower legs inward in an A shape, also known as "bowed legs." Varus deformities are typically associated with degenerative joint disease, whereas inflammatory arthropathies tend to cause valgus knee deformity. Place the dorsum of the hand on the distal leg and advance it cephalad over the fully extended knee, feeling for temperature changes. Nor-

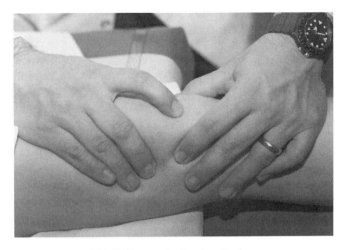

FIG. 7. Knee palpation for effusion.

mally, the knee is cooler than the rest of the leg; any increased temperature should be noted. Next, place the more cephalad examining hand on the suprapatellar bursa with the thumb and third finger of the other hand on either side of the patella. The index finger is used to press down, or ballot, the patella to feel for a significant effusion (Fig. 7). The bulge or bubble sign is present when the patient's knee has a small effusion. The examiner first applies proximal and lateral pressure on the extended knee. The synovial fluid from the medial joint space is "milked" out of this space by stroking the medial aspect of the extended knee. Then immediately the lower hand strokes up along the lateral aspect of the patella looking for a bulge, or "bubble," on the medial aspect of the knee. The medial collateral ligament is tested by bending the patient's knee slightly with a hand against the lateral joint line while the other hand applies outward pressure against the ankle (Fig. 8). The examiner feels for excessive motion or a knocking as the medial tibial plateau comes back against the medial femoral condyle. In the same manner, the lateral collateral ligament is stressed by reversing the position of the hands and applying pressure laterally and inward against the ankle. Again feel for displacement and then for the knocking back together of the lateral tibial plateau against the lateral femoral condyle. The knee should flex to 135 degrees and extend to 0 degrees (Fig. 9). The knee is externally rotated by turning the ankle outward with the lower hand, and then the process is repeated with the upper hand palpating for any locking, clicking, or crepitation. Next, the knee is internally rotated and the process repeated once again, palpating for locking, clicking, or crepitation. The entire examination is repeated for the contralateral knee. The patient is then asked to lie down and a drape is placed between the legs for proper coverage during the remainder of the examination.

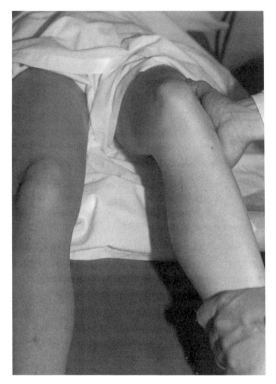

FIG. 8. Testing medial collateral ligament.

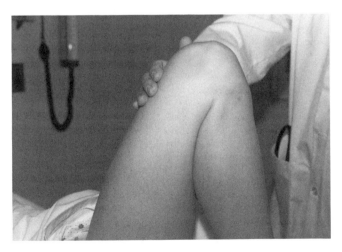

FIG. 9. Flexion of the knee.

Straight Leg Raise

This maneuver is performed by holding the posterior ankle and elevating either leg. When the patient complains of discomfort, generally at 80 degrees of flexion from the table, the examiner inquires as to the location of the pain. Tightness of the hamstring muscles behind the knee is normal and resolves when the knee is flexed. Radicular or sciatic pain usually extends down the entire leg. The patient will frequently complain of pain in the lower back and may complain of pain in the contralateral leg (positive cross leg straight leg raise test) which is most indicative of sciatic irritation. The leg may be lowered slightly and then the foot dorsiflexed to stretch the sciatic nerve to try to reproduce the sciatic pain. If the pain is not reproduced, the initial pain was likely due to hamstring stretch. If the pain is reproduced on dorsiflexion, try to locate where the pain is most severe, whether in the lumbar spine region or along the sciatic nerve. The straight leg test is performed in the same manner on the well leg. If testing the uninvolved leg produces back/sciatic pain on the contralateral (involved) side, then presumptive evidence exists for a lumbar lesion, such as a herniated disk.

Hips

To examine the hip, the examiner begins testing hip flexion by placing the upper hand beneath the normal lumbar lordosis with the lower hand lifting behind the knee. The bent knee is then raised as far as is comfortably possible, normally 135 degrees (Fig. 10). A flexion contracture is characterized by the patient's inability to extend the leg without arching the lower spine. Hip extension can be tested by

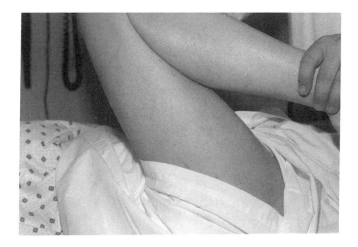

FIG. 10. Flexion of the hip.

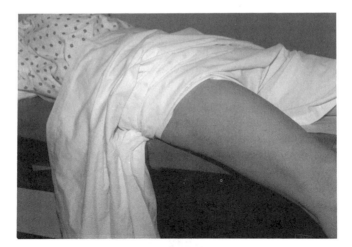

FIG. 11. Extension of the hip.

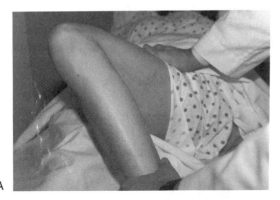

A

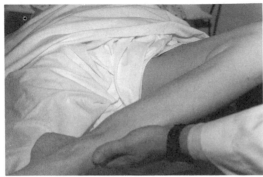

B

FIG. 12. A: Internal rotation of the hip.
B: External rotation of the hip.

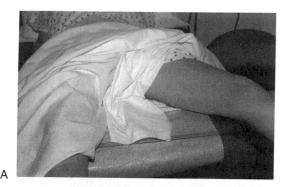

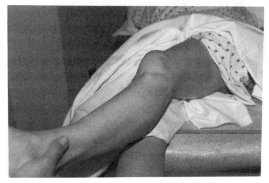

FIG. 13. A: Abduction of the hip. **B:** Adduction of the hip.

dropping the leg off the side of the table or having the patient lie prone and raise the leg (Fig. 11). Normal extension is 30 degrees. Internal and external rotation can be tested with log rolling—the leg is rolled, with the knee in full extension, first medially and then laterally. The knees are then flexed to 90 degrees and the hips are again rotated. Normal limits for rotation at the patella are 45 degrees for external rotation and 35 degrees for internal rotation (Fig. 12A and B). The location of any discomfort during these maneuvers is noted. True hip joint pain generally localizes to the groin and frequently to the anterior thigh. A more common condition is trochanteric bursitis, which causes pain in the lateral aspect of the upper thigh over the greater trochanter of the hip. The hip may then be tested for normal abduction, which is usually 45 to 50 degrees without discomfort, and adduction, which is normally 20 to 30 degrees without discomfort (Fig. 13A and B).

Ankle and Foot

The ankle is next inspected for swelling or erythema. Again palpate lightly using the dorsum of the examining hand to feel for subtle signs of warmth. The medial and lateral malleolar regions are palpated for tenderness, thickening, or effusion. The anterior joint line is palpated over the dome of the talus while moving the foot in plantar flexion, exposing more of the joint margin. The Achilles tendon insertion and then the infra-Achilles bursa is palpated with the thumb and index finger on either side of the Achilles tendon. Achilles tendinitis is common in the spondyloarthropathies (ankylosing spondylitis, psoriatic arthritis, reactive arthritis, Reiter's syndrome, inflammatory bowel–related arthritis), whereas Achilles bursitis is more common in rheumatoid arthritis. The heel is palpated and percussed for tenderness to seek a calcaneal spur or plantar fascitis. The mid-foot is then palpated over the cuboid and the styloid process of the fifth metatarsal. Next, the metatarsophalangeal joints are palpated individually with the thumb on the plantar surface over the metatarsal head and the index finger on the dorsal surface. Tenderness, subluxations, deviations, calluses, and bony changes should all be noted and recorded. It is common with the inflammatory arthritides to have cocked-up toes from subluxations at the metatarsal heads. Tenderness between the third and fourth metatarsals may indicate a Morton's neuroma. Diffuse swelling of individual digits, so-called sausage digits, are associated with the spondyloarthropathies. The plantar surface should be examined for the rash *keratoderma blenorrhagica*, which might indicate Reiter's syndrome or possibly guttate psoriasis. Toe nails may show pitting, indicating psoriasis as well. Lastly, signs of Raynaud's or any vascular abnormality must be investigated by checking pulses, capillary refill, and performing a careful neurologic examination to rule out mononeuritis multiplex, which might indicate a vasculitis.

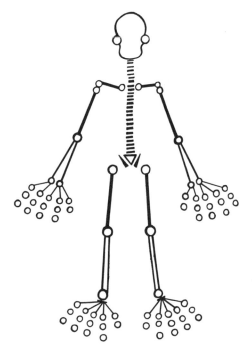

FIG. 14. Stick diagram for recording findings.

RECORDING THE FINDINGS

It is important to follow serial changes in the joint examination from one visit to the next in order to document the progression of the arthritic disease as well as to evaluate the efficacy of treatment. This may easily be accomplished by using a stick figure diagram illustrating specific joints and major muscle groups (Fig. 14). It is important to make note of both tenderness and swelling as well as to record limitations in range of motion that can then be compared with future examinations.

COMMON FINDINGS IN SELECTED CONDITIONS

Rheumatoid Arthritis

The American College of Rheumatology has defined rheumatoid arthritis as a symmetrical arthritis involving the small joints of the hands and feet, lasting longer than 6 weeks (3). Additionally, rheumatoid arthritis may involve the temporomandibular and sternoclavicular joints and potentially any joint of the extremities. Interestingly, rheumatoid arthritis spares the axial skeleton with the exception of the atlantoaxial joint (C1–2). The joint pain is present both at rest and upon motion. Morning stiffness lasts longer than 1 hour, typically improving with increased activity. Palmar erythema is an incidental but common finding. If the cricoarytenoid joint is involved, hoarseness results. Tender subcutaneous nodules most frequently occur on the extensor surface of the proximal forearm and on the Achilles tendon. Vasculitis may complicate rheumatoid arthritis, causing a purpuric skin rash or mononeuritis multiplex (frequently foot drop).

Seronegative Spondyloarthropathies

This broad category of inflammatory disease includes four distinct arthritides: psoriatic arthritis, ankylosing spondylitis, Reiter's syndrome/reactive arthritis, and the arthritis associated with inflammatory bowel disease. Each of these conditions has in common an asymmetrical peripheral arthritis, potential involvement of the sacroiliac joint, and may be associated with an enthesopathy (inflammation at the tendon insertion site). Painful anterior uveitis may complicate any of these four arthropathies.

Psoriatic Arthritis

Some unique features of psoriatic arthritis include asymmetric involvement of the sacroiliac joint, erosions of the small joints of the hands and feet, and dactylitis ("sausage digit"). Nail pitting or dystrophy and onycholysis are common clues to psoriasis even in the absence of a rash.

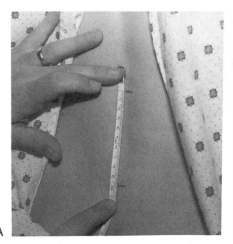 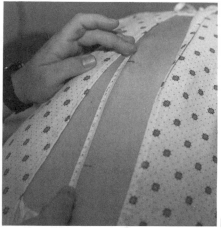

A   B

FIG. 15. A: Schober index baseline measurement. **B:** Schober index measurement with forward flexion.

Ankylosing Spondylitis

Ankylosing spondylitis is characterized by symmetric involvement of the sacroiliac joint and nonerosive, oligoarticular involvement of the large joints (knees, hips, shoulders). Physical examination shows a loss of the normal lordotic curve as well as decreased rotation and lateral flexion at the waist. Upon bending forward, the patient will compensate for the spinal fusion by flexing at the hip. Schober's test is used to measure flexion of the lumbar spine (Fig. 15A and B). This test is performed by making marks at the level of L5–S1 and then 10 cm above the first mark with the patient standing erect. Next the patient is asked to bend forward and touch his or her toes. The distance between the two marks is measured at the point of greatest forward flexion, and the result is reported as the change in excursion. With ankylosing spondylitis, lumbar excursion is often less than 3.5 cm. When the upper spine is involved, chest wall expansion is less than 3.5 cm and neck extension is decreased.

Reiter's Syndrome

Reiter's syndrome and the reactive arthritides are characterized by asymmetric involvement of the sacroiliac joint. The peripheral arthritis is erosive, oligoarticular, and typically involves the joints of the lower extremities and sometimes the wrists. The classic triad of Reiter's syndrome includes conjunctivitis, urethritis, and arthritis. Circinate balanitis and keratoderma blenorrhagicum are pathognomonic for this disease. Pericarditis and aortic regurgitation may develop. Dactylitis may also occur in Reiter's syndrome and in reactive arthritis.

Inflammatory Bowel Disease and Arthritis

The arthritis associated with inflammatory bowel disease is a nonerosive oligoarticular disease typically involving the knees, ankles, and elbows. Involvement of the sacroiliac joint is symmetrical.

Systemic Lupus Erythematosus

The skin manifestations of lupus include malar rash, discoid rash, and a more generalized photosensitive skin rash. Characterized as a nonerosive, symmetrical polyarthritis, systemic lupus erythematosus predominantly involves the small joints of the hands and feet and frequently involves the wrists, knees, ankles, elbows, and shoulders. Avascular necrosis should be considered in a lupus patient who complains of hip or knee pain. Serositis is diagnosed on physical examination by a pleural or pericardial friction rub and by rebound tenderness of the abdomen. Aortic regurgitation can develop. Seizure and psychosis are the cardinal signs of neurological involvement of lupus.

CREST and Progressive Systemic Sclerosis (Scleroderma)

The principle findings in these diseases are similar; however, they are distinguished by the extent of involvement: skin tightening proximal to the metacarpophalangeal joints, truncal skin tautness, and internal organ involvement are seen in scleroderma. Scleroderma is strictly a clinical diagnosis. CREST is a pneumonic for **C**alcinosis (may be seen involving the fingers, forearms, elbows and knees), **R**aynaud's syndrome, **E**sophageal dysmotility, **S**clerodactyly, and **T**elangiectasia (matlike, frequently seen on the face and oral mucosa). Raynaud's syndrome may be so severe in CREST/scleroderma that ulcerations of the fingertips may occur. Audible friction rubs may be heard over tendons in motion during the active stage of scleroderma. Cardiomyopathy, pulmonary hypertension, and renal failure may be consequences.

Crystalline Arthritides

Gout

Gout is a monoarticular arthritis at onset; however, with chronic recurrence it may become an asymmetric, erosive polyarthritis involving the feet, ankles, hands, wrists, and elbows. Tophi are rare these days, but may be seen at the ears and elbows. Gout is of sudden onset with maximal inflammation developing within 1 day. The two most impressive signs of gout are joint redness and pain severe enough to provoke the patient to exclaim "even the sheet hurts my toe." Factors that provoke a flare of gout include diuretics, low-dose aspirin, alcohol, starvation, exercise, rapid weight loss, diabetic ketoacidosis, trauma, and surgery. Low-grade fever may occur during an acute flare of gout.

Calcium Pyrophosphate Deposition

Calcium pyrophosphate deposition disease (CPPD) may present in one of two ways. As "pseudo-osteoarthritis," CPPD is an acute, nonerosive oligoarticular arthritis involving the knees, wrists, second and third metacarpophalangeal joints, hips, shoulders, and elbows. As pseudo-gout, CPPD is an acute, nonerosive monoarticular arthritis involving the knee or wrist.

Special Considerations

- Pain perceived in the knee may actually be referred pain due to hip pathology.
- Arthritis may precede the skin rash in psoriatic arthritis.
- Jaccoud's arthropathy (reversible ulnar deviation of the metacarpophalangeal joints) is associated with systemic lupus erythematosus and repeated bouts of rheumatic fever.
- Polyarticular gout, rheumatoid arthritis, and exuberant osteoarthritis can be difficult to differentiate.
- Diplopia in a patient with polymyalgia rheumatica or giant cell arteritis is an emergency; 50% go on to develop blindness.
- New onset polyarthritis in patients older than 50 is a clue to a possible neoplasm.
- Spondyloarthropathies are commonly associated with human immunodeficiency virus (HIV) disease. Before initiating immunosuppressive therapy, the physician should strongly consider checking HIV status. (Methotrexate therapy in HIV-positive patients can have devastating consequences.)
- When pain is out of proportion to the physical findings, consider sleep disturbances, stress, and/or depression possibly related to fibromyalgia or myofascial pain syndromes.
- Do not take the patient's history for granted when they say they do not have a rash. They are often unaware of a rash hiding in the scalp, ears, umbilicus, and upper gluteal folds, as may be seen in psoriasis.
- A complete accounting of over-the-counter medications may be very important; for instance, low-dose aspirin can precipitate gout attacks. Serum sickness, Steven-Johnson's syndrome, erythema nodosum, erythema multiforme, and vasculitic-appearing syndromes may be due to over-the-counter medications.
- Parents, grandparents, and school teachers who come in contact with children are at risk to contract arthritis-associated viral illnesses. Parvovirus is one example, causing Fifth's disease in children and a symmetrical polyarthritis in adults.
- Blood pressure is particularly important in patients with scleroderma because renal crisis is frequently life threatening.

- Any lupus patient with a fever should be evaluated immediately.
- Bilateral Bell's palsy suggests Lyme disease.
- Perforation of the ocular globe may result from long-standing, undetected scleromalacia in rheumatoid arthritis.

REFERENCES

1. Centers for Disease Control. Arthritis prevalence and activity limitations—United States, 1990. *MMWR* 1994;43:433–8.
2. Weinrich MC, Maricq HR, Keil JE, et al. Prevalence of Raynaud phenomenon in the adult population of South Carolina. *J Clin Epidemiol* 1990;43:1343:49.
3. Arnett FC, Edworthy SM, Block DA, et al. The American Rheumatism Association 1987 revised criteria for the classification of rheumatoid arthritis. *Arthritis Rheum* 1988;31:315–24.

SUGGESTED READING

Bates B. *A guide to physical examination and history taking.* Philadelphia: J.P. Lippincott, 1991:475–90.
Doherty M, Doherty J. *Clinical examination in rheumatology.* London: Wolfe, 1992:23–136.
Hoppenfeld S. *Physical examination of the spine and extremities.* Norwalk, CT: Appleton-Century-Crofts, 1976:1–104,143–262.
Polley HF, Hunder GG. *Rheumatologic interviewing and physical examination of the joints.* Philadelphia: W.B. Saunders, 1978:61–274.
Salter RB. *Textbook of disorders and injuries of the musculoskeletal system.* Philadelphia: Williams & Wilkins, 1970:9–58.
Walker HK, Hall JD, Hurst JW. *Clinical methods.* Boston: Butterworth, 1980:401–12.

Clinical Skills for Adult Primary Care
edited by M. E. Silverman and J. W. Hurst.
Lippincott-Raven Publishers, Philadelphia © 1996.

16

Examination of the Breasts

William E. Mitchell, Jr., M.D.

Piedmont Hospital, Atlanta, Georgia 30309

"Observe, record, tabulate, communicate. Use your five senses."
William Osler, quoted in Thayer LS. Osler, the teacher.
Johns Hopkins Hosp Bull 1919;30:198.

One of nine American women will develop breast cancer. Many of these cases will be found by mammography or self-examination, but mammograms are fallible and many women fail to look for and/or find cancers that can be felt by a conscientious examiner. A woman will generally assume that a breast examination by a professional will have been thorough, and more accurate than her own self-examination, and she may not perform self-examination until several months afterward. It is important, therefore, that her faith in the professional's examination be justified. None of the examination elements described below can be omitted without some risk, but an adequate routine examination of the breast may require no more than 3 or 4 minutes. On the other hand, physical examination of lumpy breasts or a woman with a nipple discharge, followed by careful recording of the findings, may take 15 to 20 minutes. Studies show that the chance of finding a subtle cancer is increased by spending more time looking for it, although "diminishing returns" probably limit the usefulness of further efforts during an apparently negative examination of 5 to 6 minutes. The examiner should know whether the patient has increased risk factors such as a family history of breast cancer or a previous biopsy result showing atypia and should approach every woman with the attitude that "there is a previously undiscovered breast cancer here somewhere and I am going to find it."

ROUTINE BREAST EXAMINATION

Timing and Sequence of the Examination

Women with no risk factors for breast cancer should have their breasts examined yearly by a professional, starting at the age of 40. Women with a family his-

TABLE 1. *Summary of steps in the breast examination*

1. Have a plan and expect to find something.
2. Inspect and compare the breasts.
3. Palpate the breasts with the patient upright, emphasizing the periareolar areas.
4. Examine each axilla and supraclavicular areas.
5. Repeat palpation with the patient supine and arms at her sides.
6. Repeat supine palpation with arms overhead.
7. Record what you found before you forget it.

tory of breast cancer or previous biopsy results showing atypia should have yearly examinations starting around the age of 30. Whether women with risk factors for breast cancer should have examinations at intervals more frequent than yearly is unsettled. At the very least, all adult women must be strongly urged to perform careful monthly breast self-examination, and their technique should be monitored by a professional.

Many women have substantial breast congestion and nodularity just before the menses, only to have it subside completely 7 to 10 days later. For these women, examinations will be most productive if scheduled 7 to 10 days after the onset of their menstrual flow. Similarly, women receiving intermittent estrogen replacement therapy should be examined at the end of the "off-estrogen" period. Conscientious application of proper techniques of inspection and palpation are the keys to discovery of many small breast cancers. To avoid omissions, it is useful to perform the same sequence in examining the breasts whether the patient is having a full general examination or is only being seen for a breast problem. It is important to have a mental checklist of the elements of the breast examination to be accomplished so that interruption or variation (such as the patient saying "Here, let me show you how I feel it best") will not lead to something being overlooked (Table 1).

The breast examination may usually be left until nothing further remains to be done while the patient is sitting. Inspection and palpation of the breast with the patient sitting can be followed immediately by examination of each axilla and completion of the examination with the patient supine. This sequencing of the breast examination reduces difficulty in correlating abnormalities found when the patient is upright compared with supine. After palpation of the breast has been completed with the patient supine, the remainder of the general physical examination can continue.

Initiation of the Examination

The patient will often be anxious but can usually be reassured by an initial calm review of any previous and current problems with her breasts. A gentle, matter-of-fact approach to examination of the breast is usually the most appropriate. If the examiner's hands are chilly, they should be warmed before actually touching the patient's skin. She should be wearing a front-opening gown or examination cape that allows either or both breasts to be inspected and examined.

Upright Examination of the Breasts

Inspection

Inspection is performed with both breasts uncovered and the patient sitting upright. The arms are first held relaxed at the patient's side, next on her hips with and without the pectoral muscles being contracted, and finally with the arms overhead. On inspection, look for asymmetry of the breast contour or the nipples, different "pointing" of the nipples, rashes or redness of the breast skin, and any dimpling or retraction with movement of the arms and contraction of the pectoral muscles. Inspection for possible dimpling or retraction may be enhanced by having the patient lean forward or by moving the whole breast toward or away from the area of suspected dimpling to accentuate it. The location of any scars should be noted and correlated with the history of previous surgeries, some of which the patient may well have forgotten.

Palpation

Before palpation is actually begun, the examiner should ask the patient whether, and where, she is aware of new abnormalities. This simple question can avoid immense embarrassment. There are two components to effective palpation. The first involves gentle movement of the examining fingers across the breast skin, searching for superficial nodules. Only rarely will a malignancy be felt best with this maneuver, but it should not be omitted. At least 95% of the palpation time should be devoted to "through-the-skin" palpation, done with index, long, and ring fingers as a unit placed flat on the breast so that palpation is done with the pads (not the tips) of all three fingers (Fig. 1). The fingers are placed on and kept firmly in contact with the breast skin, and the fingers and breast skin are moved together as a unit over the underlying breast parenchyma in a circular motion at least three or four times in each spot before moving on. Density (relative resistance to palpation) of the breast tissue, specific nodules and defects, and the ability or inability to outline underlying ribs should be noted and recorded on a diagram. Either of two basic patterns can be used to ensure that no areas are missed (Fig. 2A and B). A spiral pattern, either getting larger or smaller and centered on the nipple/areolar complex can be used. Many find a "search plane" pattern of advancing parallel lines more reproducible and reliable, but this is a matter of personal preference. Remember that breast tissue is often found as high as the second rib and laterally well into the upper axilla. In examining the nipple/areolar complex, look for nodules, nipple asymmetry, thickening, crusting, rashes, and spontaneous or elicited nipple discharge. A frequent cause of uncertainty is due to the variable

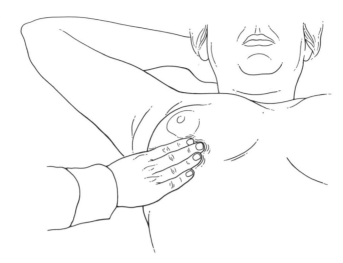

FIG. 1. The index, middle, and ring fingers as a unit are placed flat on the breast and moved in a circular motion to feel through the skin with the pads (not the tips) of the fingers.

location of the central tips of the breast lobules. These may be confused with nodules. They may be well defined, contrasting with the tissue closer to the nipple, which often consists of the very soft lactiferous sinuses. Two findings may suggest that the area in question is not a true nodule. First, some of the other lobular tips around the circumference of the areola may be similar. Also, a lobular tip will not have a defined 360 degree border; only the area closest to the nipple will have a distinct edge, and when traced outward toward the periphery of the area in question, it will blend indistinguishably into the rest of the lobule.

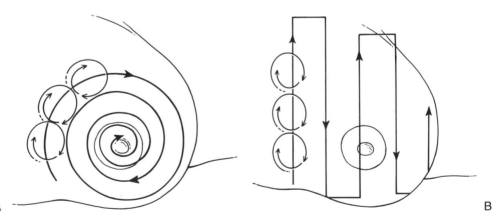

FIG. 2. A: Here a series of circular palpations cover the entire breast in a spiral pattern. **B:** Alternatively, a "search plane" pattern can be used to ensure that the entire breast is examined.

Discharge should be sought by gently squeezing the base of the nipple with two fingers, then gathering several additional centimeters of duct tissue beneath the areola and gently squeezing toward the nipple. The location of the duct(s) from which discharge is seen and the character and amount of discharge should be recorded. A small amount of crusting of the nipples without discharge is fairly common and usually of long standing. If no rash or discharge is associated with crusting, it is of no concern.

Examination of the Axilla

This is best accomplished with the patient's forearm resting relaxed and supported on the examiner's same forearm (e.g., left on left), with the examiner cupping the patient's elbow in his or her palm. The examiner places the other (right hand for left axilla) hand with the fingers extended as high into the lateral upper axilla as possible, attempting to get above any nodes embedded in the axillary fat. The tips of the index, long, and ring fingers are then held firmly together and slightly cupped and pushed toward the chest wall, capturing the axillary fat. The axillary skin is quite mobile so that the fingertips can be kept in contact with the axillary skin for the first few centimeters as the fingers move downward. The lymph nodes will be felt as they slip upward past the fingertips. This maneuver becomes increasingly uncomfortable with repetition, so it should not be done more than three or four times at one session. Note and record the number, size, tenderness, consistency, and shape of palpated nodes and determine whether they are attached to one another ("matted") or are separate and freely movable.

The supraclavicular areas also may be examined conveniently while the patient is upright. Normal nodes are occasionally palpable, but any node that is over 8 to 10 mm in size, or firm, should be noted.

Supine Examination of the Breasts

Next, with the patient supine, repeat the systematic search, first with the arms at her side and then overhead. A frequent problem area, particularly with large breasts, is at the lower border of the breasts, where the breast tissue may fold over rather than taper gradually. This may be particularly noticeable medially. Such an area is elongated, usually bilateral, and can generally be eliminated by firmly pushing the breast cephalad, thus smoothing out the inframammary fold.

Occasionally the border of the breasts, particularly laterally or high in the axilla, may be prominent, simulating a nodule. These areas will not have circumferentially identifiable borders, and on the side opposite the border the breast tissue will blend smoothly into the nearby breast.

In women with large or pendulous breasts, the breast tissue can often be flattened and made more accessible for careful examination if the breast is rolled toward the opposite side by placing a pillow beneath the same side shoulder, or by gently pulling the breast toward the opposite side with the examiner's other hand.

Normal Anatomy and Findings

The glandular tissue (parenchyma) of the breast is found in the subcutaneous tissues between the skin proper and the fascia covering the underlying pectoralis major and serratus anterior muscles, usually extending from the second to the sixth ribs and from the border of the sternum medially to the anterior half of the axilla laterally. Usually the breast parenchyma in the upper outer quadrant is prolonged into the axilla, gradually thinning and becoming indiscernible, but occasionally there will be easily palpable breast tissue lateral to the border of the pectoralis major muscle that is referred to as an "axillary tail" or "axillary breast." Such an area may attract attention because of fibrocystic disease or hypertrophy with pregnancy. The functioning breast tissue is composed of glandular tissue in 12 to 20 roughly wedge-shaped lobules, each of which is drained by a duct system under the areola, which has a central dilated area called the lactiferous sinus. The duct then narrows again as it enters the nipple. The location of the opening on the nipple of each duct corresponds to some extent to the area drained. Unfortunately, this is not completely reliable, and apparently identical adjacent duct orifices may drain parenchymal areas of widely differing sizes and shapes. The glandular tissue is surrounded by a varying amount of fat and is supported by a connective tissue framework that is attached superficially to the skin and loosely to the muscle fascia below. The more prominent of these septa are often called Cooper's ligaments. With aging, glandular tissue gradually atrophies, fatty tissue becomes more prominent, and the suspensory connective tissue framework becomes looser, resulting in a smaller, more pendulous, and usually softer breast after the menopause. These changes are reduced but not eliminated by estrogen replacement after the menopause. With pregnancy, the breasts become larger, firmer, and often more tender. Many women note that weight gain or loss is disproportionately reflected in changes in the breast size, presumably due to variation in the fat content of the breast. The glandular tissue of each lobule usually ends near the areolar border, and the tips of the lobules where the parenchyma ends may be palpable and may contrast with the somewhat emptier feel of the central subareolar/nipple area. Near the surface of the areolar skin are found the easily palpable 1- to 3-mm sebaceous glands of Montgomery. The skin of the nipple and areola is pinkish-brown in color and there is a superficial, highly reactive smooth muscle network that contracts in response to tactile stimulation and cold.

The axilla is bounded laterally by the upper arm, medially by the chest wall, and superiorly by the axillary vessels, which only rarely can be felt. The subscapular muscle group is felt posteriorly, and the pectoralis muscles are palpable anteriorly. Most of the axillary content is fat, in which are found 10 to 35 almond- or bean-shaped lymph nodes. These are usually less than 12 mm in maximum dimension but may be enlarged in response to infection or the presence of malignancies.

Abnormal Findings

Abnormalities on Inspection

Asymmetry of size alone is usually a developmental abnormality of no concern, as is the condition of "tubular" breasts in which the breasts are small and somewhat cylindrical in shape with one end of the cylinder beneath the areola. Should there be dimpling of the skin, flattening of a normally rounded breast contour, or foreshortening of one breast, a contraction of the fibrous supporting structure (Cooper's ligament) should be suspected. In the absence of a scar, such contour deformities are often due to a malignancy. A nipple or areolar rash of greater than 3 weeks' duration may be due to intraductal cancer (*Paget's disease* of the nipple), particularly if it is not associated with nursing or a rash elsewhere. A *peau d'orange* or orange skin appearance of breast skin with marked lymphedematous thickening of the skin itself and prominent depressed pores is usually associated with subdermal lymphatic obstruction by malignancy, but may be associated with benign inflammation or may occasionally be idiopathic. Significant redness of the breast skin is usually due to one of the following: *abscess*, in which case pain and tenderness are usually striking; malignancy, as with *inflammatory breast cancers*, in which over one-third of the breast skin will be reddened, tender, and thickened; local *irritation/dermatitis;* or, rarely, *vasculitis.* With the patient's arms overhead, a mild, often tender bowstringing under the skin may occasionally be seen oriented vertically and extending across the inframammary border. This is *Mondor's disease*, which is a self-limited superficial phlebitis of the thoracoepigastric vein. It is occasionally bilateral and often idiopathic, but it is sometimes associated with local injury, breast biopsy, or wearing of a tight bra.

Abnormalities on Palpation

Here the main issue is usually whether a significant nodule is present. It is normal for the breast tissue to be significantly denser in the upper outer quadrants than elsewhere; fortunately, this tends to be bilaterally similar if not identical. The most common causes of dominant nodules are gross cysts, cancer, fibroadenomas, and fibrocystic disease (Table 2). Gross cysts are rarely seen in women after the menopause unless they are associated with hormone replacement therapy. They are often multiple, usually spherical, often elastic and tender, usually well defined, and often variable during the menstrual cycle. Cancers tend to have the following characteristics: they are hard rather than soft, attached to surrounding tissue such

TABLE 2. *Comparison of gross cysts, cancers, and fibroadenomas*

	Gross cysts	Cancer	Fibroadenoma
Number	Often multiple	Single	Usually single
Shape	Spherical	Irregular	Spherical to ovoid
Tenderness	Common	Unusual	Rare
Consistency	Soft to firm	Usually hard	Firm
Definition	Usually good	Poor	Very good
Mobility	Usually good	Poor	Very good

as skin and pectoral fascia rather than being freely mobile, prevent the identification of ribs beneath them, have no mirror-image counterpart in the other breast, are irregularly shaped rather than spherical, and are basically nontender. Fibroadenomas are usually well defined, nontender, firm, mobile, and generally occur in women in their teens and 20s.

Fibrocystic disease without gross cysts is a common cause of breast nodules and includes a wide spectrum of physical findings, including pain on movement, local tenderness, and thickening and/or nodules in the breast. Fibrocystic disease is rarely hard and is never associated with redness or fixation of the skin. This condition may start in the teens, gradually worsens with age, and varies significantly with the menstrual cycle, worsening each month until the onset of the menses, after which it subsides for 5 to 10 days, only to return. After the menopause, it generally resolves unless there is continued stimulation of the breasts with hormonal replacement therapy. There are no completely reliable techniques for distinguishing localized fibrocystic disease from breast cancer other than biopsy, but (as with gross cysts) pain, tenderness, and bilaterality suggest fibrocystic disease, as does a documented variability with the menstrual cycle.

Miscellaneous Abnormalities

Gynecomastia

True gynecomastia is a visible and palpable enlargement of the male breast due to hypertrophy of the ductal tissue. This presents as a disk-shaped, discrete, tender firmness beneath the nipple and areola. Gynecomastia is almost never significantly eccentric. It is often seen transiently at puberty, where it may be bilateral or unilateral. Other situations in which gynecomastia is seen include patients with liver disease, after bilateral orchiectomy, with estrogen supplementation, and as a side effect of a long list of medications, including digitalis. When seeing a patient with gynecomastia, references should be consulted regarding the side effects of all the patient's medications. Obese men also may develop a fatty enlargement of the subcutaneous tissues in the pectoral area beneath the nipples which may mimic a female breast, but the enlargement is elongated rather than hemispherical and does not contain the ductal hypertrophy of true gynecomastia. On palpation, the fat in this area generally blends smoothly into the subcutaneous fat over the anterior chest wall.

Supernumerary Nipples

These may be associated with a miniature areola, usually resembling 4- to 12-mm raised nevi, and are seen in the "milk line" extending from the axilla to the groin. They are not functional and require no concern or treatment except rarely for cosmetic reasons.

Nipple Discharge

This is quite common and not usually related to a malignancy. Reassuring characteristics of the nipple discharge include origin from multiple ducts, bilaterality, association with recent pregnancy, lactation, recent change in hormone therapy, and association with medications such as major tranquilizers, reserpine, and methyldopa. Bilateral nipple discharge unassociated with lactation is occasionally seen with pituitary adenomas. When discharge is noted from a single duct, it should be tested for blood and a cytological examination considered. Any precipitating "trigger point" should be sought. The most likely site of origin of the discharge will usually be suggested by the location of the duct from which the discharge is seen. A rolling pressure with the fingertips should be gently and precisely used, starting 8 to 10 cm outside the areolar border, to document the location (i.e., the clock face location and distance from the nipple) at which the discharge is first elicited. Because some discharges may be scanty, it is often prudent to combine careful localization and immediate preparation of slides for occult blood and/or cytologic examination. Particular attention should be devoted to identifying any previously overlooked nodules in the area from which the discharge is elicited because the presence of such a nodule increases the likelihood of a malignancy. Nipple discharge not related to hormonal changes is generally due to mammary duct ectasia (a variation of fibrocystic disease), benign intraductal papillomas, and intraductal carcinoma. It should be remembered that although a bloody nipple discharge definitely requires histologic definition, most bloody nipple discharges are due to papilloma or ductal ectasia.

Nipple Inversion

This is generally of long standing and is rarely significant unless it has changed. If new, however, it should be considered analogous to dimpling and investigated further.

Patients with Implants

Several million women have had breast augmentation, generally with silicone-containing implants. These may be placed between the native breast tissue and the pectoralis major muscle or, more recently, beneath the pectoralis muscle. Implants may be associated with capsular formation, which leads to a very firm, often tender, spherical implant with the native breast on top of it. They also may leak, often causing a nodule adjacent to the implant. Nodules of the native breast parenchyma, whether benign or malignant, occurring in patients with implants may be easy to feel if the implant/capsule is firm, but a nodule may sink into a soft implant, making it considerably more difficult to feel. Therefore, soft (and more cosmetically satisfactory) implants require more time for proper examination and it may be possible to evaluate some nodules only by using a pincerslike grasp through the native breast to secure and identify a nodule by extracting it away from the yielding implant beneath.

Scars and Defects

Healed breast biopsy sites have various associated palpable abnormalities, the most notable of which are defects, dog-earing, and deep scarring. Defects occur when adjacent breast tissue is not reapproximated after biopsy and cause problems because the "shoulders" simulate a mass on each side of the defect. Each of these shoulders has only one edge, blending imperceptibly into nearby breast tissue on the other three sides. Dog ears occur when adjacent breast tissue is reapproximated after biopsy, causing a prominent palpable crumpling/heaping up of tissue at each end of the deep closure. Deep scarring can be seen with and without deep closure when the healing process deep in the breast is accompanied by exuberant fibrosis. It is obviously important to note and record the palpable features of all scars for future reference because cancers occurring near old scars tend to be noticed and examined via biopsy later than are nodules of similar characteristics in undistorted areas of the breast. This is probably due to patient/examiner uncertainty as to whether an irregularity near a scar is new or old. Records of how it felt on earlier examinations can be invaluable.

RECORDING THE FINDINGS

If preprinted recording sheets are not available, it is easy to draw free hand the outline of the breasts and record all findings, including scars, defects, nodules, thickening, axillary nodes, and the site of any nipple discharge. It is often useful to show this diagram to the patient and, if she is not familiar with examining her breasts, suggest that she examine herself every day for a month and make a similar diagram for her own future use. Women are much more inclined to examine their breasts if they know that a professional examination has just been performed without anything alarming being found. Daily examination for 30 days will quickly accustom a woman to what is normal for her, whereas the more traditional monthly examination never allows many women to get past the threshold of uncertainty. The common outcome of such uncertainty is abandonment of self-examination.

SUGGESTED READING

Blamey R, Evans A, Ellis I, Wilson R. *Atlas of breast cancer.* Coral Springs, FL: Merit, 1994.
Bland KI, Copeland EM. *The breast: comprehensive management of benign and malignant diseases.* Philadelphia: W.B. Saunders, 1991.
Love SM. *Dr. Susan Love's breast book.* Reading, PA: Addison-Wesley, 1991.
Teal J, Schneider P. *Straight talk on women's health.* New York: Master Media, 1993.

Clinical Skills for Adult Primary Care
edited by M. E. Silverman and J. W. Hurst.
Lippincott-Raven Publishers, Philadelphia © 1996.

17

Examination of the Female Pelvis

Sandra Adamson Fryhofer, M.D.

*Emory University School of Medicine, Atlanta, Georgia 30322
and Piedmont Hospital, Atlanta, Georgia 30309*

"Always note and record the unusual. Keep and compare your observations. Communicate or publish short notes on anything that is striking or new."

William Osler. From Thayer LS. Osler, the teacher.
Johns Hopkins Hosp Bull 1919;30:199.

Primary care physicians are expected to provide total primary care for women as well as men. By mastering the art of the female pelvic examination, the physician can provide care for the whole person.

SCREENING GUIDELINES FOR THE PELVIC EXAMINATION

The following screening guidelines are recommended. The U.S. Preventive Service Task Force recommends a Papanicolaou (Pap) smear and pelvic examination for all sexually active women and for those age 18 or older every 1 to 3 years until age 65 (1). The National Cancer Institute recommends yearly examinations for all sexually active women age 18 and older. The American Cancer Society also recommends annual examinations for women who are sexually active or over 18 (2). After a woman has had three or more consecutive satisfactory normal annual examinations, the Pap test may be done less frequently at the discretion of her physician. The frequency of screening should be based on risk factors for cervical cancer, including early onset of sexual intercourse, multiple sex partners, history of human papilloma virus, and lower socioeconomic status.

TECHNIQUES

Getting the Right Tools

Before the examination begins, it is essential to have the right tools or the examination will be an unpleasant experience for both the physician and the patient. The examiner will need the following materials:

- Light source
- Assortment of specula
- Materials needed to obtain cultures (chlamydia, gonorrhea, viral), KOH, wet prep
- Pap smear slide and fixative
- Water-soluble jelly lubricant
- Examining gloves (double-glove the hand used for the internal examination)

Types and Use of Specula

A Roman trivalve speculum was one of the first in 79 A.D. Since that time, hundreds of vaginal specula have been devised. Most primary care physicians learned to use the Graves speculum in training; however, many patients find the Graves speculum uncomfortable and prefer the Pederson speculum, which is a half inch narrower than the others. Both plastic and metal speculums are available; however, metal speculums are easier to manipulate, whereas the plastic ones seem to "pinch" more easily. The plastic speculum offers the advantage of easier viewing of the vaginal walls. A virginal speculum should be available. Sometimes it is difficult to view the cervix because the vaginal walls are occluding the view. This can occasionally happen in women who have had several children. To remedy the problem, simply snip off the end of a finger of a rubber glove, insert the speculum through the glove, and then insert the gloved speculum into the patient. The glove will hold open the vaginal walls and allow the cervix to be viewed.

Organizing the Tools

The two drawers at the end of the examining table may be used during the pelvic examination. The top drawer can be used to store clean specula, culture supplies, water-soluble jelly lubricant, Pap smear slides and fixative, and sanitary napkin pads (Fig. 1). The bottom drawer contains a large metal "cake pan" lined in disposable paper towels. Specula are placed in this pan after the examination. At the end of the day, specula can then be cleaned and autoclaved. Specula should be cleaned in a solution such as Lysol Quartenary Cleaner/Disinfectant (National Lab, Montvale, NJ), which is nonabrasive to stainless steel. While wearing gloves, use a sponge to remove debris from the speculum. Soak in 0.5 ounce of cleaner diluted in 1 gallon of water for at least 10 minutes. Rinse and dry thoroughly, then autoclave specula. The solution should be made at least daily.

Preparing the Patient for the Examination

Because of the nature of the examination, the medical history should be obtained while the patient is fully dressed before changing into an examining gown.

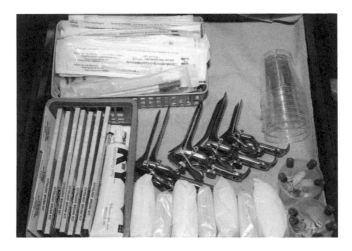

FIG. 1. Organization of drawer for pelvic examination.

One of the purposes of obtaining the history is to establish rapport with the patient to help her relax. This will add to the ease and accuracy of the examination and avoid the difficulties of examination through or against tense muscles. The patient should empty her bladder before the pelvic examination is performed. Sometimes a full bladder can be confused with a pregnant uterus or an ovarian cyst (3). Patients also appreciate an ongoing explanation of what the physician will be doing during the examination. In positioning the patient, make sure that her hips extend slightly past the end of the examining table. Adjust stirrups for patient comfort. It is often difficult for elderly patients to abduct their legs. One maneuver is to move the stirrups farther away from the patient and not as far apart. Let the patient know when you are ready to start the examination. This can be easily accomplished by gently touching the patient's arm or leg before beginning the examination. It is recommended to use the back of the hand as this is considered less familiar. Double-glove the hand to be used for the internal part of the bimanual examination, then take off the outer glove before doing the rectovaginal examination. In this way, the rectum is not contaminated with bacteria or other conditions that might be present in the vagina such as human papilloma virus.

THE EXTERNAL EXAMINATION

The external examination begins with a visual survey. Check for signs of swelling, inflammation, ulceration, and atrophy. During the external examination, the following areas should be evaluated (4):

- Vulva (in Latin, "covering")
- Clitoris (in Greek, "shut-up" or "concealed")

- Urethral meatus (in Greek, *ouros* or "drizzling rain")
- Skene's gland (paraurethral glands or lesser glands)
- Labia minora
- Labia majora
- Bartholin's glands (vulvovaginal glands or greater glands)
- Perineum (in Greek, "around evacuation")

In checking the Skene's gland, insert the index finger in the vagina, press up on the urethra, and gently milk the urethra outward to look for discharge or infection. The Bartholin's glands are checked by inserting the index finger in the vagina near the posterior end of the introitus. Palpate at the 5:00 and 7:00 o'clock positions using the index finger inside and the thumb outside the vagina. The Bartholin's glands can usually not be palpated unless there is a problem such as a cyst or abscess. A Bartholin's duct cyst can usually be felt between the fingers. Note any tenderness or discharge.

There are several benign conditions of the vulva, such as hypertrophic dystrophy, which can be treated with steroid cream, and lichen sclerosus, which is an atrophic condition that can be treated with androgen such as testosterone cream or progesterone in oil. Look for condyloma, caused by the human papilloma virus, some strains of which can predispose to dysplasia and cancer. If a suspicious area is seen, it can be helpful to place some white vinegar (3% acetic acid) on the vulva. First warn the patient that it might sting a little. Leave it on for 3 to 5 minutes and then look at the area under a magnifying glass. If it turns white, it can be an abnormal area that might need to be examined via biopsy. A high index of suspicion for vulvar cancer must be maintained. Itching is one of the most common complaints in women with vulvar neoplasia.

EXAMINATION FOR CYSTOCELE, RECTOCELE, AND UTERINE PROLAPSE

After the external examination, check for vaginal outlet support by having the patient strain down and cough while checking for bulges. Bulging from above represents a cystocele; bulging from below implies a rectocele. Check for uterine prolapse and grade it as follows:

- 1st degree, cervix in vagina
- 2nd degree, cervix at introitus
- 3rd degree, cervix and vagina at introitus

THE INTERNAL EXAMINATION (THE SPECULUM EXAMINATION)

Use warm water to lubricate the speculum. Do not use any other lubricants because they can interfere with the Pap smear and other studies. Keep the blades of the speculum away from the sensitive periurethral area. Take care not to pull pubic hairs or pinch the labia during the insertion. Before inserting the speculum, use the forefinger and middle finger to exert downward pressure on the posterior wall of the vagina. It is easiest to insert the speculum "up and down" so that the greatest width of the speculum goes from anterior to posterior. Continue to insert the speculum while turning it 90 degrees and moving it in a downward posterior motion. Open the speculum, pull back slightly, and the cervix will generally come into view. Then tighten the screw on the speculum. When looking at the cervix, make a notation of the cervical os or opening. A nulliparous cervical os is small and either round or oval; a parous cervix is slitlike. There also can be other variations as a result of childbirth. Look at the cervix for signs of redness and discharge, which can indicate infection or irritation from gonorrhea, candida, gardnerella, chlamydia, or herpes. Do the KOH and wet prep and obtain any cultures at this time. Look for any lumps and bumps. An endocervical polyp may be seen and should be examined via biopsy. Simply take a forceps and twist the polyp. It may be necessary to snip the stalk with the biopsy forceps. Then apply some Monsel's solution or a silver nitrate stick to stop the bleeding and send the specimen to the laboratory. A common variation is a Nabothian cyst, which presents as a little lump on the cervix and has a yellowish tint. This is a little gland that plugs up and appears to be a cervical pimple. Finally, look for the warty lesions of the human papilloma virus, which can be associated with cervical dysplasia.

The Pap Smear

Cervical cancer is the sixth most common cancer in women (5). Since the introduction of the Pap smear in the 1940s, the incidence and mortality of invasive cervical cancer in the United States has markedly decreased. In 1940, the incidence of cervical cancer was approximately 45,000 cases a year. In 1992, the number was down to 13,500. The incidence of invasive cervical cancer has decreased by at least 70% over the past 40 years.

The Pap smear is highly effective as a screening test. The test is insensitive but specific. False negative results have been reported. The specificity for cervical cancer is 90% to 99% (1).

According to the American Cancer Society, several instructions can be given to the patient to obtain an optimal result on the Pap smear. Treat any vaginal infection or discharge before performing the Pap smear—inflammatory cells can be confusing to the pathologist. It is best for the patient to refrain from intercourse for 24 to 48 hours before the test because some of the reactive changes can be confusing to the pathologist. Vaginal medications should not be used for 24 to 48 hours before the test because they can interfere with interpretation. It is also important not to douche within 48 hours before obtaining the Pap smear. Douching can remove abnormal cells that might give important information to the screening pathologist.

There are three basic parts of the cervix: the exocervix, which is covered with squamous cells; the endocervix covered with columnar cells; and the area between called the squamocolumnar junction, the transformation zone, or the T-zone. Although 95% of all cancers originate in the transformation zone, it is important to sample all three areas of the cervix when performing the Pap smear. Prepackaged kits of tools for performing the Pap smear are commercially available and are very convenient to use. These kits contain a glass microscope slide with a frosted end on which to pencil the patient's name, a wooden spatula for obtaining cervical and vaginal smears, a nylon-tipped cytology brush for the endocervical specimen, and a little packet of fixative. If the packet of fixative is not available, fixative can be sprayed on the slide. The can should be kept about 10 to 12 inches from the slide so that it will not blow cells off the slide.

To obtain the specimen, the wooden spatula is rotated 360 degrees on the transformation zone, making sure there is contact with the cervical mucosa during this entire turn. These cells are then wiped on one side of the glass slide. The endocervical brush is then inserted into the endocervix no further than the length of the brush and rotated 180 degrees only, to cut down on any bleeding. The endocervical brush should not be used on pregnant patients. These cells are then gently wiped on the other side of the Pap smear slide. Fixative must be sprayed using a spray fixative or squeezed on if the fixative pouch is used. If possible, fixative should be applied within 10 seconds to avoid an air-drying effect, which can interfere with slide interpretation. Cytology fixative should include a 95% ethyl alcohol–$2^{1}/_{2}$% carbowax combination. There are several styles of applying the sample to the Pap smear slide. One method is called the VCE—vaginal, cervical, endocervical—method. Some laboratories simply request that specimens obtained from the spatula and those obtained from the endocervical brush be separated.

A pathologist who can be contacted when there are questions about a smear is invaluable. By obtaining the best sample and preparing it properly, reliability and quality of this screening tool is maximized.

The Vaginal Examination

As the speculum is removed, turn the speculum around and look at the vaginal walls to inspect the vaginal mucosa. Check for color, signs of trauma, discharge, and ulcerations. Look for vaginal cancer and the cobblestone appearance of human papilloma virus.

The Bimanual Examination

The purpose of the bimanual examination is to feel the uterus, both ovaries, and other adnexal structures. It is very important to maintain visual contact with the patient. Valuable information can be obtained by observing the facial expression during this part of the examination. Begin by applying lubricant to the fingers of the hand that will be placed internally. Drop the lubricant onto the fingers. Never contaminate the tube of lubricant by touching it after touching the patient.

The bimanual examination means just what the term implies—two hands. One hand is used internally and is termed the internal or vaginal hand. The other hand is used externally and is called the external or abdominal hand. There are different opinions as to which hand, left or right, should be used as the internal hand. Some experts suggest using the dominant hand. Others prefer the nondominant hand. Some experts suggest that, no matter which hand is your dominant hand, the left hand should be used internally because the natural curve of the left hand aids in feeling around the sigmoid colon. Whichever technique seems most comfortable is generally selected.

In order to introduce the internal fingers, press downward on the perineum with two fingertips. Try to avoid the periurethral area because this area is sensitive. Continue to insert the fingers in a downward and posterior direction and turn the finger upward. Continue to insert the fingers into the vagina until the cervix is felt. Sometimes it is necessary to gain extra length of reach by placing your foot on the step of the examining table and leaning slightly forward. Bend the elbow, rest it on your knee, and use the weight against the elbow to push the fingers in a little deeper.

Examining the Cervix

Now that the cervix is within reach, palpate the surface of the cervix. The cervix should feel like the tip of a nose in consistency.

Examining the Uterus

Position the finger of the internal vaginal hand underneath the cervix and lift upward to bring the uterus closer to the abdominal wall in order to trap the uterus between the two hands.

In order to avoid common errors, never begin depression of the abdominal wall too close to the pubis. It is best to begin at the umbilicus and move downward toward the symphysis pubis. Special care should be taken not to shift the fingers of the abdominal hand frequently because this can be interpreted by the patient as poking (6). Movements should be slow and fluid, not jabbing. Identify the uterus between the hands. Try to palpate and feel with the internal or vaginal fingers. Do not depend on the abdominal fingers to feel the uterus. The function of the abdominal hand is to press the pelvic structures down so palpation can be accomplished by the internal (vaginal) fingers.

It is important to determine if the uterus is anterior (anteverted) or posterior (retroverted). Separate the vaginal fingers slightly. Move the vaginal fingers anterior or upward to palpate where the uterine cervix joins the uterine fundus. An anteverted uterus is easy to locate in this manner. If the uterus is not located, move the fingers below or posterior to the cervix. The retroverted uterus can be located in this way. Notation should be made of the shape, size, and consistency of the uterus. It is important to try to feel as much of the uterus as possible.

Examining the Adnexal Structures

The adnexal structures consist of the fallopian tubes and ovaries. Each side is examined in turn. In examining the adnexal structures, pull the fingers back slightly but do not remove them. Shift your body position to the side opposite the side of the patient that is being examined. The fingers of the internal hand should be between the cervix and the vaginal wall. Place the abdominal hand at the anterior-superior iliac spine. Move the external hand up slightly and then slightly medially and then gradually downward toward the symphysis pubis (7). Using slow, gentle pressure, the abdominal hand should be sweeping the adnexal structures toward the vaginal hand. The fingers of the vaginal hand should be turned slightly upward. Examining the ovary may be slightly uncomfortable for the patient. Now shift to the opposite side and repeat the examination. Having completed the bimanual examination, the vaginal fingers are removed.

The Rectovaginal Examination

The examiner either takes off the outer glove of the internal hand or regloves the internal hand. Again, this prevents spreading infections from the vagina to the rectum. The rectovaginal examination is not always necessary, but it should be performed if the uterus is retroverted in order to further evaluate abnormalities found on the bimanual examination, especially if malignancy is suspected or for routine colorectal screening if a patient is over 40 years of age. Begin by dropping lubricant to the fingers of the hand that will be used internally. Insert the index finger into the vagina and the middle finger in the rectum. Go through the same examination used in the bimanual examination. Careful attention should be given to examining the retroverted uterus. Carefully palpate the rectovaginal septum, the rectal mucosa, and the posterior cul de sac. Now gently remove the examining fingers. A specimen for stool guaiac testing can be applied to the testing card using residual stool from the examining glove. The examining gloves are then removed. Assist the patient in sitting up after the examination if help is needed. It is courteous to give the patient a soft tissue to aid in removal of any residual lubricant. Be sure to give the patient an explanation of the findings of the examination.

The Uterus

Normal Findings

The uterus is a pear-shaped, fibromuscular organ approximately 9 cm long, 6.5 cm wide, and 3.5 cm thick. The normal position of the uterus is anteverted and anteflexed, that is, tilted a little forward and also bent a little forward on its axis. One of five women has a retroverted uterus, which is a little more difficult to examine (8). Obstetrician-gynecologists correlate uterine size with weeks of pregnancy. General guidelines to help gauge size can be termed the 3-4-5 rule (8,9):

- 3 months = 12 weeks = just above pubic symphysis
- 4 months = 16 weeks = level of anterior-superior iliac spine
- 5 months = 20 weeks = level of the umbilicus

Abnormal Findings

Fibroids or myomas present as firm, irregular nodules. The size should be estimated. Lobulated asymmetrical enlargement is characteristic of uterine fibroids. Fibroids usually regress after the menopause, but their growth can be encouraged by hormonal therapy (7).

The Adnexal Structures

Normal Findings

The ovary is an almond-shaped structure approximately 3.5 cm long, 2.5 cm wide, and 2 cm thick. Mildly enlarged cystic ovaries are fairly common in the reproductive years. It is important to remember that the postmenopausal ovary tends to atrophy in size. As a result, it is almost impossible to palpate a normal ovary in a postmenopausal patient. Likewise, the palpation of an ovary that is "normal" for a premenopausal woman may very well represent an ovarian tumor in the postmenopausal patient (7). Fallopian tubes cannot usually be palpated. Tenderness and enlargement of the fallopian tubes should be noted (7).

Abnormal Findings

Ultrasonography is often useful in evaluating pelvic masses found on physical examination. Specifically, the use of the transvaginal probe can add to the specificity of the classical transabdominal ultrasound (10).

Pelvic Mass

In evaluating a pelvic mass, the size of 5 cm is an important number. Masses larger than 5 cm may require surgical intervention; however, cysts smaller than 5 cm often can be observed over a period of a few months and followed with ultrasound to document change (10).

Fecal Mass

A cecum filled with feces can sometimes masquerade as a pelvic mass. If this is suspected, reexamination after an enema can be helpful.

Physiologic Ovarian Cysts

Follicular cysts result when a mature follicle fails to rupture at the time of ovulation. They can range in size from 3 to 8 cm and often can resolve on their own. Sometimes a clinical trial of hormonal suppression is useful. Luteal cysts occur when blood collects within the follicle after ovulation (10).

Hydrosalpinx/Tuboovarian Abscesses

These occur as a result of an inflammatory process. In the case of a hydrosalpinx, the fimbriated end of the tube gets stuck together because of the inflammatory process, thereby trapping secretions within the tube and causing the tube to enlarge in size.

Endometriosis

Implants can be palpated on the uterosacral ligaments. They have a nodular feel. Endometrial implants can be embedded in the myometrium of the uterus and are known as adenomyosis. Adenomyosis will present as irregular thickening of the uterus. Endometriomas or large collections of endometriosis that become cystic masses can also occasionally be palpated in the pelvis.

Ectopic Pregnancy

The importance of this consideration cannot be underestimated. If in doubt, a pregnancy test is essential. To know the date of the last menstrual period is mandatory.

Dermoid Cysts

This is also termed benign teratoma and is the most common type of germ cell tumor found in women of child-bearing age. They can contain teeth, skin, fat, and hair.

Ovarian Cancer and Other Abnormalities

One of the most dreaded discoveries is ovarian cancer in the guise of a pelvic mass. In addition, such a mass could also reflect metastases from a primary neoplasm from another region. Finally, the examination can detect such congenital abnormalities as vaginal septa, double vagina, double cervix, and double uterus.

REFERENCES

1. U.S. Preventive Services Task Force. *Guide to clinical preventive services.* Baltimore: Williams & Wilkins, 1989.
2. American Cancer Society. Guidelines for the cancer related check-up: an update. 1993.
3. Ryan KJ, Berkowitz R, Barbieri RL. *Kistner's gynecology.* Chicago: Year Book Medical, 1990.
4. Kase NG, Weingold AB, Gershenson DM. *Principles and practice of clinical gynecology.* 2nd ed. New York: Churchill-Livingstone, 1990.
5. Rose PG. Cervical cancer. *Emerg Med* 1993;3:133.
6. Beacham DW, Beacham WD. *Synopsis of gynecology.* 10th ed. St. Louis: Mosby, 1982.
7. Barber HRK. Pelvic examination: step by step guide. *Hosp Med* 1980;4:52.
8. Bates B. *A guide to physical examination.* 2nd ed. Philadelphia: J.B. Lippincott, 1979.
9. Gabbe SG, Niebyl JR, Simpson JL. *Obstetrics: normal and problem pregnancies.* New York: Churchill-Livingstone, 1986.
10. Chervenak FA, Isaacson GC, Campbell S. *Ultrasound in obstetrics and gynecology.* Boston: Little, Brown, 1993.

SUGGESTED READING

Kurman RJ. *Blaustein's pathology of the female genital tract.* New York: Springer-Verlag, 1994.

Kvale JN, Kvale JK. Common gynecologic problems after age 75. *Postgrad Med* 1993;4:263–72.

Martin PL. *Handbook of office gynecology.* Orlando, FL: Grune & Stratton, 1985.

Patsner B. Uterine cancer. *Emerg Med* 1993;3:157.

Pernoll M, Benson RC. *Current obstetric and gynecologic diagnosis and treatment.* Norwalk: Appleton, 1987.

Piver MS, Hempling RE. Ovarian cancer. *Emerg Med* 1993;3:141.

Sox H. Preventive health services in adults. *N Engl J Med* 1994;22:1589–95.

Veridiano NP. Vaginal and vulvar cancer. *Emerg Med* 1993;3:149.

Walker HK, Hall WD, Hurst JW. *Clinical methods.* Boston: Butterworth, 1980.

Wynn RM. *Obstetrics and gynecology: the clinical core.* Philadelphia: Lea & Febiger, 1974.

Clinical Skills for Adult Primary Care
edited by M. E. Silverman and J. W. Hurst.
Lippincott-Raven Publishers, Philadelphia © 1996.

18

Examination of the Male Genitalia, the Prostate, and for Hernia

William M. Scaljon, M.D.

Piedmont Hospital, Atlanta, Georgia 30309

"The art of the practice of medicine is to be learned only by experience; 'tis not an inheritance; it cannot be revealed."

William Osler, quoted in Thayer WS. Osler, the teacher.
Johns Hopkins Hosp Bull 1919;30:198.

The routine examination of the male genitalia is usually reserved for the last part of the examination. Especially in children and adolescents, this can be an embarrassing and uncomfortable experience. The examiner's attitude and sensitivity to the patient is important and helpful in obtaining a satisfactory examination.

This portion of the physical examination should be stressed as much as any other part of the body. The omission or abbreviation of this examination may constitute grave consequences for the patient and the physician.

EXAMINATION OF THE PENIS

Technique

The patient is best examined standing in front of the examiner. If the individual is uncircumcised, the foreskin or prepuce should be easily retracted to expose the glans. The prepuce should be shifted forward over the glans when the inspection is completed. Palpation of the penile shaft should be performed using the thumb and first two fingers as the examiner notes the presence of any tenderness, induration, infection, or masses.

Normal Findings

Inspection of the penis shows it to be free of subcutaneous fat and generally more pigmented than the rest of the skin. The flaccid penis is nontender. Fibrous

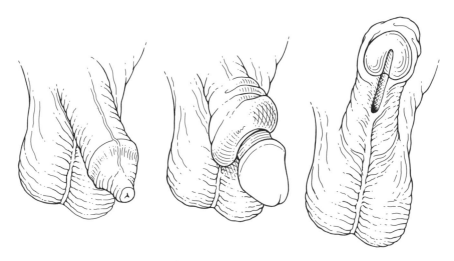

FIG. 1. Phimosis.   **FIG. 2.** Paraphimosis.   **FIG. 3.** Hypospadias.

tissue without nodularity can be felt. The urethral meatus is a pink, slitlike opening ventral to the tip of the glans.

Abnormal Findings

- Phimosis: a redundancy and contraction of the foreskin that makes the retraction of the foreskin difficult (Fig. 1). This is usually congenital or the result of recurrent infection.
- Paraphimosis: a result of the foreskin being retracted behind the glans and subsequently unable to be returned to its normal position (Fig. 2). This results in edema of the glans and foreskin.
- Balanitis: an irritation of the prepuce in uncircumcised males.
- Balanoposthitis: an inflammation of the prepuce and glans of uncircumcised males.
- Meatal stenosis: a pinpoint-sized urethral meatus resulting in a decreased urinary stream.
- Hypospadias: a congenital, abnormal ventral location of the urethral meatus (Fig. 3).
- Epispadias: a congenital dorsal location of the urethral meatus.
- Cancer/epidermoid carcinoma: a painless, ulcerated lesion noted under the prepuce in uncircumcised males (Fig. 4). Persistent penile lesions should be considered suspicious for the condition.

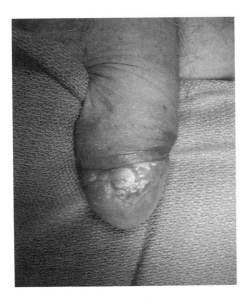

FIG. 4. Cancer of the penis.

Sexually Transmitted Diseases

- Venereal warts (*condyloma acuminata*): pinkish or brown tumorous lesions on a stalk, sometimes resembling a cauliflower, found on the glans penis and prepuce. These result from infection by human papillomavirus.
- Syphilitic chancre: a dark or reddish sore that may ulcerate, forming an indurated base with rounded, raised edges (Fig. 5). The lesion is painless.
- Herpes simplex: appears as small vesicles with a red base (Fig. 6). May be located anywhere on the penis and are usually painful.
- Peyronie's plaque: a fibrous plaque usually located in the dorsal aspect of the penis invading the fascial layer of the corporeal body (Fig. 7). This plaque creates a disfiguration curvature when the penis is in an erect position.
- Priapism: a prolonged penile erection, which is usually painful. It can be seen in individuals with leukemia and sickle cell disease.

EXAMINATION OF THE SCROTUM

Technique

As with the examination of the penis, the patient should be standing for this evaluation. Palpation of the scrotum should be performed with the thumb and next two fingers. In addition to observation and palpation of the scrotum, transillumination with a flashlight in a darkened room may outline intrascrotal masses.

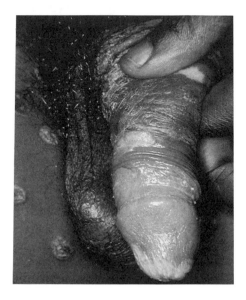

FIG. 5. Syphilitic chancre.

Normal Findings

The scrotum, just as the penis, should be more deeply pigmented than the skin of the body. The scrotal skin is folded, loose, and may vary in thickness depending on the patient's age, external temperature, and original state. Spontaneous retraction of the scrotum during the examination is the result of stimulating the cremasteric reflex. Asymmetry of the scrotum is common due to an increased length

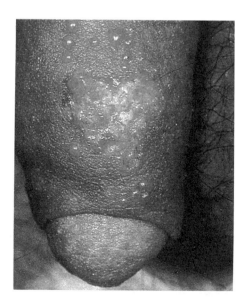

FIG. 6. Herpes simplex.

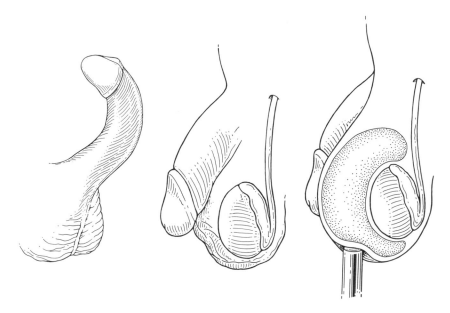

FIG. 7. Peyronie's plaque. **FIG. 8.** Normal scrotum, testes, and epididymis. **FIG. 9.** Hydrocele.

of one spermatic cord. The left hemiscrotum may then appear to be lower than the right hemiscrotum.

The two testes lie freely in the scrotal sac and are approximately 3 to 4 cm × 2 to 5 cm in size in the adult male. The testes are normally sensitive but should not be too tender to examination. The epididymis is normally located on the posterolateral aspect of the testes and should be quite firm, indiscrete, and nontender (Fig. 8). Palpation of the vas deferens should reveal a smooth tubal structure, which travels with the spermatic vessels.

Abnormal Findings

- Hemangiomas of the scrotal skin: small varicosities of the skin that may bleed spontaneously.
- Sebaceous cyst of the scrotal skin: small lumps on the scrotal skin that may contain white pearly material.
- Agenesis of testis or cryptorchism: a poorly developed scrotum. It can be suspected by an abnormal scrotal contour, an indication of either agenesis of the testis or cryptorchism. Palpation of the scrotum may not detect a testicle. Palpation of the inguinal canal may detect an undescended testicle. An atrophic testicle may indicate past mumps orchitis.

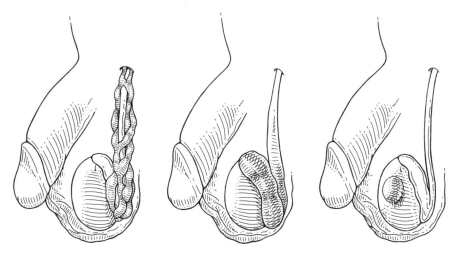

FIG. 10. Varicocele.   **FIG. 11.** Epididymitis.   **FIG. 12.** Testicular tumor.

- Hydrocele: a painless collection of fluid within the scrotum (actually within the tunica vaginalis). This can be diagnosed by placing a flashlight against the posterior aspect of the scrotum in a darkened room (Fig. 9). The examiner should be able to transilluminate the scrotum if the mass is fluid. A solid mass (testicular tumor or hernia) will not transilluminate.
- Varicocele: an abnormal dilatation of veins within the spermatic cord. This is usually due to incompetent valves in the venous system (Fig. 10). Approximately 90% of varicoceles are present in the left hemiscrotum. Palpation of the varicocele is classically described as feeling "a bag of worms." Varicoceles are the number one cause of infertility in males.
- Epididymitis: a tender, swollen mass sometimes inseparable from the testicle (Fig. 11). This is seen more commonly in adults and can be associated with urinary tract infections. Untreated, this inflammation may involve the testicle and is then classified as an epididymoorchitis.
- Torsion of the spermatic cord: an elevated testicle with a twisted spermatic cord above the testicle, commonly termed a "bell-clapper sign." There is a history of acute onset of severe testicular pain. Diaphoresis with associated nausea is common. This is mainly seen in preadolescent boys. Observation of the scrotum may demonstrate a high-riding testicle. Torsion of the spermatic cord is classified as a surgical emergency and should be attended to immediately. Clinical distinction between torsion of the spermatic cord and acute epididymitis may be determined by supporting the involved hemiscrotum in the palm of the examiner's hand. If the pain is relieved with this support, the likely diagnosis is epididymitis.
- Testicular tumors: a firm, irregular, nontender mass within the testicle (Fig. 12). This mass does not transilluminate. Careful palpation should be able to de-

termine whether the mass is intratesticular or adjacent to the testicle. In the latter case it would more likely be a benign lesion. Testicular tumors are usually noted in young males between 20 and 40 years of age. Most tumors are not tender unless rapid growth causes ischemia.

EXAMINATION OF THE PROSTATE

Technique

Examination of the prostate is best performed by having the patient stand and bend over an examining table. With a well-lubricated forefinger, the prostate is palpated through the anterior surface of the rectum (Fig. 13). The entire posterior surface of the prostate, including the upper and lateral margins and midline sulcus, should be outlined.

Normal Findings

The normal size of the prostate is similar to a walnut. The consistency is comparable with the thenar eminence of the palm. Both posterior lobes should be

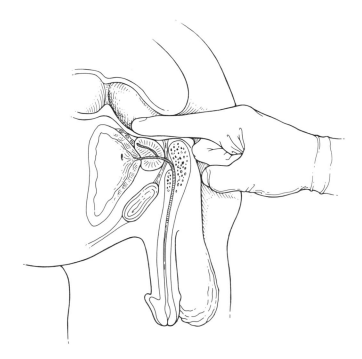

FIG. 13. Examination of the prostate.

symmetrical and smooth in consistency. In most cases, the seminal vesicles are not palpable.

Abnormal Findings

- Prostatitis: a tender prostate on palpation. A tender, fluctuant mass indicates an abscess is present. Care should be taken when performing a prostatic examination in acute prostatitis because of the possibility of producing dissemination of bacteria and subsequent septicemia.
- Chronic prostatitis: a boggy prostate with irregularity and induration. Prostatic calculi, resulting from chronic prostatitis, can be mistaken for cancer.
- Benign prostatic hyperplasia: a symmetrical enlargement of the prostate protruding into the anterior wall of the rectum with no associated induration and/or irregularities.
- Cancer: a hard, irregular prostate. Ninety percent of cancers involve the posterior lobe. Inability to identify borders of the prostate may be suggestive.

EXAMINATION OF THE INGUINAL CANAL FOR HERNIAS

Technique

An examination for an inguinal hernia(s) completes the physical examination of the male genitalia. The patient should be in a standing position and asked to

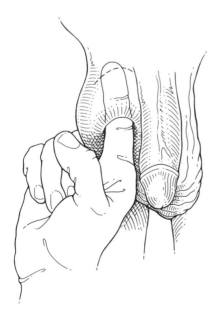

FIG. 14. Technique for examining for indirect inguinal hernia.

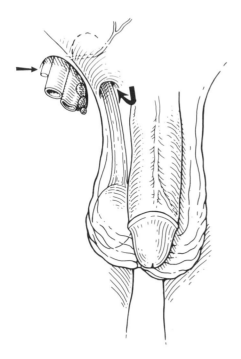

FIG. 15. Sites of hernias. Curved arrow points to external inguinal ring. Straight arrow points to femoral ring.

bear down, as if having a bowel movement. The examiner observes for any bulges in the inguinal area. Next, the patient is asked to relax. The forefinger is inserted into the inguinal canal medial to the spermatic vessels (Fig. 14). If the patient is a child, the examiner should use the little finger. The patient should then be instructed to cough; if a hernia is present, the bowel or omentum is felt against the exploring finger. An inguinal hernia is described as being indirect if it lies within the inguinal canal (Fig. 15).

The hernia also may extend into the external ring and enter into the scrotum. Indirect hernias are the most common of the abdominal hernias and are most frequently found in young men. It is not uncommon to have bilateral indirect hernias; therefore, one should examine both inguinal areas thoroughly.

Normal Findings

No bulge should be seen or felt.

Abnormal Findings

• An indirect inguinal hernia is felt as a protrusion within the inguinal canal.

- A direct inguinal hernia presents as a bulge medial to the external inguinal canal in the region of Hesselbach's triangle. It rarely enters the scrotum. This type of hernia is more common in men over the age of 40.
- The femoral hernia, which pushes through the femoral ring, is most common in women. On examination, the inguinal canal is empty of bulges.

SUGGESTED READING

Bates B. *A guide to physical examination and history taking.* 4th ed. Philadelphia: J.B. Lippincott, 1991:369–81.

Smith DR. *Smith's general urology.* 13th ed. Norwalk, CT: Appleton & Lange, 1992:40–7.

Mosby G. *A visual guide to physical examination: male genitalia, rectum and hernias* [videorecording]. 2nd ed. Westport, CT: Jacoby/Storm, 1986.

Judge RD, ed. *Clinical diagnosis: a physiologic approach.* 5th ed. Boston: Little, Brown, 1989:363–88.

Major RH. *Major's physical diagnosis: an introduction to the clinical process.* 9th ed. Philadelphia: W.B. Saunders, 1981:375–89.

Clinical Skills for Adult Primary Care
edited by M. E. Silverman and J. W. Hurst.
Lippincott-Raven Publishers, Philadelphia © 1996.

19

Examination of the Neurologic System

Douglas S. Stuart, M.D.

Piedmont Hospital, Atlanta, Georgia 30309

"As no two faces, so no two cases are alike in all respects, and unfortunately it is not only the disease itself which is so varied, but the subjects themselves have peculiarities which modify its action."

William Osler. *Aequanimitas and other addresses.*
Philadelphia: P. Blakiston & Son, 1928:130.

A well-performed neurologic examination can reliably discriminate between normality and abnormality in the central and peripheral nervous system. Although an extensive neurologic examination need only be performed when clinically indicated, a quick screening examination adds little additional effort to the routine general examination and should be considered indispensable. Considering the extraordinary cost of ancillary studies such as computed tomography and magnetic resonance imaging and the relatively low yield of these tests in the setting of a normal neurologic examination, the few minutes spent in examination can be extremely cost effective.

TECHNIQUE

A good neurologic examination begins with specific information from the history. Handedness should always be ascertained to assess hemispheric dominance. A family history and occasionally a pedigree should be obtained, given the high incidence of hereditary neurologic disease. In addition, a complete list of prescription and over-the-counter medications is necessary. In the physical examination, the carotid arteries should be palpated and auscultated in all new patients (see Chapters 12 and 13). Bruits should be assessed for asymmetry and differentiated from transmitted heart sounds. The skull should be examined for any outward evidence of trauma or previous surgery. Facial structure and expression should be noted because it may provide clues to a number of different disease states (e.g., Cushing's syndrome or Parkinson's disease).

MENTAL STATUS

It is customary to begin with an examination of the patient's mental state. Most clinicians formulate a rough assessment of this from interaction during the history. When higher integrative functions are clearly not impaired, this may be sufficient. When a quick, but objective, screening examination is desired, the Mini–Mental Status Exam is useful (1) (Table 1). When significant questions exist about a patient's intellectual performance, a formal mental status examination is important. This should begin with an assessment of the level of consciousness: hyperalert, alert, sleepy, lethargic, stuporous, or comatose. The patient should be

TABLE 1. *Mini-Mental Status Examination.*

Maximum score	Question
	Orientation
5	What is the (year) (season) (date) (day) (month)?
5	Where are we (state (county) (town) (hospital) (floor)?
	Registration
3	Name three objects, one second to say each, then ask the patient to repeat all three after you have said them. Give one point for each correct answer. Continue repeating all three objects until the patient learns all three. Count trials and record.
	Attention and calculation
5	Serial sevens. One point for each correct response. Stop after five answers. Alternatively, spell "world" backward.
	Recall
3	Ask for the three objects named in Registration. Give one point for each correct answer.
	Language
2	Name a pencil and a watch.
1	Repeat the following "No ifs, ands, or buts."
3	Follow a three-stage command: "Take paper in your right hand, fold it in half, and put it on the floor."
1	Read and obey the following: Close your eyes.
1	Write a sentence.
1	Copy a design.
Total 30	

Assess level of consciousness along a continuum

Alert	Drowsy	Stupor	Coma

From Folstein MF, Folstein F, McHugh P. Mini-mental state: a practical method for grading the cognitive state of patients for the clinician. *J Psychiatr Res* 1975;12:196–7. Reproduced by permission of author and Pergamon Press.

able to identify the location of the examination, including the hospital and room number. Knowledge of the time, month, and date should be ascertained. The patient's understanding of his or her medical situation should be appropriate, and affect and mood should be noted, particularly regarding depression and mania. Thought content should be assessed and the presence of delusions and hallucinations should be excluded.

SPEECH AND LANGUAGE

Speech and language should be formally assessed, especially in all cases of unexplained confusion. Language testing includes verbal fluency, auditory comprehension, reading, writing, and repetition. Paraphasic errors should be excluded. These may be totally nonsensical words or sound-alike words, such as substituting *grencil* for *pencil.* To exclude dysnomia, the patient should be able to name common objects in the examining room. Motor speech should be noted during the course of the history and need not be tested formally unless abnormalities seem apparent. Stock phrases, such as *Methodist Episcopal, truly rural,* or *liquid electricity,* tax the powers of articulation and are useful for testing purposes.

PARIETAL LOBE TESTS

In cases of unexplained confusion or inexplicably poor psychomotor performance, some consideration should be given to parietal lobe dysfunction. Parietal lobe testing, when performed, should screen both dominant and nondominant parietal functions. Tests of dominant parietal lobe function include calculation, finger recognition, and right-left orientation. Asking the patient to pick out the examiner's right ring finger or to make change is a quick and reliable screen of this part of the brain. The nondominant parietal lobe subserves functions such as constructional skills and spatial orientation. This can be tested by having the patient copy a complicated figure or draw a map of their home. Another simple test for the nondominant parietal lobe has the patient copy the face of a clock, properly placing the numbers and hands of the clock to denote a time specified by the examiner. The drawing should be symmetrical. Neglect of one side of the clock (usually the left) would indicate an abnormality.

MEMORY

Memory testing is not always necessary, especially in a younger patient. It should be considered routine in patients with trauma, seizures, and in the elderly. Memory testing should evaluate immediate recall, recent memory, and remote memory. Typically, three or five unrelated objects are given to the patient to remember and the examiner requests these back after 5 to 10 minutes. To be certain that these have been registered into active memory, the list should be repeated immediately or this memory test is not valid. Another useful memory test is digit span; the average adult can recite six digits backwards with little difficulty. Quick screening for remote memory could include naming past U.S. Presidents or the patient's grandchildren in chronological order.

CRANIAL NERVE EXAMINATION

The cranial nerves are generally tested in a sequential fashion immediately after the mental status examination.

Olfactory Nerve

The olfactory nerve, cranial nerve I (CN I), is rarely tested except in the case of a specific complaint of smell or taste. Each nostril should be tested separately with an aromatic substance, such as coffee, vanilla, or tobacco.

Optic Nerve

The optic nerve (CN II) is assessed in several different ways that are covered in more detail in Chapter 7. In a well-illuminated room, visual acuity should be checked in each eye using a Snellen card at a distance of 14 inches. Color perception need only be checked in cases of suspected optic nerve dysfunction and is best performed with a red object looking for unilateral "red desaturation." The pupils are then assessed for their size, shape, and symmetry. The reactivity to a bright light is confirmed both directly and consensually. In addition, a brisk constrictive response should be seen with accommodation. Visual fields should be checked, typically to confrontation. In this examination, the examiner and patient each occlude one eye and compare visual fields with the other. All four quadrants must be included to define whether hemianopsia or quadrantanopsia is present. Finally, the optic nerve head is inspected for pallor suggesting atrophy as well as for papilledema. Spontaneous venous pulsations are often difficult to see and are of limited clinical significance.

Oculomotor, Trochlear, and Abducens Nerves

Ocular motility is next assessed and encompasses the functions of the oculomotor (CN III), trochlear (CN IV), and abducens (CN VI) nerves. Eye movement should be checked in each of the eight principal directions of gaze, and any subjective sensation of diplopia should be reported. A useful way to verify alignment of consensual eye movements is to have the patient follow a penlight with their eyes and observe the location of the light reflex off the cornea. This should be symmetrical. When testing eye movements, the presence or absence of nystagmus should be noted. A few beats of nonsustained horizontal nystagmus on far lateral gaze is not unusual and should generally be considered within normal limits. Finally, the presence or absence of ptosis should be observed by comparing the level of the eyelid on the iris. The lower edge of the eyelid should be about level with the upper margin of the iris, and both sides should be symmetrical.

Trigeminal Nerve

The trigeminal nerve (CN V) has sensory, motor, and autonomic functions. The sensory examination is performed on all three divisions of this nerve: ophthalmic, maxillary, and mandibular. This may be done with a pin. The ophthalmic and maxillary divisions may be tested using a cotton swab to stimulate a corneal or nares reflex (especially useful in an intubated or comatose patient, in whom sensory loss may be otherwise not apparent). The trigeminally innervated muscles of mastication include the temporalis, masseter, and pterygoids. Masseter function is tested with the jaw tightly clenched. The belly of the muscle is palpated, and an attempt is made to open the jaw. Any wasting of the temporalis should be noted. The patient is asked to open the jaw widely, and any lateral deviation is also noted.

Facial Nerve

The facial nerve (CN VII) provides the principal motor input to the muscles of facial expression. It also subserves taste for the anterior two thirds of the tongue and sensation to the external auditory canal. Facial symmetry should be verified at rest and while smiling or grimacing. The depth of the nasolabial crease is often a subtle sign to look for because weakness will usually cause flattening in comparison with the unaffected side. Patients should be asked to close their eyes tightly. Under normal circumstances, the examiner should be unable to pry the eye(s) open. Taste may be checked using a salty or sweet water solution applied with a cotton applicator.

Vestibulocochlear Nerve

The vestibulocochlear nerve (CN VIII) provides sensory input from cochlear hearing and vestibular equilibrium centers. In a routine bedside examination, the vestibular division is difficult to assess, although nystagmus is a clue that there may be problems. The cochlear division is typically screened for auditory threshold by whispering from a distance of 2 to 3 feet on either side. The opposite ear should be occluded, and no visual clues can be given. Threshold to a 256- or 512-hertz tuning fork also can be similarly performed. The Rinne test involves placing a tuning fork on the mastoid process and then just outside the external auditory canal. Bone conduction is compared with air conduction; under normal circumstances air conduction would be appreciated approximately twice as long as bone conduction. The Weber test is performed with the tuning fork placed over the middle of the forehead. Any lateralization of the sound is abnormal and should be noted.

Glossopharyngeal and Vagus Nerves

The glossopharyngeal (CN IX) and vagus (CN X) nerves are usually tested together. A gag reflex is checked by stimulating the posterior portion of the tongue or pharynx with a tongue depressor. The glossopharyngeal nerve provides most of the afferent sensory input for the gag reflex, sensory innervation to the posterior pharynx, and taste to the posterior one-third of the tongue. The motor efferent portion of the gag reflex is carried through the vagus nerve, which subserves palatal elevation. In addition, the vagus is responsible for the swallowing reflex and also innervates the vocal cords. Hoarseness or hypophonia might suggest vagal nerve pathology. Visceral autonomic functions of the vagal nerve are usually not tested at the bedside.

Spinal Accessory Nerve

The spinal accessory nerve (CN XI) has both cranial nerve and cervical nerve root contributions. The cranial nerve portion innervates the sternocleidomastoid and superior portion of the trapezius muscle. Although shoulder shrug is one way of testing this nerve, it is fairly nonspecific because a major portion of this movement is from muscles outside of the 11th nerve territory. Instead, sternocleidomastoid function should be assessed with lateral rotation of the skull (each sternocleidomastoid will turn the head to the contralateral side). Atrophy in the neck muscles and sometimes drooping of the shoulder may be seen in injuries to this nerve.

Hypoglossal Nerve

Finally, the hypoglossal nerve (CN XII) is tested. The tongue is assessed for its bulk and symmetry. The presence of significant fasciculations should be noted, although they are commonly over-reported and usually relate to the tongue not being completely at rest. Tongue protrusion should be midline and tongue movement side to side easily performed without much associated facial motor activity.

NECK AND SPINE EXAMINATION

The neck should be examined next for signs of meningismus, increased tone, and paraspinal tenderness. This should usually be done with the patient supine and the examiner passively flexing the neck. In a screening examination, the patient may be asked to touch their chin to the chest. Sperling's sign should be tested by having the patient flex their neck laterally to one side and then the other. Cervical root pain may be brought out with this maneuver. Any evidence of significant paraspinal or spinal tenderness should be excluded with firm palpation or percussion of these areas. Passive straight leg raising should be performed to evaluate radicular pain caused by lumbosacral radiculopathy (*Lasegue's sign*). Any unusual hairy tuft over the lumbar spine that might suggest an occult spina bifida should be noted.

THE MOTOR EXAMINATION

The motor examination needs to address four different aspects of motor function: bulk, tone, strength, and any abnormal involuntary movements. To assess bulk, the patient must be properly exposed. Any asymmetry of bulk should be noted and the distribution of any obvious wasting recorded. Tone should be examined to passive range of motion. Normal resting limbs will have some slight tone and will not be entirely flaccid. Increased tone needs to be classified according to the type of hypertonia (e.g., spasticity, cogwheeling, etc.). Strength is measured in terms of absolute power and symmetry. The British Medical Research Council scale is the most commonly used grading system and assigns any given muscle a score (Table 2). The use of plus (+) or minus (−) to any of these numbers adds some flexibility to this otherwise fairly limiting scale. A good screening examination should at least evaluate deltoids, biceps, triceps, grip, finger abductions, quadriceps, hamstrings, dorsiflexors, and plantarflexors. Abnormal involuntary movements may be intermittent. It should be noted whether they are exaggerated by rest or action.

THE SENSORY EXAMINATION

A complete sensory examination will test three different modalities: spinothalamic function, dorsal column sensation, and cortical sensation. In reality, a rea-

---

TABLE 2. *Motor examination*

0	No movement
1	Trace movement
2	Movement accomplished with gravity eliminated
3	Movement against gravity
4	Able to resist some force beyond gravity
5	Normal strength

From *Aids to the examination of the peripheral nervous system.* London: Bailliere-Tindall, 1986:1. Used by permission.

sonable screening examination need only check light touch (spinothalamic) for symmetry and distal vibratory sensation in the fingers and toes (dorsal column/proprioceptive). When sensory symptoms are at issue, spinothalamic sensitivity to pinprick and discrimination between sharp and dull should be examined using a clean safety pin or some other sharp and dull object. Patterns of sensory nerve loss should be analyzed according to recognized dermatomal or peripheral nerve distribution (Figs. 1 and 2). Because of infection control issues, a new pin should be used with each patient and older instruments such as the Wartenberg wheel should be abandoned. Physicians should look for side-to-side asymmetries as well as a distal graded sensory loss. Where appropriate, a spinal cord sensory level should be estimated. Temperature sensation may be objectively assessed using test tubes of water at varying temperature, but for most purposes a subjective reporting of the sensitivity to a cold tuning fork is sufficient. In truth, it is rare for temperature testing to yield any additional information to the sensory examination; therefore, it is not usually performed under routine conditions.

Dorsal column sensitivity should be tested by assessing vibration and joint position sense. Vibratory sensation is easily assessed with a 128-hertz tuning fork applied to the interphalangeal joints in the feet and hands. The duration that a patient feels the vibration can be measured in seconds and compared side to side, or the examiner can use his or her own vibratory sensation as a control. The latter technique is generally quicker and is recommended. Joint position sense can be checked by measuring the patient's threshold to subtle alterations in finger and toe position, or, in extreme cases, to foot and hand position. As an alternative, the Romberg test is a sensitive measure of proprioceptive ability, and, when normal, usually obviates the need for further joint position sense testing. Romberg testing entails having the patient stand with feet together and eyes closed. Balance is maintained easily in the normal patient, even with a slight push from the examiner.

On occasion, the above primary sensory modalities will be normal despite clear abnormalities of the somatosensory cortex. In this situation, tests of cortical sensation may be necessary. Stereognosis is one example and can be tested at the bedside. The patient is asked, with eyes closed, to feel and then identify coins, keys, or other available objects. The impaired side is tested first to avoid giving unnecessary clues. Other cortical tests include graphesthesia (identifying numbers drawn on the hand or fingers), kinesthesia (identifying the direction of a stimulus moving up or down one of the limbs), or, to some extent, stimulus localization. The most sensitive measure of cortical sensation is two-point discrimination. This is performed using two identical pins or a pair of sharp, sterilized calipers. The normal resolution of one from two points is between 2 and 5 mm at the fingertips, 4 cm on the feet, and 8 to 12 mm on the palm.

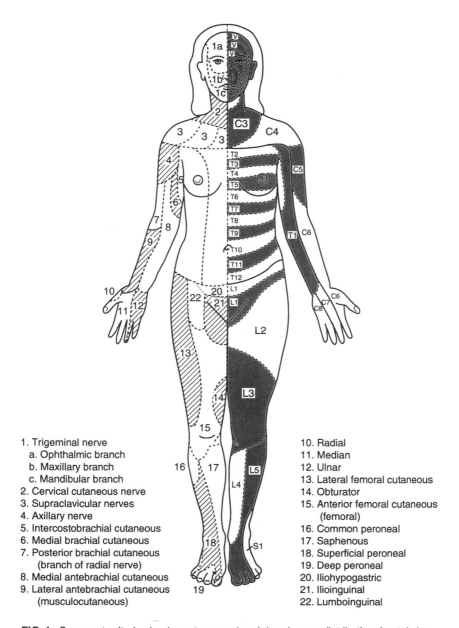

1. Trigeminal nerve
   a. Ophthalmic branch
   b. Maxillary branch
   c. Mandibular branch
2. Cervical cutaneous nerve
3. Supraclavicular nerves
4. Axillary nerve
5. Intercostobrachial cutaneous
6. Medial brachial cutaneous
7. Posterior brachial cutaneous
   (branch of radial nerve)
8. Medial antebrachial cutaneous
9. Lateral antebrachial cutaneous
   (musculocutaneous)

10. Radial
11. Median
12. Ulnar
13. Lateral femoral cutaneous
14. Obturator
15. Anterior femoral cutaneous
    (femoral)
16. Common peroneal
17. Saphenous
18. Superficial peroneal
19. Deep peroneal
20. Iliohypogastric
21. Ilioinguinal
22. Lumboinguinal

FIG. 1. Sensory territories by dermatome and peripheral nerve distribution: frontal view.

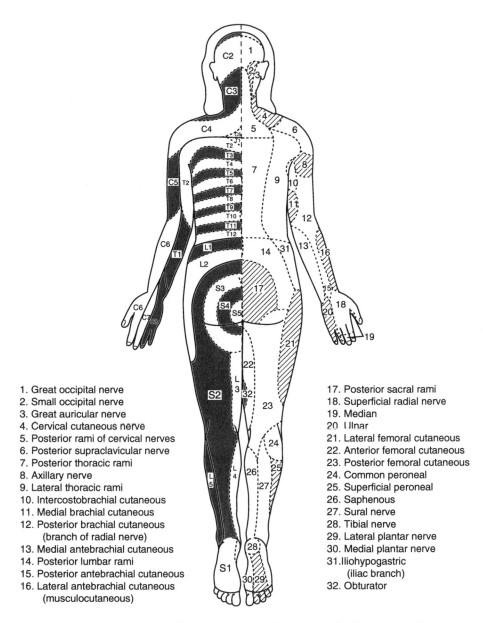

1. Great occipital nerve
2. Small occipital nerve
3. Great auricular nerve
4. Cervical cutaneous nerve
5. Posterior rami of cervical nerves
6. Posterior supraclavicular nerve
7. Posterior thoracic rami
8. Axillary nerve
9. Lateral thoracic rami
10. Intercostobrachial cutaneous
11. Medial brachial cutaneous
12. Posterior brachial cutaneous
    (branch of radial nerve)
13. Medial antebrachial cutaneous
14. Posterior lumbar rami
15. Posterior antebrachial cutaneous
16. Lateral antebrachial cutaneous
    (musculocutaneous)

17. Posterior sacral rami
18. Superficial radial nerve
19. Median
20. Ulnar
21. Lateral femoral cutaneous
22. Anterior femoral cutaneous
23. Posterior femoral cutaneous
24. Common peroneal
25. Superficial peroneal
26. Saphenous
27. Sural nerve
28. Tibial nerve
29. Lateral plantar nerve
30. Medial plantar nerve
31. Iliohypogastric
    (iliac branch)
32. Obturator

FIG. 2. Sensory territories by dermatome and peripheral nerve distribution: posterior view.

CEREBELLAR TESTING

The cerebellar examination should include tests for dysmetria of the arms and legs. Dysmetria is the uncoordinated, side-to-side motion of a moving limb as it approaches its target position. This is usually accomplished by asking patients to touch the examiner's finger at arm's length and then their own noses, going back and forth as rapidly as possible. In the lower extremities, the heel should be drawn back and forth, up and down the anterior tibia, while lying supine. Wavering to and fro or any significant past-pointing or overshooting should be considered indicative of cerebellar dysfunction. Rapid alternating movements are another important test of cerebellar function and can be performed in the upper and lower extremities quite easily. The hands may be rapidly pronated and supinated; foot tapping is a reasonable equivalent in the feet. These movements should be fairly smooth and rhythmic as opposed to the rather clumsy and arrhythmic quality seen in cerebellar disease.

GAIT

The gait examination should be assessed on an open corridor where the patient can have a sustained and fairly normal stride for at least 20 to 30 feet. The stance is assessed as well as the posture. The degree of arm swing should be symmetric. Turns should be performed and the patient asked to walk on their toes. Characteristic postures and/or gait should be recorded.

TENDON REFLEXES

Tendon reflexes are tapped sharply with a rubber reflex hammer to examine for symmetry, hyperreflexia, and hyporeflexia. Generally, it is easiest to start with the head and work down. A jaw jerk should be elicited by placing the index finger over the chin and then tapping gently while the patient holds the jaw half open and relaxed. In normal adults, a jaw jerk response is minimal. Next, the biceps (C5–6), triceps (C7–8), and brachioradialis reflexes (C5–6) are examined. Any "spread" of the reflex into adjacent muscle groups not directly involved in the reflex arc is noted and usually reflects hyperreflexia. In the lower extremities, the knee jerk (L3–4) and ankle jerks (S1–2) are tested. In all but the elderly, an absent ankle jerk is abnormal. Every effort should be made to elicit an ankle jerk, including use of reinforcement maneuvers. The *Jendrassick maneuver*, in which the patient clasps the hands together and isometrically pulls while the reflex is being elicited, is the most common reinforcement method.

A plantar reflex is usually the last reflex tested. This threshold-type response is obtained by lightly stroking the lateral aspect of the sole of the foot, from the heel to the fifth metatarsal region, and then medially to the first metatarsal. This is done with gradually increasing intensity until a response is obtained. The normal response is flexion of the toes and withdrawal of the leg. An abnormal response consists of extension of the great toe and fanning of the others. Any other response should be interpreted with caution and considered equivocal.

FRONTAL RELEASE PHENOMENA

As the last step in the routine neurological examination, it is valuable to look for so-called *frontal release signs*. These are commonly considered confirmatory signs of diffuse cerebral dysfunction, as in dementia or other degenerative diseases. However, it is common for neurologically normal elderly patients to have one or more frontal release signs without a pathological connotation. The signs that seem to have the most specificity for abnormality are the grasp reflex and the glabellar tap (*Myerson's sign*). A grasp reflex may be obtained by placing the hand or finger in the patient's palm and observing whether the patient involuntarily or irrepressibly grabs this object. The patient should then be asked to let go; in severe cases they will be unable to. The glabellar tap is performed by gently tapping over the nasion with the finger out of view so that the response is not a visual one. Compulsive and irresistible blinking is the abnormal response. Normal patients will rapidly adapt to this stimulus without further blinking.

SUMMARY OF ABNORMAL FINDINGS FOR CERTAIN NEUROLOGIC CONDITIONS

It is beyond the scope of this chapter to categorize and describe all of the abnormalities to be found during the course of the neurologic examination. Instead, the remainder of this chapter will look at several common clinical problems in neurology that might present to the primary care physician and describe the cardinal neurologic features of these diseases.

Stroke

Stroke is the most common serious illness in neurology, and a few specific elements of the neurological examination are particularly relevant. The first question to be answered in any stroke patient is whether the presentation is that of small or large vessel disease. Small vessel disease, as in hypertensive lacunar stroke, results from progressive hypertrophy of the blood vessel wall in penetrating arteries and typically presents with a pure motor or pure sensory syndrome affecting the face, arm, and leg equally. However, this is not a hard and fast rule. Large vessel disease may be cardioembolic or atherosclerotic and usually manifests cortical signs such as aphasia, apraxia, neglect, or hemianopia. When examining for stroke, the most important features to note are the presence or absence of carotid bruits, aphasia, behavioral state changes, visual field changes, anatomic distribution of weakness and/or numbness, and the presence or absence of brainstem signs. Such brainstem signs usually include one or more of the following: diplopia or ocular motility problems, nystagmus, ataxia, dysarthria, perioral numbness, or coma. In an acute infarction, the affected side may be flaccid or hyporeflexic for several hours or days before spasticity and hyperreflexia set in. Intracerebral hemorrhage and subarachnoid hemorrhage can also present as strokelike syndromes. Features these etiologies share in common include severe headache, meningismus obtundation, and severe hypertension.

Headache

Perhaps the most common neurological problem in primary care is headache. The essential features of the neurological examination are as follows: The presence of an elevated temperature or stiff neck should be excluded because of the frequent association of meningitis and headache. The mental state is important and any evidence of obtundation in the setting of headache should lead the examiner to consider either an infectious process, increased intracranial pressure, or hemorrhage. The ocular fundi should be examined carefully for the presence of papilledema, which might indicate an underlying mass lesion or idiopathic intracranial hypertension (pseudotumor cerebri). The temporal arteries should be palpated, especially in the elderly, due to the high incidence of temporal arteritis in this population.

Vertigo

Strictly defined, "vertigo" is the subjective sensation of motion when the patient is at rest, whereas "dizziness" is a broad term used interchangeably to describe everything from presyncope to ataxia. Complaints of dizziness are common, and the first decision to be made is whether the complaint relates to true vertigo, lightheadedness, or some other nonspecific disequilibrium. The neurologic examination can help differentiate peripheral (usually vestibular) causes of vertigo from the more worrisome central vertigo related to brainstem disease. During examination, nystagmus should be sought on vertical and horizontal gaze as well as in primary position. The direction of the nystagmus can sometimes be a useful localizing clue, but there are exceptions to this rule and it cannot be used exclusively. The nystagmus of peripheral vertigo (e.g., *Meniere's disease* or *benign positional vertigo*) is fatiguable and will wane with sustained eye position. A striking positional quality to the vertigo is almost always due to a peripheral condition. A mild degree of positional vertigo may be seen in central vertigo as well. The cardinal features to look for in central vertigo include the presence of associated central signs such as diplopia or dysconjugate gaze, perioral numbness, disturbances of consciousness, dysarthria, and peripheral sensory or motor impairment. If none of these features are present, it is a fairly safe assumption that the etiology of the vertigo is located peripherally. If any of these symptoms are present, the possibility of a structural brainstem process or vertebrobasilar ischemia should be considered.

Peripheral Neuropathy

There are many different kinds of peripheral neuropathy. These are classified mainly according to their distribution and the nature of their pathology (i.e., demyelinating versus axonal). The pattern of distribution may be multifocal, suggesting mononeuritis multiplex, in which single nerve territories seem to be involved in a random fashion, sparing other adjacent nerves. A more common distribution would be distal sensory-motor polyneuropathy, beginning at the feet and tips of the fingers and producing sensory and motor dysfunction in an ascending fashion. The more proximal territories are spared in this type of neuropathy, which is most commonly seen in diabetes. There are a number of other different types of peripheral neuropathy, including pure motor, pure sensory, and autonomic neuropathy, but these are somewhat less common. On examination, features suggestive of neuropathy include loss of sensation, either in a distal distribution or in a well-defined peripheral nerve or nerve root territory (Figs. 1 and 2). Most significant neuropathies will produce hyporeflexia or areflexia; the presence of hyperreflexia should cast serious doubt on the existence of an underlying neuropathy. Vibratory sensation is generally very sensitive to neuropathic changes and is commonly lost first. Distal muscular atrophy or weakness may be present, usually following the sensory disturbance by months or years. Foot drop is particularly common and may be screened for by having patients walk on their heels to bring out subtle weakness. The presence of pes cavus or hammer toes should lead to a consideration of a congenital or hereditary neuropathy, such as *Charcot-Marie-Tooth disease.* Cranial nerves are less commonly involved in peripheral neuropathy, although multiple cranial nerve palsies should lead to a search for infiltrative or inflammatory diseases affecting the skull base or the subarachnoid space (e.g., carcinomatous meningitis).

Dementia

The neurologic examination may provide certain telltale features suggestive of a progressive neurodegenerative cause of dementia versus other etiologies of cognitive decline. Obviously, the mental status examination is the most important tool, and, in a dementia evaluation, all elements of the mental state should be characterized. The vast majority of dementia syndromes will be *Alzheimer's disease* or one of the other neurodegenerative diseases, such as *Pick's disease, Lewy body encephalopathy,* or *progressive supranuclear palsy*. In particular, Lewy body encephalopathy and progressive supranuclear palsy usually have striking Parkinsonian features on examination in addition to their dementia. Pick's disease is difficult to differentiate from Alzheimer's antemortem but will occasionally have a preponderance of psychotic symptoms at onset. Immediate recall and recent memory are markedly more impaired than remote memory early in the disease. Concentration may be poor and denial is common on the part of the patient. A reliable second observer, such as a close family member, is critical in teasing out the subtle decline in higher integrative function that is frequent. Of importance in the rest of the neurological examination, one must look for signs that lead away from a diagnosis of Alzheimer's. For instance, significant eye movement abnormalities might suggest progressive supranuclear palsy or Wernicke's encephalopathy. A severe gait disorder early in the course of the dementia should cast some doubt on a diagnosis of Alzheimer's disease and promote a consideration of multiinfarct dementia or normal pressure hydrocephalus. Significant peripheral neuropathy might raise the possibility of B_{12} deficiency, thyroid disease, diabetes, or an infectious cause of dementia such as human immunodeficiency virus infection or neurosyphilis.

Coma

An extensive examination is essential for following critically ill patients with altered levels of consciousness. This should begin with an assessment of the level of consciousness as well as the degree of arousability. Arousability to voice, light tactile stimulation, and vigorous painful stimulation (as in nailbed pressure or a sternal rub) should be checked. Evidence of meningitis should be excluded by checking neck resistance. The pupils should be assessed for symmetry and reactivity. Any anisocoria should warn of an asymmetrical increase in intracranial pressure with incipient herniation. Eye movements to vestibulo-ocular stimulation should be checked with a "doll's eye" maneuver in which horizontal and vertical eye movements are observed while passive, moving the patient's head side to side or up and down. The presence of full conjugate eye movements with this maneuver is one good measure of intact brainstem function. Be aware, however, that the vestibulo-ocular reflex is suppressed in an awake patient and its absence in that situation should not be misconstrued as brainstem disease. A corneal reflex or nares reflex should be checked to assess facial sensation in unresponsive patients. The presence or absence of a gag reflex should be noted as well. Withdrawal to pain should be brisk and symmetrical—any pathological withdrawal responses, such as decortication or decerebration, should be taken to suggest diffuse cerebral disease or herniation. Reflexes, tone, and Babinski responses should be tested. Rating scales, such as the Glasgow scale, are popular but divulge little information about the actual neurological condition of any given patient. Overreliance on these scales should be avoided.

REFERENCE

1. Folstein MF, Folstein S, McHugh P. Mini-mental state: a practical method for grading the cognitive state of patients for the clinician. *J Psychiatr Res* 1975;12:189–98.

SUGGESTED READING

Barrows HS, Bennett K. The diagnostic (problem solving) skill of the neurologist. *Arch Neurol* 1972;26:273–7.

Buettner UW, Zee DS. Vestibular testing in comatose patients. *Arch Neurol* 1989;46:561–653.

Caplan LR. *The effective clinical neurologist.* Cambridge, MA: Blackwell Scientific, 1990.

Chimowitz MI, Logigian EL, Caplan LR. The accuracy of bedside neurological diagnosis. *Ann Neurol* 1990;8:78–85.

DeJong RN. *The neurologic examination.* New York: Hoeber Medical Division, Harper & Row, 1967.

Jenkyn LR, Reeves AG, Warren T, et al. Neurologic signs in senescence. *Arch Neurol* 1985;42:1154–7.

Massey EW, Scherokman B. Soft neurologic signs. *Postgrad Med* 1981;70:66–70.

Mayo Clinic & Mayo Foundation. *Clinical examinations in neurology.* Philadelphia: W.B. Saunders, 1971.

Miller JQ. The neurologic content of family practice: implications for neurologists. *Arch Neurol* 1986;43:286–8.

Snyder BD. An efficient approach to the mental status examination. *Minnesota Med* 1979;62:901–5.

Spector RH, Troost BT. The ocular motor system. *Ann Neurol* 1981;9:517–25.

Tweedy J, Reding M, Garcia C, et al. Significance of cortical disinhibition signs. *Neurology* 1982;32:169–73.

Clinical Skills for Adult Primary Care
edited by M. E. Silverman and J. W. Hurst.
Lippincott-Raven Publishers, Philadelphia © 1996.

20

Introduction to Initial Routine Laboratory Testing

Wyman P. Sloan III, M.D.

Piedmont Hospital, Atlanta, Georgia 30309

"The practice of medicine is an art, based on science."

William Osler. *Teacher and student in Aequanimitas and other addresses.*
Philadelphia: The Blakiston Company, 1932:34.

The vast array of laboratory tests and procedures accessible to the modern physician has greatly expanded our diagnostic capabilities. Yet, despite the availability of this highly sophisticated technology, the incidence of misdiagnosis has not changed appreciably over the past 20 years (1). There appears to be a disturbing trend of excessive reliance on and misuse of the clinical laboratory. The diagnostician must appreciate the fallibility and limitations of these tests and procedures (2,3). Clinical judgment serves as the foundation, and the history and physical examination should remain at the heart of the diagnostic process.

The era of managed care has introduced sweeping changes in the manner that health care will be delivered in this country. Ambulatory medicine, primary care, and preventive interventions are assuming even greater emphasis. Payors are demanding accountability in terms of health outcomes and costs of established screening strategies. The annual physical examination has been abandoned in favor of a more tailored approach targeted to populations at risk. The evidence supporting current screening recommendations is surprisingly scant and reevaluation is ongoing. For example, a recent analysis of the National Cholesterol Education Program's report on detection, evaluation, and treatment of high blood cholesterol levels suggests that the guidelines for drug treatment to lower high cholesterol levels in the average young adult is not cost effective (4) (estimated cost of $1 million to $10 million/year of life prolonged) or ethically justifiable (because of metaanalysis findings of an increase in noncoronary heart deaths among middle-aged males randomized to receive cholesterol intervention) (5). As a result, there has been a call "to change direction" and limit cholesterol screening and intervention to the minority of the population for which benefits clearly outweigh harm—those with coronary heart disease or other factors that place them at high risk (5,6).

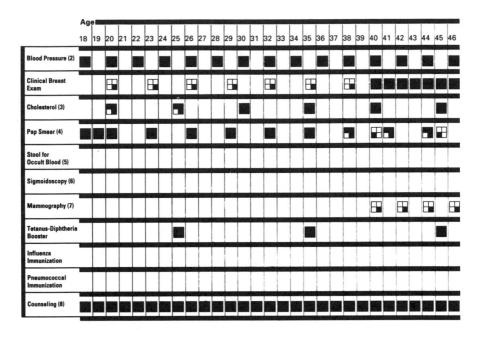

A blackened square indicates that the service is recommended. An empty square indicates that either a recommendation has been made to not provide the service or that no recommendation has been made for or against the service by the particular authority. The placement and spacing of squares indicate a suggested age range and frequency for testing rather than actual ages at which services should be provided.

ACP	USPSTF
CTF	OTHER

ACP — American College of Physicians
USPSTF — US Preventive Services Task Force
CTF — Canadian Task Force on the Periodic Health Examination
Other — Immunization Recommendations – CDC Immunization Practices Advisory Committee.
Cholesterol Recommendations – National Cholesterol Education Program Panel on Detection, Evaluation, and Treatment of High Blood Cholesterol in Adults.
Hypertension Recommendations – Joint National Committee on Detection, Evaluation, and Treatment of High Blood Pressure.
Cancer Screening Recommendations – American Cancer Society.

FIG. 1. Preventive care guidelines for asymptomatic, low-risk adults: recommendations from various North American health organizations. From Eddy (7). Used by permission of the American College of Physicians.

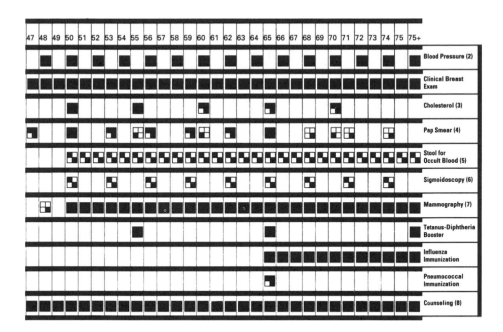

1. This list shows selected, age-specific preventive care services recommended by at least one of the ACP, CTF, or USPSTF, which should be offered to persons who do not have a family history, symptoms, signs, or other diseases that place them at increased risk for preventable target conditions. All authorities stress the importance of determining each person's unique risks for preventable disease in order to individualize preventive care. Strategies for the selective provision of a wider range of services to persons at low and increased risk for particular target conditions are found in Tables 2 through 5.

2. The CTF recommends screening at least every 5 years and at every clinical encounter. Others agree or suggest screening every 2 years.

3. The CTF recommends periodic serum cholesterol testing in men between the ages of 35 and 59 years. The USPSTF recommends determinations in middle-aged men and suggests that testing of young men, women, and the elderly may be clinically prudent.

4. ACP and USPSTF do not recommend a Papanicolaou smear for women over 65 years of age who have had consistently normal smears in the previous decade. CTF suggests Papanicolaou smears every 3 years before 35 years of age and every 5 years to 74 years of age, after two normal annual smears following the onset of sexual activity.

5. CTF and USPSTF concluded that there is insufficient evidence to recommend for or against fecal occult blood testing.

6. ACP recommends sigmoidoscopy every 3 to 5 years or air contrast barium enema every 5 years. Neither the CTF nor the USPSTF recommends for or against screening sigmoidoscopy.

7. American Cancer Society recommends annual or biennial mammography for women from 40 to 49 years of age.

8. ACP, USPSTF, and CTF emphasize that all adults should be routinely counseled about tobacco use, nutrition, exercise, sexual behavior, substance abuse, injury prevention, and dental care.

FIG. 1. Continued.

A number of organizations have established preventive care guidelines, and their recommendations are summarized in Fig. 1. Most of these tests can be performed at the time of random clinical encounters and do not require special appointments. Service can be provided by physicians, nurses, physician associates, or other physician extenders. Finally, recommendations are necessarily flexible and clinical judgment remains paramount. The chapters that follow are intended to present a current perspective on the value of tests that are commonly considered routine and often ordered for screening purposes on a periodic examination.

REFERENCES

1. Kirch W, Schafii C. Reflections on misdiagnosis. *J Int Med* 1994;235:399–404.
2. Woolf SH, Kamerow DB. Testing for uncommon conditions: the heroic search for positive test results. *Arch Intern Med* 1990;150:2451–7.
3. Ober PK. Uncle Remus and the cascade effect in clinical medicine: Brer rabbit kicks the tar-baby. *Am J Med* 1987;82:1009–13.
4. NCEP Expert Panel. Report of the national cholesterol education program expert panel on detection, evaluation, and treatment of high blood cholesterol in adults. *Arch Intern Med* 1988;148:36–69.
5. Hulley SB, Newman TB, Grady D, et al. Should we be measuring blood cholesterol levels in young adults? *JAMA* 1993;269:1416–9.
6. Hulley SB, Walsh JMB, Newman TB. Health policy on blood cholesterol—time to change directions. *Circulation* 1992;86:1026–8.
7. Eddy DM. *Common screening tests.* Philadelphia: American College of Physicians, 1991.

Clinical Skills for Adult Primary Care
edited by M. E. Silverman and J. W. Hurst.
Lippincott-Raven Publishers, Philadelphia © 1996.

21

The Biochemical Profile

Bruce F. Walker, M.D.

Piedmont Hospital, Atlanta, Georgia 30309

The biochemical profile may be defined as a systematic panel or battery of tests performed using large-volume, automated chemistry instruments for the purpose of detecting, documenting, excluding, or managing disease. The composition of typical biochemical profiles may approach 18 or more different analyses.

USES AND INDICATIONS OF THE BIOCHEMICAL PROFILE

Outpatient/Ambulatory Care Setting

The general biochemical profile is not indicated for routine screening and assessment of health status in asymptomatic adults (1). Although there are implications for disease prevention, health maintenance, and early intervention in asymptomatic patients, the biochemical profile is not designed to be used as a screening test. Efficient use of a screening test requires knowledge of the prevalence of disease in a particular population (2). Therefore, its use must be guided by clinical and historical findings.

Selected components that are indicated for screening asymptomatic adults include the following (3):

- Total cholesterol at least once every 5 years.
- Glucose (fasting or after an oral glucose challenge) in patients at increased risk for diabetes mellitus.
- Creatinine, with or without blood urea nitrogen, to detect progressive renal insufficiency in at-risk patients.
- Screening for abnormalities of serum calcium in asymptomatic patients is controversial and not recommended because there is questionable benefit in detecting cases of clinically silent primary hyperparathyroidism.
- In the absence of specific clinical signs and symptoms, screening for abnormalities of alkaline phosphatase, uric acid, aspartate aminotransferase, lactate dehydrogenase, total protein, albumin, and electrolytes is not recommended.

Preadmission Testing

General biochemical profiles are not indicated for routine elective admission to the hospital. Selective use may provide important baseline data and guide initial management. Minimum testing recommendations for preoperative patients are as follows (4):

- Glucose and creatinine in patients over 40 years of age.
- Glucose, creatinine, and a complete blood count in patients over age 60.
- Potassium in patients on diuretics or undergoing bowel preparation.

Inpatient Testing

Serial biochemical profiles may be used to monitor disease, assess response to treatment, and detect complications. The frequency of testing must be guided by the clinical setting. Specific organ panel testing may be more efficient and is available in most hospital laboratories.

Nursing Home/Chronic Care Home Setting

The general biochemical profile should be limited to monitoring, follow-up, and diagnostic purposes in severely impaired residents. Its use in screening may not be warranted (5).

Pitfalls and Limitations of the Biochemical Profile: Unwanted Tests

Biochemical profiles in common practice today often contain unwanted, "piggy-backed" tests. Abnormal results of these unwanted tests may lead to a long, expensive, and fruitless workup, termed the Ulysses syndrome (6). Like Ulysses after the Trojan War, the patient and physician pass through a lengthy, adventuresome journey before returning to the previous state of departure. Tests with a low expectation of abnormality in a given patient should not be ordered. As the prevalence of disease decreases, the positive predictive value of a test also decreases. Thus, a seemingly innocent encounter may lead to a "Tar Baby" phenomenon, in which a cascade of misleading, frustrating, and costly tests is the result (7). Selective ordering of only those tests targeted to address clinical data will eliminate some of these unwanted analyses and the potential for unexpected abnormal test results.

THE UNEXPECTED TEST RESULT

Inherent limitations in reference values may be a source of the unexpected test result. Reference values may be defined as a set of values of a measured quantity obtained from a population in a specified state of health (8). By convention, this generally refers to all values within the 95% limits (mean ± 2 standard deviations) in the chosen population. Population characteristics (age, sex, physiologic variation) and laboratory characteristics (specimen handling, methodology) influence the reference range. Assuming independence of the measured tests, the probability that at least one of n constituents will fall outside of its 95% reference interval is $1 - (0.95)^n$. Table 1 demonstrates that the likelihood of an abnormality increases in proportion to the number of tests ordered. Using this assumption, the 20-test biochemical profile has a 64% chance of one or more abnormal results in a population of healthy patients (9).

Other causes of the unexpected test result include patient preparation, laboratory error, drug-metabolite interferences, and other disease states not initially considered.

General Approach to the Unexpected Test Result

- Notify the laboratory and request a verification. The same sample should be repeated.
- A new sample may be obtained with consideration given to patient preparation and specimen handling.
- Use the correct reference interval.
- Validate appropriateness for age, sex, physiologic conditions, and laboratory methodology.
- Consider using a broader (99%) reference range.
- Consider possible drug-metabolite interferences.
- Consider differential diagnoses.
- Consider additional follow-up studies, as appropriate, based on clinical data and the degree of abnormality.

TABLE 1. *Probability of a healthy person having abnormal results in a biochemical profile using mean ± 2 standard deviations as reference values*

No. of tests	% Probability that at least one test result will be abnormal
1	5
6	26
12	46
20	64

From Winkel P, Statland BE. Interpreting laboratory results: reference values and decision making. In: Henry JB, ed. *Clinical diagnosis and management by laboratory methods.* 18th ed. Philadelphia: W.B. Saunders, 1991:50. Used by permission of W.B. Saunders Company.

REFERENCES

1. Speicher CE, Smith JW Jr. *Choosing effective laboratory tests.* Philadelphia: W.B. Saunders, 1983.
2. Watts NB. Medical relevance of laboratory tests. *Arch Pathol Lab Med* 1988;112:379–82.
3. Cebul RD, Beck JR. Biochemical profiles: applications in ambulatory screening and preadmission testing of adults. In: Sox HC Jr, ed. *Common diagnostic tests.* 2nd ed. Philadelphia: American College of Physicians, 1990:343–66.
4. Narr BJ, Hansen TR, Warner MA. Preoperative laboratory screening in healthy Mayo patients: cost effective elimination of tests and unchanged outcomes. *Mayo Clin Proc* 1991;66:155–9.
5. Kim DE, Berlowitz DR. The limited value of routine laboratory assessments in severely impaired nursing home residents. *JAMA* 1994;272:1447–52.
6. Rang M. The Ulysses syndrome. *Can Med Assoc* 1972;106:122–3.
7. Ober KP. Uncle Remus and the cascade effect in clinical medicine. *Am J Med* 1987;82:1009–13.
8. Winkel P, Statland BE. Interpreting laboratory results: reference values and decision making. In: Henry JB, ed. *Clinical diagnosis and management by laboratory methods.* 18th ed. Philadelphia: W.B. Saunders, 1991:49.
9. Winkel P, Statland BE. Interpreting laboratory results: reference values and decision making. In: Henry JB, ed. *Clinical diagnosis and management by laboratory methods.* 18th ed. Philadelphia: W.B. Saunders, 1991:50.

Clinical Skills for Adult Primary Care
edited by M. E. Silverman and J. W. Hurst.
Lippincott-Raven Publishers, Philadelphia © 1996.

22

Lipoprotein Screening

Mark E. Silverman, M.D.

*Emory University School of Medicine, Atlanta, Georgia 30322
and Piedmont Hospital, Atlanta, Georgia 30309*

Hyperlipidemia is strongly associated with an increased risk of myocardial infarction and death related to coronary artery disease (1,2). Reduction in total serum and low-density lipoprotein (LDL) cholesterol has been shown to decrease this risk (2,3). Although causal effects and benefits are unproven, studies have shown that diet and/or lipid-lowering drugs can decrease the formation of atherosclerotic plaque, cause regression of already formed plaque, and improve endothelial-mediated vasomotor response of the atherosclerotic vessel (1,4). The National Cholesterol Education Program has recommended the following testing guidelines (3):

PATIENTS WITH NO APPARENT DISEASE

Total cholesterol and high-density lipoprotein (HDL) cholesterol should be measured once every 5 years in all adults 20 years of age or older.

PATIENTS WHO HAVE BORDERLINE HIGH-RISK LDL (130–150 MG/DL) ON INITIAL SCREENING

Repeat lipoprotein analysis yearly.

PATIENTS WITH LDL-CHOLESTEROL ±160 MG/DL OR CLINICAL ATHEROSCLEROTIC DISEASE

Initially, a fasting lipoprotein analysis is conducted on at least two occasions. Follow-up measurements should be made 6 months after a trial of dietary therapy and 6 to 8 weeks after drug therapy.

REFERENCES

1. Levine GN, Keaney JF, Jr, Vita JA. Cholesterol reduction in cardiovascular disease—clinical benefits and possible mechanisms. *N Engl J Med* 1995;332:512–21.
2. LaRosa JC. Cholesterol and cardiovascular disease: how strong is the evidence? *Clin Cardiol* 1992; 15(suppl III):2–7.
3. National Cholesterol Education Program. Detection, evaluation, and treatment of high blood cholesterol in adults. Second report, NIH Publication No. 93-3095, September, 1993.
4. Treasure CB, Klein JL, Weintraub WS, et al. Beneficial effects of cholesterol-lowering therapy on coronary endothelium in patients with coronary artery disease. *N Engl J Med* 1995;332:481–7.

Clinical Skills for Adult Primary Care
edited by M. E. Silverman and J. W. Hurst.
Lippincott-Raven Publishers, Philadelphia © 1996.

23

Routine Complete Blood Count

Robert S. Allen, M.D.

Piedmont Hospital, Atlanta, Georgia 30309

The complete blood count (CBC), including a total white cell count and differential, hemoglobin, hematocrit, mean corpuscular volume, and platelet count, can be very helpful in uncovering unsuspected primary hematological as well as systemic disorders, in confirming diagnoses, following up response to treatment, and as a baseline for future comparison.

PATIENTS WITH NO APPARENT HEMATOLOGIC DISEASE

The CBC should be obtained at the time of the routine physical examination. It should not be part of the laboratory evaluation in patients who present for a specific problem that does not suggest a hematological abnormality.

The normal total white count is frequently quoted as 5,000 to 10,000/dl (1). The total white count includes neutrophils, lymphocytes, monocytes, eosinophils, and basophils. The normal neutrophil count is 2,500 to 7,500/dl (1). It should be noted that African Americans may have a neutrophil count as low as l,500/dl, so that the normal total white count in African Americans may easily be as low as 3,000/dl (1). The normal lymphocyte count ranges between 1,000 and 4,000/dl (1). The normal hemoglobin in men varies between 14.0 and 17.7 gm/dl and between 12.0 and 15.7 gm/dl in women (1). It is often not well recognized that there is some reduction in the normal lower limit of hemoglobin in people as they grow older. For this reason, minimal anemia in elderly individuals may simply reflect a slight reduction in the bone marrow function associated with aging. The normal platelet count ranges between 150,000 and 400,000/mm³ (1).

Visual examination of the peripheral smear is not indicated routinely in an individual who is asymptomatic and has a normal CBC. Review of the peripheral smear is important in evaluating thrombocytopenia because platelet clumping can result in a spuriously low platelet count. This condition, referred to as pseudothrombocytopenia, is simply a benign laboratory manifestation seen in certain individuals whose platelets clump after being collected in an ethylenediaminetetraacetic acid–coated tube.

PATIENTS WITH ABNORMAL FINDINGS ON INITIAL CBC

An elevated neutrophil count is seen most commonly in infection but can be seen with other inflammatory conditions and primary hematological disorders. Neutropenia is most commonly seen as a result of certain infectious conditions and as a result of medications, particularly chemotherapy.

Lymphocytosis is seen most commonly with viral infections and with chronic lymphocytic leukemia. Lymphocytopenia is a well-described complication of human immunodeficiency virus infection, and the serial measurement of the total lymphocyte count as well as the ratio of helper to suppressor cells is a valuable longitudinal study in this population of patients.

The mean corpuscular volume is helpful in evaluating anemia. The normal value ranges from 80 to 100 μm^3 (1). Microcytosis is seen most commonly with iron deficiency and thalassemia. Sideroblastic anemia and anemia of chronic disease are less common causes of microcytosis. Macrocytosis may be seen with hemolytic anemia due to the increased size of reticulocytes and often as a result of alcohol intake. Macrocytic anemias in elderly individuals raise the question of a myelodysplastic syndrome, and macrocytosis is seen commonly as a result of B_{12} or folic acid deficiency.

Thrombocytosis occurs commonly with iron deficiency anemia and in inflammatory conditions. Less commonly, thrombocytosis is secondary to a primary hematological disorder; this is especially likely if the platelet count is above $1,000,000/mm^3$ (1). Thrombocytopenia is seen frequently with immune thrombocytopenic purpura, hypersplenism, and as a result of medications, particularly chemotherapeutic agents.

The differential white count is helpful in evaluating an abnormal white count. Abnormal white cells are suggestive of a primary hematological disorder. Abnormal morphology of the red cells can be seen with hypochromia and microcytosis accompanying iron deficiency, in patients with liver disease who demonstrate target cells, in patients with a microangiopathic process with fragmented red cells, and in patients with hemoglobinopathies. The examination of the platelets on the blood smear is helpful in distinguishing between thrombocytopenia secondary to a consumptive disorder such as immune thrombocytopenic purpura, in which the platelets are large, and thrombocytopenia secondary to a production defect such as a medication effect, in which the platelets are of normal size.

The CBC is important in assisting in the evaluation of patients who present with the symptoms of anemia, such as dyspnea on exertion, decreased energy, and orthostasis. The white count should be evaluated in patients who have signs or symptoms suggestive of an infectious process, and the platelet count should be obtained in patients with bruising, bleeding, or other signs suggestive of a coagulopathy.

The CBC should be serially followed in patients who are anemic in order to document a response to therapy. Neutrophilia noted in a patient who is obviously infected does not require a routine check to document its return to normal; however, an otherwise unexplained neutrophilia does require a follow-up CBC. Neutropenia should be followed serially because a granulocyte count below 1,000/dl on a prolonged basis predisposes to an infection. Thrombocytosis is followed to document control of the platelet count in a reasonable range. Thrombocytopenia is serially measured; a platelet count below 20,000/mm^3 (1) demands immediate attention; a platelet count below 50,000/mm^3 (1) may require an intervention in a chronic thrombocytopenic state such as immune thrombocytopenic purpura.

HEMATOLOGIC DISEASES THAT CAN BE PRESENT WITH A NORMAL CBC

The CBC can be normal in the early stages of all forms of anemia; however, the development of microcytosis or macrocytosis with a normal hemoglobin may assist in the early detection of an anemic process. The total white count may be normal in a primary hematological condition such as leukemia; however, the evaluation of the differential and review of the peripheral blood smear will often detect abnormal cells so that the illness can be detected at an earlier stage. The early stages of immune thrombocytopenias may easily have a platelet count in the low-normal range; however, even a minimally chronically depressed platelet count in the range of 130,000 to 140,000/mm^3 (1) should be evaluated.

HEMATOLOGIC DISEASES THAT CAN BE ELIMINATED WITH A NORMAL CBC

The normal CBC can eliminate a primary hematological illness in individuals who present with a variety of symptoms. A normal hemoglobin rules out anemia as the cause of dyspnea on exertion or decreased energy. The normal white count is often useful in suggesting a noninfectious process as the cause of a febrile illness or acute abdomen, and a normal platelet count is useful in evaluating patients who present with clinical coagulopathies. It should be noted that qualitative platelet disorders can cause serious platelet dysfunction in patients with a normal platelet count so that a bleeding time should always be obtained in this clinical situation.

REFERENCE

1. Williams WJ, Beutler E, Erslev AJ, et al. *Hematology.* 4th ed. New York: McGraw-Hill, 1990.

SUGGESTED READING

Beck WS. *Hematology.* 5th ed. Cambridge, MA: The MIT Press, 1991.
Colman RW, Hirsh J, Marder VJ, et al., eds. *Hemostasis and thrombosis.* 2nd ed. Philadelphia: J.B. Lippincott, 1987.

Clinical Skills for Adult Primary Care
edited by M. E. Silverman and J. W. Hurst.
Lippincott-Raven Publishers, Philadelphia © 1996.

24

Urinalysis

Jerry D. Cooper, M.D.

Piedmont Hospital, Atlanta, Georgia 30309

Study of the urine as a means of detecting disease has been described since the beginning of medicine. Originally these descriptions were limited to gross observation of certain properties of urine. Modern urinalysis also involves a macroscopic examination of the urine, including color and specific gravity. In addition, a reagent strip (dipstick) is now used to provide semiquantitative estimates of protein, glucose, and blood. More recently, reagent strip tests have been added for bacteriuria (nitrite test) and pyuria (leukocyte esterase test). Dipstick urinalysis refers to these reagent strip tests, which are the most commonly used in screening urinalysis. More elaborate urine reagent strips are also available commercially in a variety of conformations, including tests for ketones, bilirubin, and urobilinogen. These additional studies add little to the usefulness of the dipstick urinalysis in screening general populations. The comments in this section are limited to use of urinalysis as a screening tool. Detailed descriptions of the technical aspects of urinalysis and application in specific disease states may be found in standard texts (1).

Urinalysis also includes microscopic examination of the sediment of a centrifuged urine specimen to detect, confirm, and quantify red blood cells, white blood cells, renal epithelial cells, casts with specific reference to type and number, crystals, yeast, bacteria, and other formed elements. Microscopic examination of the urine sediment is not included in the dipstick urinalysis used for general population screening.

Microscopic examination of urine sediment is a powerful tool in selected populations, such as those with known renal disease.

During the past several decades, the concept of the periodic health evaluation, known variously as the annual physical, interval examination, or annual checkup, has increased in popularity. More recently, selectivity in the use of various diagnostic maneuvers has been advocated with tailoring of health diagnostic services to specific populations. Specific recommendations incorporating these concepts have been published by certain groups, including the U.S. Preventive Services Task Force (2) and the American College of Physicians (3). Their guidelines will be included in the recommendations given in this summary of the use of urinalysis in adult primary care. There are variations in preventive care guidelines among these and other authorities. The differences in these screening recommendations may be understood through reflection on the targets, objectives, and rationale of the major studies. These differences may be troubling to the adult primary care physician who finds it necessary to act on these recommendations.

Decisions regarding screening in these circumstances are best made on the basis of the physician's knowledge of the medical history and circumstances of the patient population under his or her care. Current recommendations regarding screening urinalysis are suggested for the following groups of patients.

PATIENTS WITH NO APPARENT DISEASE

U.S. Preventive Services Task Force

Use dipstick urinalysis to screen for asymptomatic bacteriuria, hematuria, and proteinuria in all people over age 60.

American College of Physicians

Recommended against screening for bacteria.

PATIENTS SUSPECTED OF A DISEASE OR AT INCREASED RISK

U.S. Preventive Services Task Force

Screen for bacteriuria in people with diabetes and pregnant women at periodic intervals.

American College of Physicians

Recommended against screening.

PATIENTS WITH KNOWN DISEASE

In patients with documented disease, the use and frequency of dipstick urinalysis is guided by the clinical circumstances of the patient. Microscopic examination of the urine sediment is also usually performed in patients with known disease including the following:

- Diagnosis and follow-up of infections of the genitourinary (GU) tract
  Lower genitourinary tract infections (cystitis, prostatitis)
  Upper genitourinary tract infections (pyelonephritis)
- Known renal disease
- Diabetes mellitus
- Hypertension
- Other systemic medical conditions with known associated genitourinary or renal components

WHAT RENAL DISEASE MAY BE PRESENT WITH A NORMAL URINALYSIS?

The most common renal disease that may be present with a normal screening urinalysis is early diabetic nephropathy. Standard urine screening methods may not be sufficiently sensitive to detect the slight elevation in urinary protein excretion that is the best early marker of diabetic nephropathy. More sensitive methods of detection involving timed urine collections are necessary to detect microalbuminuria, defined as 30 to 300 mg/day or 20 to 200 µg/min of urinary protein excretion on at least two of three timed measurements. Patients with the following conditions should be screened annually for microalbuminuria (4):

- Insulin-dependent diabetes mellitus of greater than 5 to 10 years' duration
- Diabetes mellitus with a family history of renal disease or hypertension

REFERENCES

1. Brenner BM, Rector FC. *The kidney.* 4th ed. Philadelphia: W.B. Saunders, 1991:937–50.
2. U.S. Preventive Services Task Force. Screening for asymptomatic bacteriuria, hematuria, and proteinuria. In: *Guide to clinical preventive services.* Philadelphia: Williams & Wilkins, 1989:155–61.
3. Hayward RA, Steinberg EP, Ford DE, et al. Preventive care guidelines. *Ann Intern Med* 1991;114: 758–83.
4. Striker G. Report on a workshop to develop management recommendations for the prevention of progression in chronic renal disease. *J Am Soc Nephrol* 1995;5:1537–40.

Clinical Skills for Adult Primary Care
edited by M. E. Silverman and J. W. Hurst.
Lippincott-Raven Publishers, Philadelphia © 1996.

25

Chest X-Ray Film

William R. Kenny, M.D.

Piedmont Hospital, Atlanta, Georgia 30309

THE VALUE OF THE ROUTINE CHEST X-RAY

The routine chest X-ray film is no longer considered a necessary part of a yearly examination on well persons. Even the inclusion of a chest X-ray film on hospital admission or preoperative evaluation has been questioned by the American College of Physicians (1). A 1990 American College of Physicians publication, *Common Diagnostic Tests*, states the following:

> Although admission and preoperative chest radiographs are able to detect unexpected or occult abnormalities in a patient otherwise asymptomatic for chest disease, the findings of a routine chest radiograph rarely affect patient management or enhance patient care. In addition, the false-positive or false-negative results that may arise from routine chest radiographs may lead to unnecessary diagnostic tests or unwarranted reassurance. The history and physical exam and the clinical judgment of the physician will determine the need for a chest radiograph (2).

The World Health Organization (3), the U.S. Department of Health and Human Services (4), and specialty societies (5) have published guidelines abandoning the "routine chest X-ray film" because multiple published studies have shown an extremely low yield of important abnormalities on screening chest radiographs, even in large populations of smokers.

The historical reason that chest X-ray films became incorporated into all hospital admissions and all preoperative evaluations for major surgery was the high incidence of clinically silent pulmonary tuberculosis. Despite recent increases in tuberculosis, the patients at risk today would almost always be identified by history or physical findings. (Positive human immunodeficiency virus status and history of intravenous drug use are two high-risk categories for tuberculosis today.) The application of cost-effective methods to the ordering of chest radiographs suggests that patients should be selected because of the physician's clinical suspicion of chest or heart disease or in a setting such as prethoracic surgery, in which postoperative chest complications might occur.

Although yearly chest X-ray films in asymptomatic individuals are clearly contraindicated, there is a rational reason for a baseline study on new patients, especially if no old films are available. Although the incidence of abnormalities in such individuals is low, a few conditions might be found that could influence future care.

COMMON OR IMPORTANT DISEASES AND ABNORMALITIES THAT MIGHT BE RECOGNIZED ON THE CHEST X-RAY FILM OF ASYMPTOMATIC INDIVIDUALS

- Occult lung carcinoma or early metastatic disease
- Cardiomegaly or abnormal cardiac configuration
- Anomalous pulmonary or systemic vasculature
- Mediastinal adenopathy from sarcoidosis or lymphoma
- Thymoma, teratoma, congenital lung cysts, or anomalous lobar divisions (azygos lobe)
- Aortic aneurysm (including dissection)
- Early pulmonary sarcoidosis or other interstitial processes
- Small pleural effusions or small pneumothoraces

IMPORTANT DISEASES OR PROCESSES THAT MAY NOT BE DETECTED ON ROUTINE CHEST X-RAY FILMS

- Early to moderately advanced chronic obstructive lung disease
- Aortic aneurysm (including dissection)
- Small pneumothoraces (exhalation films may emphasize tiny pneumothoraces)
- Mild valvular heart disease
- Hypertrophic heart disease
- Small neoplasms or those hidden by other structures
- Early interstitial diseases such as *Pneumocystis carinii* pneumonia and idiopathic pulmonary fibrosis
- Mild lymphadenopathy
- Cardiac tumors

ILLNESSES THAT MIGHT BE SUSPECTED FROM THE HISTORY OR PHYSICAL EXAMINATION THAT CAN GENERALLY BE EXCLUDED BY A GOOD QUALITY CHEST X-RAY FILM

- Pneumonia
- Congestive heart failure
- Severe valvular heart disease
- Lung metastases (possibly excluding early lymphangitic spread, which can be subtle)

* Pneumothorax
* Pleural effusions
* Free peritoneal air
* Large pericardial effusion

Studies from the Mayo Clinic (6), Johns Hopkins (7), and Memorial Sloan-Kettering (8) performed to determine the value of screening smokers (all studies were limited to men) with chest X-ray films and sputum cytologies for early lung cancer were widely interpreted as providing strong evidence that screening for lung cancer did not decrease death rates. However, recent analysis of these studies shows that screened patients were more likely to be diagnosed in an early stage of lung cancer with a greater resectability rate (46% versus 32%) and greater 5-year survival rate (33% versus 15%) (9). Now it is felt that although massive screening efforts are not economically productive or feasible, patients at risk of lung cancer should be followed closely and a yearly chest film may be justified in this setting.

Preoperative chest X-rays represent another area of controversy. No well-designed, prospective study has ever been done to determine what criteria (age, site of surgery, preexisting illnesses, etc.) are needed to justify preoperative X-rays.

Some preliminary guidelines have been published suggesting which patients should have a chest film preoperatively (10):

* Patients with suspected or known chest disorders that could complicate the perioperative period
* Patients having surgery involving the chest cavity
* Patients having surgery in sites close to the chest such as standard cholecystectomy
* Patients with heart disease

CHEST X-RAY FILMS IN OLDER PATIENTS

Advanced age is not always an indication for preoperative chest X-rays, but because there is a higher incidence of symptoms and signs of chest disease in the elderly, many should have an X-ray film before receiving a general anesthetic. This decision is usually decided by community standards of care or physician judgment (11).

REFERENCES

1. Tape TG, Mushlin AI. *The utility of routine chest x-rays. Common diagnostic tests.* Philadelphia: American College of Physicians, 1990:78–98.
2. American College of Physicians. *Common diagnostic tests, use and interpretation.* Philadelphia: American College of Physicians, 1990:398.
3. WHO Scientific Group on the indications for and limitations of major x-ray diagnostic investigations. *A rational approach to radiographic investigations.* Geneva: World Health Organization, 1983:7-28 (WHO Technical Report Series No. 689).

4. National Center for Devices and Radiological Health. *The selection of patients for x-ray examinations: chest x-ray screening examinations.* Rockville, MD: Food and Drug Administration, 1983, HHS Publication No. (FDA) 83-8204.

5. American College of Radiology. *Referral criteria for chest x-ray examinations. (Policy statement).* Chicago: American College of Radiology, 1982.

6. Fontana RS, Sanderson DR, Woolner LB, et al. Lung cancer screening. The Mayo program. *J Occup Med* 1986;28:746–50.

7. Tockman MS. Survival and mortality from lung cancer in a screened population. The Johns Hopkins study. *Chest* 1986;89(suppl):324–5.

8. Melamed MR, Flehinger BJ, Zaman MB, et al. Screening for early lung cancer. Results of the Memorial Sloan-Kettering study in New York. *Chest* 1984;86:44–53.

9. Strauss GM, Gleason RE. Screening for lung cancer reexamined. A reinterpretation of the Mayo lung project randomized on lung cancer screening. *Chest* 1993;103(suppl):337–41.

10. Mendelson DS, Khilnani N, Wagner LD, et al. Preoperative chest radiography: value as a baseline for comparison. *Radiology* 1987;165:341-43.

11. Sewell JM, Spooner LL, Dixon AK, et al. Screening investigations in the elderly. *Aging* 1981;10:165–8.

Clinical Skills for Adult Primary Care
edited by M. E. Silverman and J. W. Hurst.
Lippincott-Raven Publishers, Philadelphia © 1996.

26

Electrocardiography

J. Willis Hurst, M.D.

Emory University School of Medicine and Hospital, Atlanta, Georgia 30322

At the outset it must be emphasized that primary care physicians must be skilled in the interpretation of electrocardiograms. Primary care physicians are exposed to electrocardiography during their training period, and many books are available for those who need personal refresher courses in the subject. Accordingly, this chapter *is not* the place for a lengthy discussion of the subject. This chapter *is* the place where the indications for an electrocardiogram should be discussed. Therefore, the electrocardiogram will be discussed in terms of the patients who should have an electrocardiogram recorded routinely, the types of heart disease that could be present when the electrocardiogram is normal, and the types of heart disease that can be eliminated when the electrocardiogram is normal.

IN WHICH PATIENTS SHOULD AN ELECTROCARDIOGRAM BE RECORDED?

The American College of Cardiology/American Heart Association Guidelines for Electrocardiography (1992) address this problem (1). The guidelines suggest the following:*

Indications for an Electrocardiogram in Patients with No Apparent Heart Disease

- To evaluate patients over 40 years of age
- To evaluate patients before administering a noncardiac drug that is known to affect the heart
- To evaluate individuals before an exercise stress test
- To evaluate persons of any age who are in occupations that require cardiovascular fitness or who are responsible for the safety of the public

---

*Adapted and used with permission of the American Heart Association.

- Some physicians recommend that an electrocardiogram be made to evaluate those individuals who plan to participate in competitive sports

Indications for an Electrocardiogram in Patients Who Are Suspected of Having Heart Disease or Are at an Increased Risk of Developing Heart Disease

- A baseline electrocardiogram should be recorded
- An electrocardiogram should be made before the administration of noncardiac drugs known to affect the heart
- An electrocardiogram is indicated prior to a surgical procedure
- A follow-up electrocardiogram should be made when there are new clinical signs of heart disease
- A follow-up electrocardiogram should be made in 1 to 5 years in patients who do not have new signs of heart disease. More frequent follow-up is needed in children less than 2 years of age
- An electrocardiogram is not indicated more often than once a year when there are no new clinical findings in this group of patients

Indications for an Electrocardiogram in Patients with Known Heart Disease

- A baseline electrocardiogram is indicated
- An electrocardiogram is indicated before beginning a new treatment that affects the heart and electrocardiogram
- Follow-up electrocardiograms should be made in patients with a change in clinical findings; with implanted pacemakers; and after an interval of time appropriate for the condition
- Before a surgical procedure

WHAT TYPES OF HEART DISEASE CAN BE PRESENT WHEN THE ELECTROCARDIOGRAM IS NORMAL?

- The resting electrocardiogram is normal in most patients who have angina pectoris caused by coronary atherosclerosis. The electrocardiogram is "nondiagnostic" in about half of the patients with myocardial infarction when they initially arrive at an emergency clinic (2).
- The electrocardiogram is commonly normal in patients with mild aortic or mitral valve disease. It is normal in some patients with moderately severe aortic or mitral valve disease. The electrocardiogram is usually abnormal when the patient has severe aortic or mitral valve disease.

- The electrocardiogram is commonly normal in patients with slight systemic hypertension. It is likely to be abnormal in patients with long-standing moderate or severe elevation of systemic blood pressure.
- The electrocardiogram may be normal in patients with dilated or hypertrophic cardiomyopathy but is more commonly abnormal.
- The electrocardiogram may be normal in patients with congenital heart disease, including patent ductus arteriosus, interventricular septal defect, coarctation of the aorta, and bicuspid aortic valve.
- The electrocardiogram may be normal in patients who give a history of pericarditis.
- Left ventricular hypertrophy can be present when the electrocardiogram is normal.
- Heart failure may be associated with a normal electrocardiogram when there is diastolic myocardial dysfunction due to coronary atherosclerotic heart disease.
- A history of cardiac arrhythmia may be associated with a normal electrocardiogram.

WHAT TYPES OF HEART DISEASE CAN BE ELIMINATED WHEN THE ELECTROCARDIOGRAM IS NORMAL?

Patients with an ostium secundum or ostium primum atrial septal defect, tetralogy of Fallot, transposition of the great vessels, tricuspid atresia, severe aortic and mitral valve disease, dilated or hypertrophic cardiomyopathy, severe and long-standing hypertension, and severe long-standing pulmonary artery hypertension rarely, if ever, have a normal electrocardiogram.

Finally, the value of correlating the findings in the electrocardiogram of each patient with the other clinical data that have been collected from each patient must be emphasized. This is the only way to learn diagnostic electrocardiography and more importantly, it is the only way to appreciate the significance of an abnormality found in the electrocardiogram.

REFERENCES

1. A Report of the ACC/AHA Task Force on Assessment of Diagnostic and Therapeutic Cardiovascular Procedures (Committee on Electrocardiography). ACC/AHA guidelines for electrocardiography. *Circulation* 1992;85:1221–8.
2. Gibler WB, Lewis LM, Erb RE, et al. Early detection of myocardial infarction in patients with chest pain; nondiagnostic ECG; serial CK-MB samples in the emergency department. *Ann Emerg Med* 1990;19:1315–66.

SUGGESTED READING

Hurst JW. The electrocardiogram. In: *Cardiovascular diagnosis: the initial examination.* St. Louis: Mosby Year Book, 1993:191–425.
Hurst JW. *Ventricular electrocardiography.* New York: Gower Medical, 1991.
Hurst JW. *Cardiac puzzles.* St. Louis: Mosby Year Book, 1995.

Clinical Skills for Adult Primary Care
edited by M. E. Silverman and J. W. Hurst.
Lippincott-Raven Publishers, Philadelphia © 1996.

27

Exercise Electrocardiography

Mark E. Silverman, M.D.

*Emory University School of Medicine, Atlanta, Georgia 30322
and Piedmont Hospital, Atlanta, Georgia 30309*

The prevalence and fear of coronary artery disease and the grave possibility of sudden death or myocardial infarction in asymptomatic patients has led to the widespread use of routine exercise electrocardiography, often demanded by the patient. Like all screening tests, this approach carries a high cost and low yield when the prevalence of the disease is low (1,2). In addition, an exercise test is imperfect, with a mean sensitivity of 68% (range 23% to 100%; lowest in single-vessel disease, highest in multivessel disease) and a mean specificity of 77% (range 17% to 100%) when ST segment depression is used as the sole criterion for the diagnosis (3). The specificity is lower in women under 50 years of age than it is in men (2). The positive predictive value of an abnormal test can vary from 20% to 90% depending on the population of patients (4). However, the predictive value of a negative test is high (77% to 99%) (4–6). As yet, there is no evidence that asymptomatic patients with coronary disease will benefit from therapy (7). In addition, many patients who have an infarction or who die suddenly experience an acute coronary occlusion related to an unstable plaque that occupies 50% or less of the luminal diameter until the acute event (4). This would not likely be detected beforehand by routine exercise testing. In symptomatic middle-aged patients (especially men over 60), the likelihood of double, triple, and left main vessel stenosis is much higher and the value of exercise testing correspondingly increases (1). These considerations have led to the following recommendations.

INDICATIONS FOR AN EXERCISE ELECTROCARDIOGRAM IN ASYMPTOMATIC PEOPLE (NO CHEST PAIN), WITHOUT APPARENT HEART DISEASE OR RISK FACTORS

Exercise testing is not recommended for routine health screening because the risk of infarction and sudden death is low, the results can be misleading, and the testing may bring about psychologic stress, harmful effects on insurance rating, and unwarranted, more expensive testing (4,7).

INDICATIONS FOR AN EXERCISE ELECTROCARDIOGRAM IN INDIVIDUALS WHO ARE ASYMPTOMATIC BUT HAVE ONE OR MORE RISK FACTORS FOR CORONARY DISEASE

The prevalence of coronary disease is increased in this population, although the overall yield of exercise testing remains low and there is no evidence that intervention makes a difference in mortality. Exercise electrocardiography is frequently used in diabetics, patients with hypercholesterolemia (cholesterol: HDL ratio exceeding 6.0), and those with a family history of coronary disease; it is controversial as to whether it should be performed routinely (2,7).

INDICATIONS FOR AN EXERCISE ELECTROCARDIOGRAM IN PEOPLE AGE 50 OR OVER WHO ARE EMBARKING ON A VIGOROUS EXERCISE PROGRAM

Cardiac arrest is much more likely to occur during vigorous exercise than at rest. The absolute risk is low, however, and it remains uncertain if screening is justified, although it is commonly performed, especially if there is a risk factor such as diabetes, smoking, family history, or hypercholesterolemia. It is not justified in individuals under age 50 in the absence of risk factors or symptoms (7).

INDICATIONS FOR AN EXERCISE ELECTROCARDIOGRAM IN PEOPLE WHO ARE IN HIGH-RISK OCCUPATIONS THAT POSE A RISK TO OTHERS SUCH AS PILOTS AND BUS DRIVERS

This area lacks information. Testing is frequently obtained but is not considered mandatory (6,7).

INDICATIONS FOR AN EXERCISE ELECTROCARDIOGRAM IN PATIENTS WHO HAVE CHEST PAIN THAT IS SUGGESTIVE BUT NOT DIAGNOSTIC FOR ANGINA PECTORIS

When the pretest probability that the patient's chest discomfort is angina pectoris is estimated to be 50% to 70%, an exercise electrocardiogram may be useful in firming up the diagnosis (2). This applies to men at any age and women after age 50. Women under age 50 who have chest discomfort suggesting the possibility of angina pectoris have an increased likelihood of a falsely positive exercise electrocardiogram (1). A more definitive test, such as a thallium stress test, dobutamine stress echocardiogram, or positron emission tomography scan is recommended (8–10).

WHEN IS AN EXERCISE ELECTROCARDIOGRAM CONTRAINDICATED IN PATIENTS WITH CHEST DISCOMFORT?

Patients with definite stable angina pectoris have a pretest probability of 90% that coronary artery disease is present. An exercise electrocardiogram offers little in regard to diagnosis. A coronary arteriogram should be considered.

Patients with unstable angina pectoris should not be exercised. A coronary arteriogram is safer and provides more important information.

INDICATIONS FOR AN EXERCISE ELECTROCARDIOGRAM IN PATIENTS AFTER A MYOCARDIAL INFARCTION (INCLUDING POSTTHROMBOLYTIC THERAPY)

There is excellent evidence that an exercise electrocardiogram after a myocardial infarction confers important prognostic information that can be used to risk-stratify patients (2,4). In addition, important functional information is obtained that can be useful in recommending an exercise program. Testing is recommended within several weeks of the infarction (2). The frequency of subsequent testing has not been determined but is often yearly.

WHAT TYPES OF HEART DISEASE CAN BE PRESENT WHEN AN EXERCISE ELECTROCARDIOGRAM RESULT IS NEGATIVE?

Mild to severe coronary disease may exist even when a maximal exercise test is normal. Noncoronary heart disease, including patients with left ventricular dysfunction, may be present with normal exercise capacity.

WHAT TYPES OF HEART DISEASE CAN BE ELIMINATED WHEN THE EXERCISE ELECTROCARDIOGRAM RESULT IS NEGATIVE?

No types of heart disease can be eliminated absolutely when the stress test is negative (normal).

WHAT TYPES OF HEART DISEASE CAN CAUSE A FALSELY POSITIVE EXERCISE ELECTROCARDIOGRAM?

- Left ventricular hypertrophy
- Valvular heart disease (including mitral valve prolapse)
- Wolff-Parkinson-White syndrome
- Left bundle branch block
- Cardiomyopathy
- Congenital heart disease
- Pericardial disease

WHAT TYPES OF NONHEART PROBLEMS CAN CAUSE A FALSELY POSITIVE EXERCISE ELECTROCARDIOGRAM?

- Digitalis
- Hypokalemia
- Anemia
- Hyperventilation
- Excessive double product
- Electrolyte abnormalities

REFERENCES

1. Steingart RM, Scheur J. Refining the estimated likelihood of coronary artery disease presence or absence. In: Hurst JW, ed. *The heart.* 7th ed. New York: McGraw-Hill, 1990:357–8.
2. Fletcher GF, Balady G, Froelicher VF, et al. Exercise standards. *Circulation* 1995;91:580–615.
3. Gianrossi R, Detrano R, Mulvihill, et al. Exercise-induced ST depression in the diagnosis of coronary artery disease: a meta-analysis. *Circulation* 1989;80:87–98.
4. Bodenheimer MM. Risk stratification in coronary disease: a contrary viewpoint. *Ann Intern Med* 1992;116:927–36.
5. Froelicher VF, Myers J, Follansbee WP. Screening apparently healthy individuals. In: *Exercise and the heart.* 3rd ed. St. Louis: Mosby, 1993.
6. Fuller T, Movahed A. Current review of exercise testing: application and interpretation. *Clin Cardiol* 1987;10:189–200
7. Sox HC, Jr, Littenberg B, Garber AM. The role of exercise testing in screening. *Ann Intern Med* 1989;110:456–68.
8. Task force. Guidelines for cardiac radionuclide testing: report of the American College of Cardiology/American Heart Association Task Force. *J Am Coll Cardiol* 1995;25:521–47.
9. Kotter TS, Diamond GA. Exercise thallium-201 scintigraphy in the diagnosis and prognosis of coronary artery disease. *Ann Intern Med* 1990;113:684–702.
10. Poldermans D, Fioretti PM, Boersma E, et al. Dobutamine-atropine stress echocardiography and clinical data for predicting late cardiac events in patients with suspected coronary artery disease. *Am J Med* 1994;97:119–25.

Clinical Skills for Adult Primary Care
edited by M. E. Silverman and J. W. Hurst.
Lippincott-Raven Publishers, Philadelphia © 1996.

28

Sigmoidoscopy

Randy J. Yanda, M.D.

Piedmont Hospital, Atlanta, Georgia 30309

Flexible sigmoidoscopy has largely replaced the rigid sigmoidoscope as the instrument of choice for examination of the rectum and distal colon. In general, flexible sigmoidoscopy has a two to three times higher yield than rigid sigmoidoscopy when examining for neoplastic lesions. Patient acceptance is also greater due to less discomfort.

The flexible sigmoidoscope is available in 30- and 60-cm lengths. Sigmoidoscopy can be performed by well-trained primary care physicians as well as specialists. A simple bowel preparation of one or two phosphate enemas 1 hour before the procedure is usually adequate. Flexible sigmoidoscopy is useful in screening patients for colonic neoplasia or for evaluating patients with symptoms referable to the lower gastrointestinal tract.

INDICATIONS FOR FLEXIBLE SIGMOIDOSCOPY IN PATIENTS WITH NO APPARENT DISEASE

Sigmoidoscopy is generally accepted as a screening test for colon cancer. Routine screening should be done in patients over the age of 50. Screening sigmoidoscopy should be performed every 3–5 years. Screening should start for patients over the age of 40 who are at increased risk for colon cancer. This includes patients with a history of breast, endometrial, or ovarian cancer or who have a first-degree relative with colon cancer. If a patient has a first-degree relative who developed colon cancer at an early age or has more than one first-degree relative with colon cancer, then screening colonoscopy rather than sigmoidoscopy should be performed. Prospective, randomized trials are not yet available that demonstrate that screening flexible sigmoidoscopy is beneficial, but two case-control studies suggest that mortality from colon cancer is reduced in patients who have undergone screening sigmoidoscopy.

INDICATIONS FOR FLEXIBLE SIGMOIDOSCOPY IN PATIENTS WITH SUSPECTED DISEASE

- To evaluate a patient with a change in bowel habits.
- To evaluate a patient with suspected anorectal bleeding.
- To evaluate a patient with localized left lower quadrant abdominal pain.
- To evaluate chronic diarrhea.

INDICATIONS FOR FLEXIBLE SIGMOIDOSCOPY IN PATIENTS WITH KNOWN DISEASE

Flexible sigmoidoscopy is useful to monitor disease activity and to evaluate response to treatment in patients previously diagnosed with inflammatory bowel disease involving the distal colon or rectum.

WHAT TYPES OF DISEASE CAN BE PRESENT WHEN THE FLEXIBLE SIGMOIDOSCOPY IS NORMAL?

- Flexible sigmoidoscopy is normal in patients with Crohn's disease when only the small intestine and/or the proximal colon is involved.
- A normal sigmoidoscopy does not exclude colon cancer or polyps that may be present in the colon beyond the reach of the scope.
- The colonic mucosa appears normal during sigmoidoscopy in patients with chronic diarrhea related to microscopic and collagenous colitis. The diagnosis is made on microscopic examination of mucosal biopsy samples.

WHAT TYPES OF DISEASE CAN BE ELIMINATED WHEN THE FLEXIBLE SIGMOIDOSCOPY IS NORMAL?

- Inflammatory bowel disease involving the rectum and distal colon.
- Colorectal cancer involving the area of colon examined with the sigmoidoscope.

SUGGESTED READING

Bond JH. Colorectal cancer: screening. *Pract Gastroenterol* 1994;18:533–7.
Newcomb PA, Norfleet RG, Storer BE, et al. Screening sigmoidoscopy and colorectal cancer mortality. *J Natl Cancer Inst* 1992;84:1572–5.
Selby JV, Friedman GD, Quesenberry CP, et al. A case-control study of screening sigmoidoscopy and mortality from colorectal cancer. *N Engl J Med* 1992;326:653–7.
Sox HC. Preventive health services in adults. *N Engl J Med* 1994;330:1589–95.

Clinical Skills for Adult Primary Care
edited by M. E. Silverman and J. W. Hurst.
Lippincott-Raven Publishers, Philadelphia © 1996.

29

Fecal Occult Blood Testing

Randy J. Yanda, M.D.

Piedmont Hospital, Atlanta, Georgia 30309

Numerous tests for the detection of occult fecal blood are available. Guaiac, a colorless leuco-dye that becomes colored in the presence of hemoglobin and hydrogen peroxide, has long been used to detect blood and remains the most widely used type of fecal blood test. Hemocult and Hemocult II (Smith Kline Diagnostics, Sunnyvale, CA) are quantitative tests most often used in controlled trials of fecal occult blood testing and are the ones generally recommended in clinical practice. These tests are simple, inexpensive, highly portable, and easy to perform.

The reactivity of the qualitative tests makes their clinical interpretation difficult. There is no consistent fecal hemoglobin level above which the guaiac tests become positive or below which they become negative. Diet must be carefully controlled because certain fruits and vegetables (radishes, turnips, cantaloupes, bean sprouts, cauliflower, broccoli, grapes) have peroxidaselike activity and can produce a false-positive test result (1). Fecal hydration before the addition of the peroxide catalyst markedly increases the sensitivity of the test but at the expense of specificity.

Newer tests, such as the Hemoquant (Smith Kline Biosciences, Van Nuys, CA), also have been developed. The Hemoquant is a quantitative assay based on the conversion of hemoglobin to fluorescent porphyrins. It is extremely sensitive and not affected by dietary peroxidase. This assay is not yet widely available for clinical use.

INDICATIONS FOR FECAL OCCULT BLOOD TESTING ON PATIENTS WITH NO APPARENT DISEASE

Fecal blood testing for the early detection of colorectal cancer is recommended yearly in patients over the age of 50 (2). Six slides should be made by the patient over 3 days. Occult blood screening is based on the assumption that the detection of occult bleeding by an asymptomatic colon cancer will result in reduced mortality in the population screened. The sensitivity for fecal occult blood testing for colon cancer is reported to be 50% to 92% (3,4). A recent large, prospective controlled study has shown that cancers detected at screening tend to be at an earlier stage than those found in the control group (5). This resulted in a statistically significant reduction in mortality of 33% in patients who were screened annually (5).

Fecal occult blood screening in patients already at increased risk for colon cancer, such as a strong family history of colon cancer, familial polyposis, chronic ulcerative colitis, and a history of previous colon cancer, is probably not appropriate. The focus in these patients should be on structural studies such as colonoscopy or barium enema.

INDICATIONS FOR FECAL OCCULT BLOOD TESTING IN PATIENTS WITH SUSPECTED DISEASE

- To evaluate a patient with a change in bowel habit.
- To evaluate a patient with chronic diarrhea.
- To evaluate a patient with unexplained weight loss.
- To evaluate a patient with a new anemia.

INDICATIONS FOR FECAL OCCULT BLOOD TESTING IN PATIENTS WITH KNOWN DISEASE

Fecal occult blood testing is not useful in monitoring patients with known disease, due to its variable sensitivity and specificity.

WHAT TYPES OF DISEASE CAN BE PRESENT OR EXCLUDED WHEN THE FECAL BLOOD TEST IS NEGATIVE?

Fecal occult blood testing generally should be used as a screening test for disease rather than as a test to exclude disease. A disease is less likely if the occult blood test is negative, but it cannot be excluded.

REFERENCES

1. Macrae FA, St. John JB, Catigiore P, et al. Optimal dietary conditions for hemocult testing. *Gastroenterology* 1982;82:899.
2. Sox HC. Preventive health services in adults. *N Engl J Med* 1994;330:1589–95.
3. Bond JH. Colorectal cancer: screening. *Pract Gastroenterol* 1994;18:533–7.
4. Selby JV, Friedman GD, Quesenberry CP, et al. Effect of fecal occult blood testing on mortality from colorectal cancer. *Ann Intern Med* 1993;118:1–6.
5. Mandel JS, Bond JH, Church TR, et al. Reducing mortality from colorectal cancer by screening for fecal occult blood. *N Engl J Med* 1993;328:1365–71.

Clinical Skills for Adult Primary Care
edited by M. E. Silverman and J. W. Hurst.
Lippincott-Raven Publishers, Philadelphia © 1996.

30

Mammography

William E. Mitchell, Jr., M.D.

Piedmont Hospital, Atlanta, Georgia 30309

Screening mammograms are performed to discover occult breast cancers before they can be detected by physical examination. There are many reasons other than screening to perform mammograms. The discussion that follows does not deal with the proper use or timing of mammograms in evaluation of specific breast problems. Like all mammograms, screening mammograms should be performed at a certified facility and read by skilled mammographers who have a substantial mammogram caseload weekly.

Many studies have been conducted to determine the benefit of screening mammograms; unfortunately there is no solid consensus on which to base recommendations (1–3). It is firmly established that screening mammograms do save lives by detection of very early breast cancers, but there are valid concerns about cost, radiation exposure, and inconvenience. A useful approach recently introduced into practice is based on categorization of a woman's inherent risk factors for the development of breast cancer and the likelihood of nonmammographic early detection of such cancer in her particular situation. Use of such an approach should incorporate frank discussion with the patient about the reason for the recommendation on the frequency of screening mammography in her individual case.

WOMEN WITH RISK OR DIAGNOSTIC DELAY FACTORS FOR BREAST CANCER

A woman who has had a previous breast cancer, atypia on a previous breast biopsy, a family history of a first-degree relative (mother or sister) with breast cancer, or a long uninterrupted history of menstrual periods, including an early menarche and a delay in the first pregnancy, probably has a significant increased risk of breast cancer (Table 1).

Also of some importance, certain factors may delay the discovery of a breast cancer by the patient or her health-care professional. These factors include very large breasts, lumpy or otherwise difficult-to-examine breasts, infrequent or incomplete breast self-examination, or no yearly examination by a professional. Any

TABLE 1. *Factors affecting risk and delay in diagnosis of breast cancer*

Risk of developing breast cancer is increased by
    Previous breast cancer
    Atypia on previous biopsy
    Family history of breast cancer in first-degree relative
    Menarche at less than 12 years of age and no pregnancy by 35 years of age
Delay in diagnosis of breast cancer may be increased under the following conditions
    Does not examine herself thoroughly each month
    Does not have examination by health care professional yearly
    Has very large breasts
    Has lumpy/difficult-to-examine breasts

of these factors could delay the discovery of an early breast cancer, making discovery by mammography all the more important. Therefore, women who are at increased risk of developing breast cancer or who have increased likelihood of delay in the diagnosis of breast cancer should have more frequent mammograms. For women who do have increased risk or delay factors, a mammogram at age 35 would probably be appropriate, followed by a repeat baseline at 40, mammograms at 2-year intervals between 40 and 49, at yearly intervals between 50 and 69, and at 2-year intervals after the age of 70 (Table 2).

WOMEN WITHOUT RISK OR DIAGNOSTIC DELAY FACTORS FOR BREAST CANCER

On the other hand, women who do not have increased risk or increased delay factors probably do not need mammograms as frequently as they have been recommended in the past. A reasonable recommendation for women who do not have increased risk and have no delay factors would be a baseline mammogram at age 40, no mammograms from age 40 to 49 in the absence of specific indications,

TABLE 2. *Recommended frequency of screening mammograms*

Age (yr)	More frequent screening, due to presence of any risk or delay factor from Table 1	Less frequent screening, due to absence of all risk and delay factors from Table 1
35	Baseline screening mammogram	None
40	Repeat baseline screening mammogram	Baseline screening mammogram
40 to 49	Every 2 years	None
50 to 69	Yearly	Every 2 years
70 and over	Every 2 years	Undetermined; either every 2 years or none

mammograms at 2-year intervals between ages 50 and 69, and (probably) no mammograms after the age of 70.

REFERENCES

1. Kattlove H, Liberati A, Keeler E, Brook R. Benefits and costs of screening and treatment for early breast cancer. *JAMA* 1995;273:142–8.
2. Kerlikowske K, Grady D, Robin S, et al. Efficacy of screening mammography. *JAMA* 1995;273:149–54.
3. Sox H. Preventive health services in adults. *N Engl J Med* 1994;330:1589–95.

Clinical Skills for Adult Primary Care
edited by M. E. Silverman and J. W. Hurst.
Lippincott-Raven Publishers, Philadelphia © 1996.

31

Prostate-Specific Antigen

Mark E. Silverman, M.D.

*Emory University School of Medicine, Atlanta, Georgia 30322
and Piedmont Hospital, Atlanta, Georgia 30309*

Prostate cancer is now the leading cause of nonskin cancer in American men, surpassing lung cancer (1). In 1994 there were an estimated 200,000 new cases (1). The risk of prostate cancer is 3% to 4% in men over age 50, with the prevalence increasing seven times between ages 50 and 70 years (2). Although the disease is well-known to remain indolent, about 38,000 men with prostate cancer will die yearly of the disease (1). Because the combination of a digital rectal examination and a prostate-specific antigen (PSA) is sensitive in detecting early prostate cancer, the American Cancer Society and the American Urological Association have endorsed an annual PSA in men 50 years and over and a routine rectal examination beginning at age 40 (3). When an abnormal rectal examination and an elevated PSA is followed by an ultrasound-guided biopsy, the rate of cancer detection is increased by 70% (3). This promising yield for early detection has brought about a seeming epidemic of prostatic cancer, which has led to a sixfold increase in the rate of radical prostatectomy (1,4). However, a careful appraisal of the cost-benefit of routine testing has led to a criticism of this approach for the following reasons (2,5):

- There is no controlled scientific evidence that early detection of prostatic cancer definitely improves survival rates from radical surgery, radiation, or cryoablation (5).
- There is a significant risk associated with radical prostatectomy, including complete incontinence in 10% and bothersome incontinence in 30% to 40%; impotence in 20% to 75%; and a mortality of 0.1% to 2% (2,3). Rectal injury, infection, bleeding, obturator nerve injury, ureteral injury, pulmonary infarction, myocardial infarction, and chronic proctitis are other possible complications.
- Only a few days in average life expectancy are gained for men 50 to 70 years of age who have had a radical prostatectomy, and this is more than counterbalanced by a net loss in quality-adjusted life expectancy (2,3,5).

- One PSA screening for all American men between ages 50 and 70 would cost about $28 billion (4). The cost-effective ratio is $113,000 to $729,000 per incremental life-year saved.
- The PSA has a high rate of false-positive results, up to 70% in patients with prostatic hypertrophy (2). A PSA of 4 to 10 does confer a 25% chance of cancer; a PSA of 10, 70% (2). The common result of a PSA of 4 to 9 brings considerable anxiety and indecision to both the patient and the physician.

Because the unproven benefits of an aggressive approach to reduce prostatic cancer mortality may be outweighed by considerable morbidity and cost, the Canadian Task Force on the Periodic Health Examination (6), the U.S. Preventive Services Task Force, the International Union Against Cancer, and others have weighed against routine screening. Therefore, at this time, they recommend that testing should be individualized and that the potential risks made fully known to the patient (2,3).

REFERENCES

1. Potolsky A, Miller BA, Albertsen PC, et al. The role of increasing detection in the rising incidence of prostate cancer. *JAMA* 1995;273:548–52.
2. Check WA. Physicians haggle over prostate screening and strategies for managing cancer, BPN. *ACP Observer* 1994;14:1,13,14.
3. Catalona WJ. Management of cancer of the prostate. *N Engl J Med* 1994;331:996–1004.
4. Krahn MD, Mahoney JE, Eckman MH, et al. Screening for prostate cancer: a decision analytic view. *JAMA* 1994;272:773–80.
5. Kramer BS, Brown ML, Porok PC. Prostate cancer screening: what we know and what we need to know. *Ann Intern Med* 1993;119:914–23.
6. Canadian Task Force on the Periodic Health Examination. Periodic health examination, 1991 update: 3. Secondary prevention of prostate cancer. *Can Med Assoc J* 1991;145:413–23.

Clinical Skills for Adult Primary Care
edited by M. E. Silverman and J. W. Hurst.
Lippincott-Raven Publishers, Philadelphia © 1996.

32

Pulmonary Function Testing by Office Spirometry

William R. Kenny, M.D.

Piedmont Hospital, Atlanta, Georgia 30309

THE VALUE AND LIMITATIONS OF OFFICE SPIROMETRY

Pulmonary function testing is widely used in the diagnosis and management of patients with known or suspected disorders of respiration. Such testing is especially valuable in identifying obstructive and restrictive processes such as asthma and interstitial lung diseases and in following the progress of pulmonary impairment (1). Spirometry with or without bronchodilator response can be done easily and with good quality control with equipment readily available for a primary care office. Computerized devices will analyze the data, and some equipment will offer an interpretation based on established normal values (2).

IMPORTANT VALUES MEASURED ON SPIROMETRY

- FVC, forced vital capacity
- FEV_1, forced expiratory volume in 1 second
- $[FEV_1 : FVC]$%, ratio of FEV_1 to FVC, multiplied by 100
- FEF 25–75, average airflow during the mid-half of the FVC, also known as the mid-flow rate
- MVV, maximum voluntary ventilation

Interpretation of pulmonary function tests is based on predicted values obtained on extensive cross-sectional population studies of nonsmokers in unpolluted environments (3,4). Relevant variables used to interpret pulmonary function are the patient's age, height, and sex. In the office setting, reliable studies can be obtained on most patients if the technician is trained to coach the patient and reproduce matching values on several repeated forced vital capacity maneuvers.

This discussion will primarily address routine tests, including pre- and post-bronchodilator spirometry, which can easily be performed in a primary care physician's office. The indications for more complete testing, such as lung volumes, diffusing capacity (DLCO), and bronchoprovocation will also be mentioned.

STANDARD USES OF PULMONARY FUNCTION TESTING

- Detection and quantification of respiratory disease (5)
- Evolution of disease
- Response to therapy
- Preoperative evaluation (to identify high-risk patients or evaluate resectability) (6)
- Assessment of disability (7)

DETECTING AND QUANTIFYING LUNG DISEASES

The detection of significant chronic obstructive lung disease in smokers or asthmatics with minimal or no symptoms is common when pulmonary function tests are used appropriately as a screening tool in those patients who have risk factors (8). Objective evidence of respiratory impairment can be a valuable tool in counseling patients to quit smoking, especially those who have been falsely reassured by years of "normal" chest X-ray films and physical examinations (9).

Although simple spirometry is often diagnostic in patients with persistent cough or dyspnea, which is unexplained on physical examination or chest radiograph, more sensitive tests may be needed if spirometry is normal.

CONDITIONS THAT MAY NOT BE DETECTED ON OFFICE SPIROMETRY

- Cough-variant asthma or bronchial reactivity without wheeze. This type of asthma may require a bronchoprovocation test, as with methacholine, to identify it (10).
- Early infectious or immunological interstitial diseases, such as *Pneumocystis carinii* pneumonia and idiopathic pulmonary fibrosis. These conditions may require a diffusing capacity (DLCO) or lung volume measurements to detect subtle abnormalities in respiratory function to explain cough, dyspnea, or fever (11).

EVALUATING RESPONSE TO THERAPY AND DISEASE PROGRESSION

Flow rates are useful for monitoring obstructive lung diseases. The vital capacity is one of the indicators of restrictive diseases such as sarcoidosis and other interstitial diseases. Although office spirometry is helpful, additional tests, including lung volumes, DLCO, and arterial blood gases, may be necessary for monitoring interstitial and restrictive lung diseases.

PREOPERATIVE TESTING

Pulmonary function testing before surgery is appropriate in any patient with cough, sputum production, or dyspnea and certainly before elective lung resection (12). Preoperative evaluation also can include baseline arterial blood gas measurements, lung volumes, and DLCO. If abnormalities are detected, therapy to improve lung function may be indicated and regional anesthesia also may be used to avoid pulmonary complications. The risk of thoracic surgery with resection of lung tissue can be partially determined by spirometry, but in some cases exercise testing or perfusion scans of the lungs may be needed to predict the patient's postoperative performance status (13).

DISABILITY EVALUATION

Occupational or environmental exposures may result in short-term, recurring, or permanent lung conditions that alter pulmonary function. Asbestos exposure, for example, causes a series of progressive abnormalities. Initially, bronchial obstructive changes are detected; later, as the condition slowly progresses, restriction of lung volume and impairment of oxygen transfer occurs. Exposure to chemical fumes may result in chemical pneumonia and scarring or even a long-term increase in bronchial reactivity as an acquired asthmatic condition. Pulmonary function testing is also useful to evaluate disability for insurance benefits in asthma, chronic bronchitis, and emphysema (14).

REFERENCES

1. Dawson A. Spirometry. In: Wilson AF, ed. *Pulmonary function testing: indications and interpretations*. Orlando: Grune & Stratton, 1985:14–6.
2. Maguire GP, Kleinhenz ME. How—and why—to use spirometry in your office. *J Respir Dis* 1994; 15:759.
3. Morris JF, Koski A, Johnson LC. Spirometric standards for healthy nonsmoking adults. *Am Rev Respir Dis* 1971;103:57–67.
4. Crapo RO, Morris AH, Gardner RM. Reference spirometric values using techniques and equipment that meet ATS recommendations. *Am Rev Respir Dis* 1981;123:659–64.
5. Crapo RO. Pulmonary function testing. *N Engl J Med* 1994;331:25–30.
6. Zibrak JD, O'Donnell CR, Marton KI. Preoperative pulmonary function testing. American College of Physicians position paper. *Ann Intern Med* 1990;112:793–5.
7. Kilburn K, Warshaw R. Pulmonary function testing for occupational epidemiology and disability. In: Wilson AF, ed. *Pulmonary function testing, indications and interpretations*. Orlando: Grune & Stratton, 1985:329–37.

8. Ferrante E, Muzzolon R, Fuso L, et al. Bronchial asthma: still an inadequately assessed and improperly treated disease. *J Asthma* 1994;31:117–21.
9. Morris JF, Temple W. Spirometric "lung age" estimation for motivating smoking cessation. *Prev Med* 1985;14:655–62.
10. Chai H, Farr RS, Froelich LA, et al. Standardization of bronchial inhalation challenge procedures. *J Allergy Clin Immunol* 1975;56:323.
11. Forster RE. Diffusion of gases. In: Fenn WO, Rahn, eds. *Handbook of physiology: Respiration.* Vol. 1. Washington, DC: American Physiological Society, 1965:863.
12. Zibrak JD, O'Donnell CR, Marton KI. Preoperative pulmonary function testing: American College of Physicians position paper. *Ann Intern Med* 1990;112:793–5.
13. Olen GN, Block AJ, Tobias JA. Prediction of postpneumonectomy pulmonary function using quantitative macroaggregate lung scanning. *Chest* 1974;66:13–6.
14. Kilburn KH. Pulmonary reactions to organic materials. *Ann NY Acad Sci* 1974;221:183–91.

Subject Index